Diamond and Dalessio's The Practicing Physician's Approach to Headache

Diamond and Dalessio's The Practicing Physician's Approach to Headache

Sixth Edition

Edited by
Merle L. Diamond, M.D., F.A.C.E.P.

Associate Director
Diamond Headache Clinic
Chicago, Illinois

Glen D. Solomon, M.D., F.A.C.P.

Medical Director
Merck & Company, Inc.
Pepper Pike, Ohio

W.B. SAUNDERS COMPANY

A Division of Harcourt Brace & Company
Philadelphia / London / Toronto / Montreal / Sydney / Tokyo

W.B. SAUNDERS COMPANY
A Division of Harcourt Brace & Company

The Curtis Center
Independence Square West
Philadelphia, Pennsylvania 19106

Library of Congress Cataloging-in-Publication Data

Diamond and Dalessio's The practicing physician's approach to headache.—6th ed. / [edited by] Merle L. Diamond, Glen D. Solomon.

p. cm.

Rev. ed. of: The practicing physician's approach to headache / edited by Seymour Diamond, Donald J. Dalessio. 5th ed. c1992.

Includes bibliographical references and index.

ISBN 0–7216–6999–9

1. Headache. I. Diamond, Merle L. II. Solomon, Glen D. III. Diamond, Seymour. IV. Dalessio, Donald J. [DNLM: 1. Headache. WL 342 D536 1999]

RC392.P73 1999

616.8′491—dc21

DNLM/DLC 98–7039

DIAMOND AND DALESSIO'S THE PRACTICING PHYSICIAN'S APPROACH TO HEADACHE ISBN 0–7216–6999–9

Printed in the United States of America.

Last digit is the print number: 9 8 7 6 5 4 3 2 1

To my father, Seymour Diamond, M.D., whose hard work and commitment to his patients have inspired this work and my career in medicine, and to my mother, Elaine Diamond, for her continued support and care.

To Donald Dalessio, M.D., an esteemed colleague and mentor, for his encouragement and enlightenment.

To my husband, David Barack, D.D.S., and my children—Max, Michael, Jacob, and Katie—for their love, support, and indulgence.

M.L.D.

To my wife, Cynthia, without whose support, guidance, and love this book would not have been possible, and to my dog, Tony, who daily reminds me of the meaning of quality of life.

G.D.S.

Contributors

JOHN G. ARENA, Ph.D.
Medical College of Georgia, Augusta
Department of Veterans Affairs, Augusta, Georgia
Biofeedback, Relaxation Training, and Other Psychological Treatments for Chronic Benign Headache

EDWARD B. BLANCHARD, Ph.D.
Distinguished Professor of Psychology, State University of New York at Albany; Co-Director, Center for Stress and Anxiety Disorders, Albany, New York
Biofeedback, Relaxation Training, and Other Psychological Treatments for Chronic Benign Headache

DONALD J. DALESSIO, M.D.
Consultant in Neurology, Scripps Clinic; Chairman of Medicine Emeritus, Green Hospital of Scripps Clinic, La Jolla, California
Traction and Inflammatory Headache and Cranial Neuralgias

MERLE L. DIAMOND, M.D., F.A.C.E.P.
Associate Director, Diamond Headache Clinic, Chicago, Illinois
Coexisting Migraine and Tension-Type Headaches (Mixed Headache Syndrome); Emergency Treatment of Headache; Headache Syndromes in Children and Adolescents: Diagnosis and Management; Physical and Neurological Examination of the Patient with Headache; Taking a Headache History; Tension-Type Headache

SEYMOUR DIAMOND, M.D.
Adjunct Professor of Pharmacology and Molecular Biology, Finch University of Health Sciences/Chicago Medical School, North Chicago; Director, Diamond Headache Clinic, Chicago, Illinois
Hormonal Headaches; Migraine Headache

PAUL N. DUCKRO, Ph.D.
Professor, Department of Community and Family Medicine, Saint Louis University Health Sciences Center; Director, Chronic Headache Program, Saint Louis Behavioral Medicine Institute, St. Louis, Missouri
Psychological Assessment of the Headache Patient

ARTHUR H. ELKIND, M.D.
Clinical Assistant Professor of Medicine, New York Medical College, Valhalla; Director, Elkind Headache Center, and Attending Physician, Mount Vernon Hospital, Mount Vernon, New York
Post-traumatic Headache

MITCHELL S. ELKIND, M.D.
Fellow, Cerebrovascular Disease and Neuroepidemiology, Columbia-Presbyterian Medical Center, New York, New York
Post-traumatic Headache

FREDERICK G. FREITAG, D.O.
Affiliate Instructor, Department of Family Medicine, Midwestern University/Chicago College of Osteopathic Medicine, Downers Grove; Associate Director, Diamond Headache Clinic, Chicago, Illinois
Headache Clinics and Inpatient Treatment Units for Headache

R. MICHAEL GALLAGHER, D.O., F.A.C.O.F.P.
Professor and Vice Dean, University of Medicine and Dentistry of New Jersey, School of Osteopathic Medicine; Director, University Headache Center, Stratford, New Jersey
Medication Overuse and Dependency in the Headache Patient

ROBERT S. KUNKEL, M.D., F.A.C.P.
Clinical Assistant Professor of Medicine, Pennsylvania State University College of Medicine, Hershey, Pennsylvania; Member, Cleveland Clinic Headache Center, The Cleveland Clinic Foundation, Cleveland, Ohio
Complicated and Rare Forms of Migraine

DAVID LEWIN, M.D.
Associate Radiologist at the Borg Imaging Group, Rochester, New York
Neurodiagnostic Imaging in the Investigation of Headache

TODD LEWIS, D.O.
Department of General Internal Medicine, The Cleveland Clinic Foundation, Cleveland, Ohio
Cluster Headache

DAVID G. LITAKER, M.D., M.Sc.
Assistant Professor, Department of Internal Medicine, Ohio State University School of Medicine, Columbus; Staff Physician, The Cleveland Clinic Foundation, Cleveland, Ohio
The Impact of Headache from the Patient's Perspective

RUSSELL C. PACKARD, M.D., F.A.C.P.
Adjunct Professor of Psychology (Psychiatry), University of West Florida, Pensacola, Florida
Psychiatric Management of the Headache Patient

JORDAN M. PRAGER, M.D.
Associate Professor of Clinical Radiology, Northwestern University Medical School, Chicago; Chief, Neuroradiology Section, Evanston Hospital, Evanston, Illinois
Neurodiagnostic Imaging in the Investigation of Headache

ALAN M. RAPOPORT, M.D.
Assistant Clinical Professor, Yale University School of Medicine, New Haven; Director, Inpatient Headache Unit, Greenwich Hospital, Greenwich, Connecticut
Cerebrovascular Disease and Headache

A. DAVID ROTHNER, M.D.
Director, Child Neurology, The Cleveland Clinic Foundation, Cleveland, Ohio
Headache Syndromes in Children and Adolescents: Diagnosis and Management

ROBERT E. RYAN, Jr., M.D.
Assistant Clinical Professor, Department of Otolaryngology, St. Louis University School of Medicine; Director, Ryan Headache Center, Chesterfield; Executive Director, Unity Health Research, St. Johns Mercy Medical Center, St. Louis, Missouri
Otorhinolaryngological Causes of Head and Facial Pain

GLEN D. SOLOMON, M.D., F.A.C.P.
Medical Director, Merck & Company, Inc., Pepper Pike, Ohio
Classification and Mechanism of Headache; Cluster Headache; Coexisting Migraine and Tension-Type Headaches (Mixed Headache Syndrome); Headache Syndromes in Children and Adolescents: Diagnosis and Management; The Impact of Headache from the Patient's Perspective; Physical and Neurological Examination of the Patient with Headache; Taking a Headache History; Tension-Type Headache

ROBERT L. TOMSAK, M.D., Ph.D.
Clinical Associate Professor of Ophthalmology and Neurology, Case Western University School of Medicine, Cleveland; Lakeland Eye Surgeons and Consultants, Lorain, Ohio
Headaches of Ocular Origin

THERESA TSCHANNEN, Ph.D.
Psychologist, M.A. Orcutt, Ph.D. & Associates, Columbus, Ohio
Psychological Assessment of the Headache Patient

Preface

to the Sixth Edition

With the sixth edition, the life of this book now spans 26 years. As a book ages in this manner, especially as it matures through multiple editions, it acquires a character of its own. In a sense the book perseveres, taking on an elusive attribute that is so easy to talk about and so hard to achieve. Good things do last. That this volume remains useful to three generations of physicians is a source of pride to us.

Early on we conceived this book as a practical text, a "working text" as we described it in the first edition. Some theory is discussed, but since much of headache theory is speculative, we have preferred not to place our emphasis there. We have instead concentrated on diagnosis and therapy—how to get the job done—a practical text for the clinician.

The current edition follows the last by seven years. Much is new. The editors have changed, as have some contributors. Their fresh ideas and concepts will invigorate the text and allow it to gather new momentum.

Finally, the reader may be assured that all of us who write here have passed many patients with headache through our hands. This book is founded on clinical experience, for which there is no substitute.

MERLE L. DIAMOND, M.D.
GLEN D. SOLOMON, M.D.

Acknowledgments

We would like to thank Ray Kersey of W.B. Saunders for his diligence and forbearance in the preparation of this text. Special thanks to Mary Franklin, whose hard work, editorial skill, and dedication contributed greatly to this volume.

MERLE L. DIAMOND, M.D.
GLEN D. SOLOMON, M.D.

NOTICE

Contents

1

The Impact of Headache from the Patient's Perspective

David G. Litaker, M.D.

Glen D. Solomon, M.D.

Introduction

Headache is a condition that affects millions of Americans in the course of their daily lives. Accounting for 9 million visits annually to primary care physicians in the United States, headache represents one of the most common problems for which individuals seek medical advice and treatment.[1] In addition to its economic impact on medical costs, headache can result in absence from the workplace and leads to impaired productivity in many individuals. Outside the workplace, headache may interfere with social activities and interpersonal relationships and have a dramatic effect on perceptions of quality of life.[2, 3] The societal impact of headache as it relates to self-perceived quality of life and social functioning is described and discussed.

Perception of Quality of Life in Individuals with Headache

Quality of life is a multidimensional concept that has been measured in many settings through the use of a variety of methods. In general, health-related quality of life (HRQOL) is a parameter that is assessed on the basis of the perceptions of individuals regarding different aspects of their overall functional status and well-being. Measurement of HRQOL has been increasingly useful in supplementing traditional clinical outcomes in the determination of the effectiveness of headache treatment and selected interventions.[4–13] Because treatments for headache have become more sophisticated and costly, the use of an end point that reflects patient perception of effect is both attractive and relevant in an increasingly consumer-oriented medical marketplace.

The subjective nature of headache and the lack of either physical findings or increased mortality have left clinicians without an objective standard by which to judge the impact of headache on individuals or society. Two general approaches have been used to "objectify" the impact of headache on the individual. The first is the use of generic instruments that measure overall functional status and well-being without reference to disease-specific symptoms. A second approach focuses on the use of disease-specific health questionnaires that are used to assess symptoms or attitudes about specific illnesses. During the past decade, several instruments of both types have been used with some success in patients with headache to demonstrate the impact of headache and the effect of treatment interventions from the patient's perspective.

Measurements of Quality of Life in the Treatment of Headache

Standardized surveys have been used for many years to measure functional status and well-being in patients with a broad range of medical problems. Careful study in the methods of HRQOL determination, however, has led to the identification of specific dimensions that have been incorporated into instruments subsequently subjected to extensive validity and reliability testing. For example, the Short

Form 36 Health Survey (SF-36), which is one of the more commonly used measures of HRQOL, has been widely used in clinical practice and extensively tested and validated in patients with chronic disease[14, 15] and headache.[16, 17]

The SF-36 consists of patient self-ratings for 36 items that measure eight health concepts, including physical functioning, social functioning, mental health, vitality, emotional health, bodily pain, and role functioning (impairment in both physical and emotional functioning due to disability) (Table 1–1). An additional measure of health transition has been included to assess an individual's perception of change in overall health status over time.[18]

By using quality of life and medical data for a nationwide sample of 9385 adults, profiles for several common chronic medical conditions have been described and compared with data for patients without chronic conditions.[14] Typically, patients with specific medical conditions perceive unique areas in which their quality of life is different from that of unaffected individuals. HRQOL profiles, which have come to be known as the measurable "health burden" of a medical illness, not only appear to be unique to specific conditions but also have a cumulative effect when multiple conditions are present.

The health burden for migraine has been compared with that of other illnesses through the use of a generic HRQOL instrument to determine its relative impact on quality of life (Fig. 1–1). After adjustment for factors that might affect patient perceptions (e.g., age, gender, and comorbid illness),[19] patients with headache report significant impairment in all dimensions of HRQOL compared with nonheadache patients (see Fig. 1–1). In a comparison of migraineurs with individuals with other chronic conditions, quality of life is greatly reduced, especially in the dimensions reflecting bodily pain, social functioning, vitality, and role functioning.[17] The use of the SF-36 in these comparative studies appears to support two conclusions. The clear differences in functional status among headache sufferers, especially migraineurs, appear to be comparable to those among individuals with conditions that might otherwise be considered more debilitating, such as angina, depression, or arthritis. Second, compared with the general US population, patients with migraine demonstrate significant morbidity in several areas that are used to measure functional status and well-being.

Other instruments have been developed to assess the specific effects of headache on well-being, functional status, and functioning in social situations. Unlike generic HRQOL surveys, disease-specific instruments are designed to measure aspects of quality of life that are most likely to be affected by a medical condition of interest. Elements of functional status that would be relevant in the study of migraine, for example, include the extent to which a patient's ability to conduct normal activities at the workplace or in social situations is changed by headache. Because the effect of headache is greatest on role function, questions regarding physical status (ability to walk, climb stairs, or perform other daily activities) typically would be excluded from headache-specific instruments. Examples of disease-specific instruments in common use in headache research include the Henry Ford Hospital Headache Disability Index[20] and the Migraine Quality of Life Questionnaire (MQOLQ).[21]

Instruments that reflect the impact of a

Table 1–1 Dimensions of Quality of Life in the SF-36 Health Survey

Domain	Number of Items	Definition
Physical functioning	10	Capacity to perform a variety of common physical activities
Role physical	4	Degree to which physical health interferes with usual daily activities
Bodily pain	2	Body pain during past 4 weeks
General health	5	Overall assessment of health in general
Vitality	4	General energy, level of fatigue in past 4 weeks
Social functioning	2	Extent to which health interferes with normal social activities
Role emotional	3	Extent to which emotional problems interfere with usual daily activities
Mental health	5	General mood or affect in past 4 weeks
Health transition	1	Change in health status in the past year

Adapted from Ware JE, Snow KK, Kosinski M, Gandek B, eds. SF-36 Health Survey: Manual and Interpretation Guide. Boston, MA: The Health Institute, New England Medical Center; 1993.

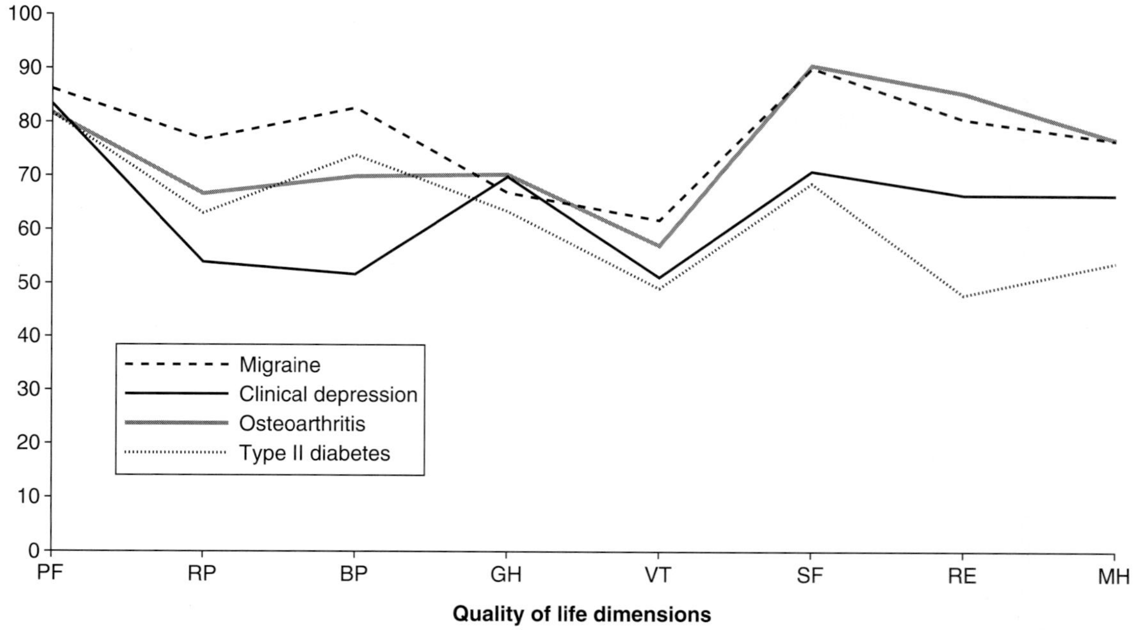

Figure 1–1 Adjusted SF-36 scores in patients with migraine and other conditions. PF, physical functioning; RP, role physical; BP, bodily pain; GH, general health; VT, vitality; SF, social functioning; RE, role emotional; MH, mental health. (Data from Osterhaus JT, Townsend RJ, Gandek B, et al. Measuring the functional status and well-being of patients with migraine headache. Headache 1994;34:340.)

single condition on quality of life allow an assessment of the unique limitations or restrictions on health not usually included in generic surveys. This approach may also allow a more sensitive assessment of the effects of treatment or longitudinal variations in patients' perceptions of quality of life during the course of disease or the degree to which an individual adjusts his or her expectations about quality of life as a result of a chronic illness. In contrast, generic instruments allow comparisons of health-related quality of life among differing populations and permit adjustment for the effects of important covariates such as age, sex, and other comorbid conditions. For this reason, many researchers prefer to combine data from both generic and disease-specific instruments to obtain the most complete assessment of the direct effects of these conditions at the patient level.

Variations in the Impact of Headache on Quality of Life

Solomon et al[22] demonstrated that chronic headache disorders differ in their effects on various aspects of well-being and functional status. As with many chronic diseases, the subtypes of headache result in unique quality-of-life profiles that distinguish them from each other (Fig. 1–2). Cluster headache, for example, has been associated with the greatest amount of pain and relatively little impairment in physical functioning, whereas chronic tension headache results in a marked impairment in mental health and a generalized reduction in functioning.[22] These differences in functional status among different headache types support the concept that each of the headache diagnoses represents a unique entity rather than a continuum of headache. An understanding of these differences may permit more focused treatment that results in improvement in both symptoms and quality of life.[22]

A longitudinal assessment of the effect of headache on health-related quality of life also demonstrates that reduction in health perceptions is not simply limited to the time of the attack. Dahlof and Dimenas[23] demonstrated that migraine patients perceive more emotional distress, less vitality, and disturbances in both sleep and general contentment between headache attacks compared with individuals unaffected by migraine.

Severity of pain also appears to correlate closely with the magnitude of the impact of

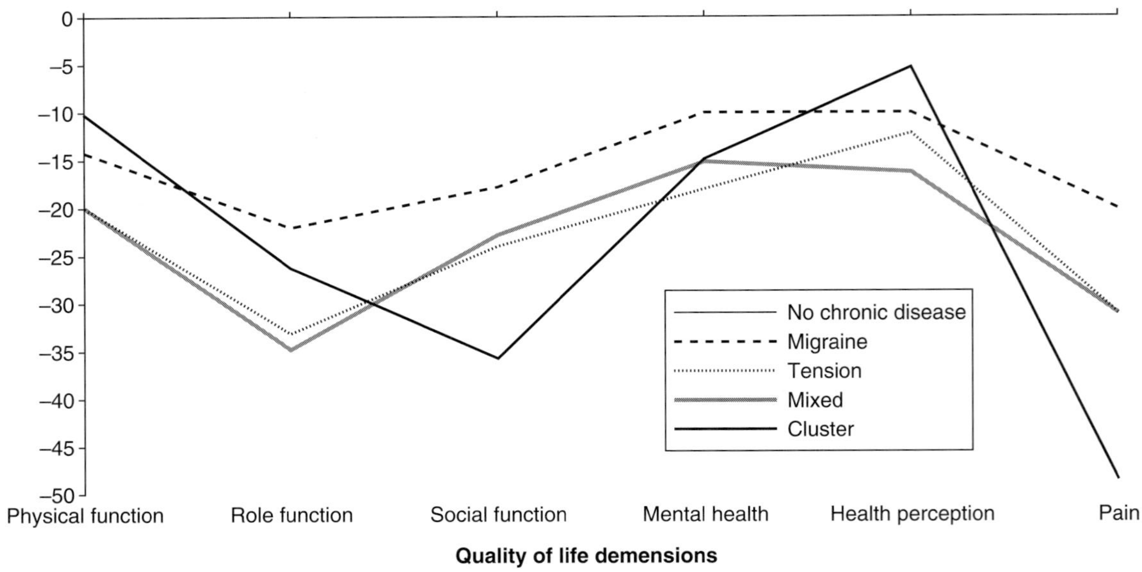

Figure 1–2 Comparison of standardized SF-20 scores by headache diagnosis. (Adapted from Solomon GD, Skobieranda FG, Gragg LA. Does quality of life differ among headache diagnoses? Analysis using the Medical Outcomes Study Instrument. Headache 1994;34:145.)

headache on individual functioning; Osterhaus et al[17] documented a relationship between the degree of headache severity and perception of quality of life (Fig. 1–3). Lipton et al[24] also demonstrated that disability from headache correlates positively with pain intensity. These observations suggest that disability and perceptions of quality of life are at least loosely interrelated and appear to be associated with severity of headache in a dose-response manner.

Impact of Headache on Social Functioning

In addition to impairment in health-related quality of life reported by headache sufferers, recent studies indicate a significant impact of headache on social functioning. In a population-based survey in Canada, Edmeads et al[2] reported that half of migraine sufferers discontinued normal activities during their attacks, and nearly one third required bedrest.

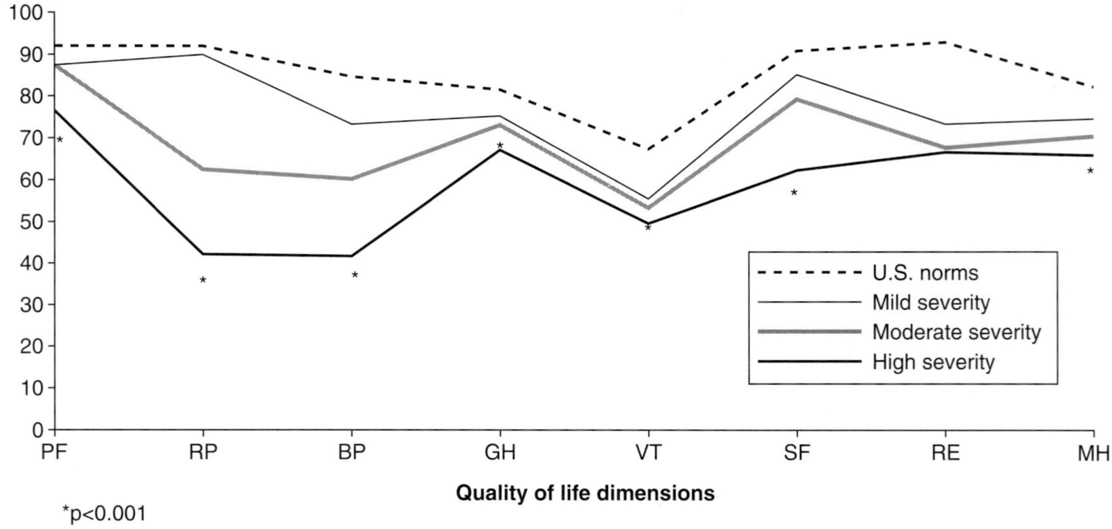

Figure 1–3 Comparison of adjusted mean SF-36 scores by self-reported migraine severity. (Data from Osterhaus JT, Townsend RJ, Gandek B, et al. Measuring the functional status and well-being of patients with migraine headache. Headache 1994;34:341.)

In more than 70% of headache sufferers in this survey, interpersonal relationships were impaired and regular activities were limited during 78% of migraine attacks. In a study in which the degree of disability associated with migraine was assessed, functional disability and the need to discontinue or cancel normal activities during attacks of headache were common and resulted in perceived decrements in social functioning.[3]

As stated, headache has a negative effect on the emotional and physical aspects of quality of life as measured with the Role Function Score of the SF-36. This finding is particularly meaningful because role functioning has been generally considered the best measure of an individual's ability to work. In migraineurs, the ability to participate in leisure activities is also impaired and may contribute to difficulties in relationships with social contacts at home and in the workplace. Dahlof and Dimenas[23] postulated that the apprehension evoked by fear of future symptoms placed symptom-free migraineurs at a higher risk than control subjects for developing additional medical problems that might further jeopardize physical or emotional status.

Effects of Headache Treatment on Quality of Life and Social Functioning

Despite the prevalence and impact of headache, there are remarkably few published data on the effects of headache therapy on quality of life. This may reflect the general paucity of outcome-oriented studies in the past decade or a lack of confidence in the use of an instrument that is based on patient report as a study end point. Regardless of the cause, a few studies have demonstrated that many instruments are adequately sensitive to change in HRQOL perceptions over time to permit an accurate assessment of treatment effect on functional status and well-being.[5, 9, 10, 11, 25]

Acute changes in patient well-being were first reported by Dahlof and Bjorkman[8] in their use of the Minor Symptom Evaluation Profile in patients with migraine who received treatment with diclofenac-K, a nonsteroidal anti-inflammatory drug. Individuals receiving this agent described significantly greater improvement in general measures of well-being compared with those receiving placebo. This study has not been repeated with other instruments, nor has this instrument been tested as extensively as others in the evaluation of drugs or treatment effectiveness.

In a study of patients with chronic headache, Skobieranda et al[26] used the SF-20 to determine changes in quality of life after the first 6 months of treatment at an outpatient tertiary care headache center. Treatment was individualized and included both prophylactic and abortive therapy. Although there were no significant improvements in the dimensions of quality of life after 6 months of treatment, 52% of patients reported an improvement in pain scores. The authors concluded that a number of factors may have led to the failure to detect adequate differences in quality of life after treatment, including heterogeneity of the intervention, insensitivity of the instrument over short periods of study, and sample bias related to the type of patients studied at a tertiary care referral center. Subsequent studies have focused on single treatment strategies (either abortive or preventive), specific headache types, and study periods of adequate length to allow the detection of clinically meaningful responses.

In migraine, the impact of prophylactic medication on quality of life is limited to a single study by Solomon, et al,[7] who evaluated quality of life during 7 months of treatment with flurbiprofen, a nonsteroidal anti-inflammatory drug. The authors reported an improvement in role functioning (headache interference with work) corresponding with reductions in headache frequency and intensity and a beneficial effect on quality of life that was sustained over the duration of the study. The results of this 15-patient, unblinded observational study suggest that the benefit of prophylactic therapy can be quantified with generic quality-of-life scales. Whether these changes in HRQOL reflect medication effect or a regression of these scores toward population means cannot be answered using this study design but is an important focus of future research efforts.

Documentation of the long-term effect of abortive therapy in migraine is limited to a single agent but is consistently found in several studies.[4, 5, 9–11, 25, 27] In each report, the effect on HRQOL by sumatriptan, a selective serotonin receptor agonist, indicated that sumatriptan, whether administered orally or subcutaneously, significantly enhanced key dimensions of HRQOL regardless of measure used (generic versus disease specific). Across the studies in which the SF-36 was used, social functioning scores improved most consistently with sumatriptan, although health perception, vitality, bodily pain, mental health, and role functioning scores also increased. D'Allens et al.[25] observed that changes in HRQOL are first detectable within 3 months and are sustained for at least 1 year after the initiation of treatment in most individuals. Comparative evaluations that are based on participants' perceptions of functional status and well-being after exposure to other interventions will be useful in developing headache treatment strategies associated with the greatest effect and longest duration.

Educational programs, individually or as part of a comprehensive treatment program, also appear to have detectable effects on patients' sense of well-being. A recent evaluation in which the effect was examined of a comprehensive migraine treatment program on 30 patients with migraine or mixed headache demonstrated treatment approaches that combined patient education with medical management contributed to enhanced self-efficacy and confidence in participants' ability to manage their headaches.[12] Other studies have confirmed that enhanced self-efficacy through education about headache and headache treatments results in individuals' ratings of such program benefits as equal to or higher than preventive or abortive treatments in contributing to treatment success.[27]

Conclusions

As one of the most common presenting pain complaints, headache affects the lives and livelihood of millions of Americans. Studies have documented areas in which the impact of headache on well-being and functional status is the greatest. Although it is difficult to measure the pain associated with headache objectively, several instruments developed over the past two decades allow insight into the effect of headache on individuals' perceptions of quality of life and social functioning. In the absence of objective clinical end points, the use of patient-derived measures relating to quality of life is essential in defining the effectiveness of therapy on the individual's life, family, and employment. Although research in this area is at a relatively early stage, several studies indicate the possibility of reducing the considerable impact of headache on well-being and functional status through the use of effective treatments or disease management strategies. Future studies in which the differential effects of newer, more effective pharmaceutical agents, education, and alternate treatment strategies in specific headache types are compared will be useful in defining methods to reduce the impact of headache and improve the quality of life and social functioning of those with headache.

References

1. Cypress B. Headache as the reason for office visits. National Ambulatory Medical Care Survey, United States. NCHS Advance Data 1981;67:1–6.
2. Edmeads J, Findlay H, Tugwell P, et al. Impact of migraine and tension-type headache on lifestyle, consulting behaviour, and medication use: A Canadian population survey. Can J Neurol Sci 1993;20:131–137.
3. Pryse-Phillips W, Findlay H, Tugwell P, et al. A Canadian population survey on the clinical, epidemiologic and societal impact of migraine and tension-type headache. Can J Neurol Sci 1992;19:333–339.
4. Solomon GD, Skobieranda FG, Genzen JR. Quality of life assessment among migraine patients treated with sumatriptan. Headache 1995;35:449–454.
5. Jhingran P, Cady RK, Rubino J, et al. Improvements in health related quality of life with sumatriptan treatment for migraine. J Fam Pract 1996;42:36–42.
6. Miller DW, Osterhaus JT, Hirsh JD, et al. Quality of life assessment among migraineurs treated with sumatriptan: Preliminary findings. Headache 1993;33:278. Abstract.
7. Solomon GD, Kunkel RS. Long-term use of flurbiprofen in migraine prophylaxis. Headache 1992;32:269–270. Abstract.
8. Dahlof C, Bjorkman R. Diclofenac-K (50 and 100 mg) and placebo in the acute treatment of migraine. Cephalagia 1993;13:117–123.
9. Beall D, Cohen J, Miller D, et al. An interim analysis of the use of subcutaneous sumatriptan in a managed care setting: Effects on health-related quality of life, impact on health care resource use, and clinical efficacy. Pharmacotherapy 1995;15:385. Abstract.
10. Adelman J, Sharfman M, Johnson R, et al. Impact of oral sumatriptan on health-related quality of life and productivity in health care professionals with migraine: An interim analysis. Pharmacotherapy 1995;15:387.

11. Bullinger M, Bruggenjurgen B. Quality of life assessment among migraineurs under current treatment and after three months treatment with sumatriptan. Presented at the European Federation of Neurological Societies, Berlin, December 1993.
12. Scopp AL, Peters KS. Patient rating of trigger elimination effectiveness in comprehensive migraine treatment program. Headache 1992;32:269. Abstract.
13. Litaker DG, Solomon GD, Genzen JR. Impact of sumatriptan on care utilization and costs of care in migraineurs. Headache 1996;36:538–541.
14. Stewart AL, Greenfield S, Hays RD, et al. Functional status and well-being of patients with chronic conditions. Results from the Medical Outcomes Study. JAMA 1989;262:907–913.
15. Stewart AL, Hays RD, Ware JE. The MOS Short-Form General Health Survey: Reliability and validity in a patient population. Med Care 1988;26:724–735.
16. Solomon GD, Skobieranda FG, Gragg LA. Quality of life and well being of headache patients: Measurement by the Medical Outcomes Study Instrument. Headache 1993;33:351–358.
17. Osterhaus JT, Townsend RJ, Gandek B, et al. Measuring the functional status and well-being of patients with migraine headache. Headache 1994;34:337–343.
18. McHorney CA, Ware JE, Raczek AE. The MOS 36-item Short Form Health Survey (SF-36): II. Psychometric and clinical tests of validity in measuring physical and mental health constructs. Med Care 1993;31:247–263.
19. Tarlov AR, Ware JE, Greenfield S, et al. The Medical Outcomes Study: An application of methods for monitoring the results of medical care. JAMA 1989;262:925–930.
20. Jacobson GP, Ramadan NM, Aggarwal SK, Newman CW. The Henry Ford Hospital Headache Disability Inventory (HDI). Neurology 1994;44:837–842.
21. Hartmaier SL, Santanello NC, Epstein RS, Silberstein SD. Development of a brief 24-hour migraine-specific quality of life questionnaire. Headache 1995;35:320–329.
22. Solomon GD, Skobieranda FG, Gragg LA. Does quality of life differ among headache diagnoses? Analysis using the Medical Outcomes Study Instrument. Headache 1994;34:143–147.
23. Dahlof C, Dimenas E. Migraine patients experience poorer subjective well-being/quality of life even between attacks. Cephalalgia 1995;15:31–36.
24. Lipton RB, Stewart WF, Von Korff M. Migraine impact and functional disability. Cephalalgia 1995(suppl 15):4–9.
25. D'Allens H, Richard A, Bertin L, et al. Responsiveness assessment of a specific quality of life questionnaire for migraineurs (QVM). Qual Life Res 1994;3:72. Abstract.
26. Skobieranda FG, Solomon GD, Gragg LA. Quality of life changes in headache patients following six months of outpatient treatment: Use of the Medical Outcomes Study Instrument. Headache 1993;33:283. Abstract.
27. VandenBree MB, Passchier J, Emmen HH. Influence of quality of life and stress coping behaviour on headaches in adolescent male students: An explorative study. Headache 1990;30:165–168.

2

Classification and Mechanism of Headache

Glen D. Solomon, M.D.

Introduction

Headache is the most common pain complaint for which patients are seen in outpatient medical practices and the seventh most common reason for medical visits in the United States. The problem of headache generates 18.3 million outpatient physician visits per year in the United States.[1] Knowledge of headache and its variants therefore is essential to the medical practitioner.

Although headache is common in clinical practice and only infrequently associated with organic disease, headache may be the presenting complaint in catastrophic illness, such as cerebral hemorrhage, meningitis, or brain tumor. To ignore the symptom of headache may risk the life of the patient. Headache may be intense whether its source is benign or malignant.

A rational approach to any condition requires an understanding of the classification and pathogenesis of the disorder.

Classification and Mechanism of Headache

The classification of any disease is difficult, and the disorder "headache" posesses particular hardship. The primary headache disorders constitute a group of syndromes of uncertain pathophysiology with a complete absence of laboratory or radiographic tests that could be used for diagnostic criteria. The headaches of a patient may change over his or her lifetime in both quantity and quality. Patients may have multiple types of headache. Although "pure" forms of headache exist, many patients experience transitional forms of headache.

The most comprehensive classification scheme for headache was developed by the International Headache Society (IHS) and published in 1988.[2] This 96-page tome provides an in-depth diagnostic classification of more than 100 types of headache divided into 13 groups. The IHS classification has become the standard for diagnosing patients for research purposes, and virtually all new headache studies use these diagnostic criteria. The diagnostic criteria for migraine, tension-type, and cluster headache are shown in Table 2–1.

The clinical usefulness of the IHS criteria in medical practice has been questioned by both primary care and headache specialists. Diamond and Dalessio[3] designed a simple, clinically useful classification scheme for headache. They divide headache into three groups: vascular, tension-type, and traction and inflammatory headaches (Table 2–2).

Vascular headache includes migraine with aura (classic migraine) and without aura (common migraine); hemiplegic, basilar, and ophthalmoplegic migraine; cluster headache; and the cluster headache variants (chronic paroxysmal hemicrania, idiopathic stabbing headache, exertional headache), toxic vascular headache, and hypertensive headache. Common to all these headaches is the tendency to vasodilation; whether the vasodilation causes the headache or is merely an epiphenomenon is unknown. Vasoconstriction also may occur and may be responsible for the painless sensory and motor auras that precede the migraine. *Toxic vascular headache* refers to a headache evoked by a systemic vasodilation produced by fever, alcohol ingestion, poisons, hypoxemia, high altitude, carbon monoxide poisoning, and vasodilating

Table 2–1 International Headache Society Diagnostic Criteria

Migraine Without Aura

A. At least five attacks fulfilling B through D
B. Headache lasting 4 to 72 hours
C. At least two of the following characteristics:
   1. Unilateral location
   2. Pulsating quality
   3. Moderate or severe intensity
   4. Aggravation by walking stairs or similar routine physical activity
D. During headache at least one of the following:
   1. Nausea and/or vomiting
   2. Photophobia and phonophobia

Chronic Tension-Type Headache

A. Average headache frequency ≥15 days per month for ≥6 months fulfilling criteria B through D
B. At least two of the following pain characteristics:
   1. Pressing/tightening quality
   2. Mild or moderate severity
   3. Bilateral location
   4. No aggravation by walking stairs or similar routine physical activity
C. Both of the following:
   1. No vomiting
   2. No more than one of the following: Nausea, photophobia, or phonophobia

Cluster Headache

A. At least five attacks fulfilling B through D
B. Severe unilateral orbital, supraorbital, and/or temporal pain lasting 15 to 180 minutes untreated
C. Headache is associated with at least one of the following signs, which must be present on the side of the pain:
   1. Conjunctival injection
   2. Lacrimation
   3. Nasal congestion
   4. Rhinorrhea
   5. Forehead and facial sweating
   6. Miosis
   7. Ptosis
   8. Eyelid edema
D. Frequency of attacks: from one every other day to eight per day

medications, such as nitrates. Under the IHS classification, toxic vascular headache would include headache induced by acute substance use or exposure, headaches associated with noncephalic infections, and headache associated with metabolic disorder.

The *tension-type* or *muscle contraction headache* is the most common form of headache in Western populations. Tension-type headache is typically described as a bandlike pressure headache without associated symptoms. This headache most commonly occurs as an episodic discomfort that responds well to over-the-counter medications and rarely requires physician intervention. When it occurs chronically, as it does in 3% of the population,[4] it can markedly impair the patient's quality of life. Chronic tension-type headache can be a common somatic manifestation of depression and occurs frequently in patients with fibromyalgia and chronic fatigue syndrome.

When chronic tension-type headache occurs in patients with frequent migraine attacks, the terms *mixed headache syndrome, chronic daily headache,* and *transformed migraine* often are used. Because there is no evidence that migraine "transforms" into chronic tension-type headache and because tension-type headache itself often is a chronic daily headache, the term *mixed headache syndrome* is used here. None of these terms are included in the IHS classification, in which migraine and tension-type headache would be listed separately with their frequencies noted.

Traction and *inflammatory headache* includes most of the organic or secondary causes of headache; these include headache evoked by organic diseases of the skull or its components, including the brain, meninges, arteries, veins, eyes, ears, teeth, nose, and paranasal sinuses. The term *traction headache* describes the often nonspecific headache seen with mass lesions of the brain, including tumors, hematomas, abscesses, and brain edema. Headaches from subarachnoid hemorrhage, meningitis, sinusitis, and disorders of the teeth and joints of the jaw and neck are included in the traction and inflammatory

Table 2–2 Classification of Headache

Vascular Headache

- Migraine
  - With aura (classic)
  - Without aura (common)
  - Complicated
    - Hemiplegic
    - Ophthalmoplegic
    - Basilar artery
- Cluster
- Toxic vascular
- Hypertensive

Tension-Type (Muscle Contraction) Headache

- Depressive equivalents and conversion reactions
- Chronic anxiety states
- Cervical osteoarthritis
- Chronic myositis

Traction and Inflammatory Headaches

- Mass lesions
- Diseases of the eye, ear, nose, throat, and teeth
- Arteritis, phlebitis, and cranial neuralgias
- Occlusive vascular disease
- Atypical facial pain
- Temporomandibular disease

group. The cranial neuralgias are included in this grouping because the neuritic pain that characterizes these conditions is associated with specific abnormalities of the function of the central nervous system.

The management of the traction and inflammatory headache or the neuralgias generally involves specific treatment for the associated underlying disease. These patients may require extensive investigation, neuroimaging, and consultations with ophthalmologists, otolaryngologists, dentists, neurologists, or neurosurgeons.

All the conditions mentioned above and listed in the classification of headache are discussed in detail in subsequent chapters.

Anatomy of Pain

Pain is generally thought of as having two components: a fast, localized sensation carried by myelinated A-delta fibers that respond to mechanical (i.e., sharp) or thermal stimulation and a slower, more unpleasant and diffuse sensation carried by unmyelinated C-fibers.

Nociceptive fibers enter the spinal cord through the dorsal horn; synapse in laminae I, II, and V of the spinal cord; and ascend as the spinothalamic tract. The spinothalamic tract consists of the neospinothalamic and the paleospinothalamic tracts. The neospinothalamic tract ascends to the thalamus, terminates in the ventral posterolateral nucleus, and projects to the somatosensory cortex. The neospinothalamic tract provides information on the quality, intensity, and location of the painful stimulus. The paleospinothalamic tract is polysynaptic, with many interactions with the reticular system and periaqueductal gray. It terminates in the medial, intralaminar, and posterior thalamic nuclei and then projects diffusely to limbic and subcortical areas. The paleospinothalamic tract, unlike the neospinothalamic tract, is not topographically organized and does not project to the somatotopically organized cerebral cortex. Thus, pain impulses carried by the paleospinothalamic tract are perceived as diffuse, whereas pain impulses carried by the neospinothalamic tract are highly localized.

The first component of pain—the sharp, localized sensation—is initiated by mechanothermal nociceptors, transmitted to the spinal cord via myelinated A-delta fibers, and carried by the neospinothalamic tract to the thalamus and cortex. The second component of pain—the prolonged, burning, poorly localized "hurt"—is initiated by C-polymodal nociceptors, transmitted to the spinal cord via unmyelinated C-fibers, and carried by the paleospinothalamic tract to the reticular system, limbus, and subcortex. Because of these projections to reticular and limbic systems, the second component of pain is associated with the arousal and emotional aspects of pain.

Pain regulation also involves two descending nerve pathways that modulate pain intensity. The descending system shares several relay stations with the ascending pain pathway. In effect, it serves as a "gate" to regulate the amount of pain information that is allowed to travel beyond the relay points in the spinal cord. The sympathetic nervous system can amplify the perception of pain carried through sensory nerves. In addition, the opioid system is organized such that there are a multiplicity of sites at which opioids, either endogenous or pharmacological, might modify nociception.[5]

First, peripheral nerve endings are accessible to opioids in systemic circulation, such as β-endorphin and proenkephalin A.[5] The primary afferent nociceptor is a bipolar neuron with its centrally directed process innervating the central nervous system and its peripherally directed process innervating tissues such as skin and joints. Opioid receptors, synthesized in the cell body of the neuron, are transported not only centrally but also peripherally. Stimulation of these peripheral opioid receptors may raise the stimulation (pain) threshold of the nociceptor terminal and inhibit the release of pain-producing inflammatory mediators (i.e., substance P) from the peripheral terminals of the primary afferent nociceptors.[6]

Second, the dorsal horn of the spinal cord is the primary processing site of the primary afferent nociceptive information. It is rich in dynorphin and enkephalin.

Third, the midbrain, brainstem, and thalamus are relay stations for nociceptive information ascending to the cerebral cortex. These structures are rich in dynorphin and enkephalin, and receive β-endorphin innervation from the hypothalamus.

Fourth, the limbic system and the cortex produce the emotional dimension of pain, are very rich in dynorphin and enkephalin neurons, and have β-endorphin input.[5]

Anatomic Substrate of Headache

The pain-sensitive structures of the head include the skin of the scalp and its blood supply and appendages; the muscles of the head and neck; the great venous sinuses and their tributaries; parts of the dura mater at the base of the brain; the dural arteries; the intracerebral arteries; the fifth, sixth, and seventh cranial nerves; and the cervical nerves. The cranium, the brain parenchyma, much of the dura and pia mater, the lining of the ventricles, and the choroid plexuses are not sensitive to pain.

In general, pain pathways for structures above the tentorium cerebelli are contained in the trigeminal nerve. Pain from these structures is referred to the frontal, temporal, and parietal regions of the skull. Pain pathways for structures below the tentorium cerebelli are contained especially in the glosopharyngeal and vagus nerves, as well as the upper cervical spinal roots. Pain from these structures is usually felt in the occipital region of the head, although radiation to the frontal and temporal regions can occur.

Pathogenesis of Migraine

Despite years of research, there is still a great deal that is not known about the pathogenesis of migraine. According to the original theory of Wolff,[6a] migraine is a vascular disease initiated by cerebrovascular spasm, whereas others have believed migraine to be of neural origin. Recent theories have suggested that spreading neuronal depression, as described by Leão,[6b] may be the cause of migraine with aura.

Research on cerebral blood flow has convincingly shown that dilatation of intracranial and extracranial arteries is a prominent feature of migraine in the headache phase in both patients with and without aura. In addition, pharmacologically induced constriction of the dilated arteries relieves migraine headache.[7]

A clinically relevant model of migraine pathophysiology should explain these vascular findings and several phenomena noted by both clinicians and patients:

- Migraines can be triggered by a large number of stimuli, including diet, sleep changes, weather changes, and hormonal changes.
- Migraine has a circadian rhythm similar to that of several diseases of abnormal vasomotor tone (vasoconstriction), including myocardial infarction, angina pectoris, and ischemic stroke.[8]
- Sleep is effective in aborting many migraines.
- Cerebral blood flow is decreased during migraine aura.
- There is both a generalized systemic vasoconstriction and a local cerebrovascular vasodilatation on the side of the head pain during a migraine attack.[9]
- Serotonin is released by platelets during a migraine.
- Calcitonin gene-related peptide (CGRP)[10] and probably substance P[11] are elevated during the migraine attack.

The trigeminovascular migraine model used to explain the above phenomena incorporates the following concepts:

1. Like other "visceral" organs, the brain has a pain system to signal tissue injury. The trigeminovascular system exists to protect the brain against insults such as ischemia, toxins, or intrinsic disease, just as angina pectoris protects the heart against ischemia.[12]

2. The trigeminal nerve can be stimulated by both electrical (neuronal) and chemical activators, including prostaglandins, serotonin, and histamine.[13] Migraine triggers work either directly to alter these chemical mediators (i.e., estrogens altering prostaglandins during menses) or through neural mediators (i.e., rapid eye movement [REM] sleep eliminates serotonin release from the dorsal raphe nucleus).

3. When stimulated, the trigeminal nerve releases substance P and CGRP into dural and meningeal blood vessels. The release of substance P causes the degranulation of mast cells and the attraction of polymorphonuclear leukocytes. This leads to the mast cell release of histamine and platelet release of serotonin, with resulting vasodilatation and exudation of plasma into the tissues. The resulting inflammation and swelling of the blood vessels represent the "sterile arteritis" described by Wolff half a century ago.

4. The neurogenic inflammation and release of substance P cause both distention of cranial arteries and headache pain.

Although the initiating event in migraine is still uncertain, it is believed that vasoconstriction induces cerebral ischemia, which activates the trigeminal nerve. Through antidromic conduction in the trigeminal nerve, substance P and CGRP are released from small-diameter sensory afferents. These neuropeptides are released into the meningeal and dural blood vessels, initiating vasodilatation, plasma extravasation, and the release of histamine from mast cells and serotonin from platelets. The pain of migraine is likely caused by sensitization from substance P of polymodal nociceptors (unmyelinated C-fibers) that course with the arteries.[13] Because the effect of substance P on nociceptors is faster than the development of sterile inflammation and vasodilation, the onset of migraine pain may precede the vasodilation of the cerebral vasculature.

How does this model explain the clinical experience of migraine? Trigger factors either have direct actions on vasomotor tone (e.g., tyramine in certain foods), or mediate neurochemical release (e.g., weather changes affect serotonin levels, sleep alters serotonin release from the dorsal raphe nucleus, stress modifies catecholamine levels). Vasoconstriction, platelet changes, and neurochemical mediators can initiate cerebral ischemia and activate the trigeminovascular system.

Increases in platelet activity and catecholamine levels, as well as increased serotonin release from the dorsal raphe, occur in the early morning hours.[8] All of these may trigger the trigeminovascular system, either directly or through vasoconstriction-induced ischemia. This may explain the circadian rhythm of migraine.

REM sleep inhibits the release of serotonin from the dorsal raphe nucleus. Sleep may abort a migraine attack by inhibiting the serotonin-mediated stimulation of the trigeminovascular system.

Serotonin Receptors

One of the major advances in improving our knowledge of migraine pathophysiology and therapy is related to the recent understanding of serotonin (5-HT) receptors. There are at least five serotonin receptor subtypes: 5-HT_{1A}, 5-HT_{1D}, 5-HT_{1C}, 5-HT_2, and 5-HT_3. The location and functional significance of each of the subtypes are under study.

A number of drugs used to treat migraine are known to be serotonin agonists or antagonists; these include methysergide, cyproheptadine, pizotifen, and amitriptyline. Drug interactions with specific 5-HT receptor subtypes may be the basis for their efficacy in both acute and prophylactic treatment of migraine.

5-HT_{1D} receptors were characterized in 1987 and are widespread in the human brain. Several studies have implicated this receptor in the constriction of cerebral blood vessels and arteriovenous anastomoses.[14] Several effective abortive agents in migraine, including dihydroergotamine (DHE) and sumatriptan, have potent activity at the 5-HT_{1D} receptor site. Prophylactic migraine drugs interact minimally with 5-HT_{1D} receptor sites in human brain.[14]

The 5-HT_{1D} receptor agonists have been shown to block trigeminovascular neurogenic inflammation, but they will not prevent inflammation caused by systemic substance P.[15] This suggests that these agents work by blocking substance P release from perivascular trigeminal nerve fibers via receptors located prejunctionally.

The 5-HT_{1A} receptor has been shown to mediate serotonin-induced contractions of the basilar artery in dogs. In addition, 5-HT_{1A} receptor agonists inhibit raphe cell firing.[14] Several antimigraine drugs have moderate or high affinity for the 5-HT_{1A} receptor, including methysergide, pizotifen, DHE, sumatriptan, propranolol, and timolol. Other migraine prophylactic drugs, such as amitriptyline, atenolol, and verapamil, have little potency at this site. No obvious correlation appears to exist between drug affinity for this receptor and potency in terms of migraine relief.[14]

The 5-HT_2 receptor has been shown to mediate smooth muscle contraction in many vascular beds. Serotonin, probably via 5-HT_2 receptors, can stimulate the production of prostacyclin and other products of arachidonic acid metabolism in smooth muscle cells. Theoretically, 5-HT_2 antagonists are able to inhibit serotonin from inducing an arachidonic acid–derived inflammatory state. The value of this inhibition is limited to prophylaxis because once the inflammatory reaction is initiated, the 5-HT_2 antagonists would be of little benefit.[14] A number of potent 5-HT_2 antagonists have been shown to be effective prophylactic agents for migraine, including methysergide, cyproheptadine, pizotifen, amitriptyline, and verapamil. Diltiazem and B-blockers are inactive at this receptor site.[14]

5-HT_{1C} receptors share similar pharmacological characteristics with 5-HT_2 receptors.

Currently available prophylactic drugs for migraine do not differentiate between the two receptors. It is possible that the mechanism of action of prophylactic agents in migraine may be by antagonism of the 5-HT_{1C} receptor rather than the 5-HT_2 receptor.[14]

5-HT_3 receptor antagonists have potent antiemetic effects. Some of these agents, such as metoclopramide, have activity in the acute treatment of migraine.[14]

Peroutka[14] summarized the hypothetical role of serotonin subtypes in migraine therapy by stating that acute migraine relief is generated by agonist activity at 5-HT_{1D} or 5-HT_{1A} receptors, or both, whereas prophylactic activity was dependent on antagonist activity at 5-HT_2 or 5-HT_{1C} receptors, or both.

To put this receptor data into the context of the trigeminovascular (neurogenic inflammation) model of migraine, agonists of 5-HT_{1D} or 5-HT_{1A} receptors may act prejunctionally on the trigeminal nerve to inhibit release of substance P, CGRP, or both.

Migraine prophylaxis would occur if antagonism of the 5-HT_2 or 5-HT_{1C} receptors prevented serotonin-induced cerebral vasospasm and concomitant ischemia, which may activate the trigeminal nerve. A second possible mechanism might involve the inhibition of arachidonic acid metabolism and inflammation by 5-HT_2 receptors antagonists.

Medications that block the stimulation of the trigeminovascular system, substance P release, or neurogenic inflammation can be used to treat migraine. Agents that stop substance P of CGRP release (i.e., sumatriptan, ergotamine) or neurogenic inflammation (i.e., nonsteroidal anti-inflammatory drugs) are useful for abortive migraine therapy, whereas agents that inhibit trigeminovascular stimulation (i.e., β-blockers, calcium blockers, antidepressants, nonsteroidal anti-inflammatory drugs, methysergide) are useful for migraine prophylaxis.

Pathogenesis of Tension-Type and Mixed Headache

The pathophysiology of tension-type headache is even less well understood than that of migraine. Episodic tension-type headache is commonly caused by increased nociception from strained muscles, as occurs with inadequate rest or poor posture, or from increased muscle tension, as occurs with stress. Increased pain impulses may cause an increased sensitivity of neurons of the trigeminal tract, and pain then may propagate itself to some extent.[16] Recurrent bouts of tension-type headache may lower the threshold for new episodes by altering the myofascial tissues, potentiating nociceptive neurons, or decreasing the activity of the antinociceptive system. It is probable that episodic tension-type headache is predominantly a disorder of peripheral mechanisms, whereas chronic tension-type headache reflects a central pain disturbance.

Chronic tension-type headache appears to be one of a group of disorders marked by low levels of brain serotonin. Patients with chronic tension-type headache commonly report symptoms of constant headache, generalized myalgias and arthralgias, difficulty in initiating and maintaining sleep, chronic fatigue, carbohydrate craving, decreased libido, irritability, and disturbed memory and concentration.[17] This disorder is similar to the disease depression; however, in chronic tension-type headache, anhedonia is not present, the mood disturbance is less marked or may be absent, and the primary symptom is headache pain. It also resembles the disease fibromyalgia, with generalized myofascial pain and sleep disturbance.

Many patients with mixed headache syndrome have a history of migraine beginning in their teens or early 20s, with the development of daily, tension-type headaches between the ages of 35 and 45. It is less common for patients to present with both migraine and daily headaches beginning at the same time. Because many of these patients have had a long history of migraine, they are well versed in the use of vasoconstrictor and analgesic medications. When their headaches cease being intermittent and become daily, patients with this syndrome often resort to frequent or excessive analgesic or vasoconstrictor use. The use of excessive medication can lead to habituation and the problems of rebound headaches.

One theory of the pathophysiology of mixed headache syndrome is based on the concept of serotonin depletion. Serotonin depletion causes increased pain sensitivity and arousal.[18] Symptoms common in patients with the proposed serotonin-depletion syndrome include chronic daily headaches, sleep disturbances (initial or late insomnia or both), mood disorder (dysthymia or depression or both), carbohydrate craving, decreased libido, premenstrual syndrome in women, and difficulties with memory and concentration. Other conditions associated with low levels of serotonin may include fibromyalgia, depression, alcoholism, and premenstrual syndrome.

This theory proposes that patients with mixed headache syndrome initially have migraine headaches. Migraine attacks are marked by acute decreases in brain and plasma serotonin levels. Between attacks, the serotonin levels return to normal. After a number of years, some migraine sufferers develop chronically low levels of serotonin. Over several years, the level of serotonin in the brain drops below a critical level, and symptoms of serotonin depletion emerge. These patients develop chronic tension-type headaches as a manifestation of their chronically low serotonin levels and continue to have migraine attacks caused by intermittent acute falls in brain serotonin.

Pathogenesis of Cluster Headache

Cluster headache is defined as a syndrome of unilateral orbital headache associated with multiple signs and symptoms; these include conjunctival injection, lacrimation, nasal congestion, rhinorrhea, forehead sweating, miosis, ptosis, and eyelid edema.[19, 20] Moskowitz[21] proposed that the anatomic locus of pathology for cluster headache is the superior pericarotid cavernous sinus. This hypothesis was based on the unique convergence of fibers from the ophthalmic trigeminal division, maxillary division (a small branch of the orbitociliary nerve), superior cervical ganglion controlling pupil and lid function, and sphenopalatine ganglion. Using single-photon emission computed tomography SPECT scanning, Gawel and Ichise[22] reported inflammatory changes in the cavernous sinus during cluster cycles that resolved during remissions. It is likely that this inflammation is sufficiently severe to obliterate venous outflow and interrupt ipsilateral sympathetic fibers that traverse the cavernous internal carotid artery wall to innervate the eye, upper eyelid, forehead, and orbital and retro-orbital vessels.[23] Pain is transmitted from related veins and arteries by trigeminal and greater superficial petrosal afferents and is exacerbated or initiated by vasodilation of sensitized arteries and veins.

References

1. Linet MS, Stewart WF, Celentano DD, Ziegler, D, et al. An epidemiologic study of headache among adolescents and young adults. JAMA 1989;261:2211–2216.
2. Headache Classification Committee of the International Headache Society. Classification and diagnostic criteria for headache disorders, cranial neuralgias, and facial pain. Cephalalgia 1988;8(suppl 7):1–96.
3. Diamond S, Dalessio DJ. Classification and mechanisms of headache. *In* Diamond S, Dalessio DJ, eds. The Practicing Physician's Approach to Headache, 5th ed. Baltimore: Williams & Wilkins; 1992:1–2.
4. Rasmussen BK, Jensen R, Schroll M, Olesen J, et al. Epidemiology of headache in a general population: A prevalence study. J Clin Epidemiol 1991;44:1147–1157.
5. Milan MJ. Multiple opioid systems and pain. Pain 1986;27:303–347.
6. Edmeads J. Bringing treatment to a head. Headache 1991;31:695.

6a. Wolff HG. Headache and Other Head Pain, 2nd ed. New York: Oxford University Press, 1963.

6b. Leão AAP. Spreading depression of activity in the cerebral cortex. J Neurophysiol 1944;7:359–390.

7. Olsen TS. The myth about spreading oligemia in migraine. Headache 1993;4:318–321.
8. Solomon GD. Circadian rhythm and migraine. Cleve Clin J Med 1992;59:326–329.
9. Iversen H, Nielsen T, Olesen J, et al. Arterial responses during migraine headache. Lancet 1990;336:837–839.
10. Goadsby P, Edvinsson L, Ekman R. Extracerebral levels of circulating vasoactive peptides during migraine headache. Cephalalgia 1989;9(suppl 10):292–293. (Abstract)
11. Goadsby P, Edvinsson L, Ekman R. Release of vasoactive peptides in the extracerebral circulation of humans and the cat during activation of the trigeminovascular system. Ann Neurol 1988;23:193–196.
12. Moskowitz M. The visceral organ brain: Implications for the pathophysiology of vascular head pain. Neurology 1991;41:182–186.
13. Moskowitz MA. Brain mechanisms in vascular headache. Neurol Clin 1990;8:801–815.
14. Peroutka S. Developments in 5-hydroxytriptamine receptor pharmacology in migraine. Neurol Clin 1990;8:829–839.
15. Buzzi MG, Moskowitz MA. The antimigraine drug sumatriptan specifically blocks neurogenic plasma extravasation from blood vessels in dura mater. Br J Pharmacol 1990;99:202.
16. Olesen J, Schoenen J. Synthesis. *In* Olesen J, Tfelt-Hansen P, Welch KMA, eds. The Headaches. New York: Raven Press; 1993:495.
17. Solomon GD. Pharmacology and use of head-

ache medications. Cleve Clin J Med 1990;57:627–635.
18. Harvey JA, Schlosberg AJ, Yunger LM. Behavioral correlates of serotonin depletion. Fed Proc 1975;34:1796–1801.
19. Couch JR. Cluster headache: Characteristics and treatment. Semin Neurol 1982;2:30–40.
20. Diamond S, Solomon GD, Freitag FG. Cluster headache. Clin J Pain 1987;3:171–176.
21. Moskowitz M. Cluster headache: Evidence for a pathophysiologic focus in the superior pericarotid cavernous sinus plexus. Headache 1988;28:584–586.
22. Gawel MJ, Ichise M. The cavernous sinus in cluster. *In* The Migraine Trust, from the Ninth Annual Migraine Trust International Symposium, September 7–10, 1992.
23. Hardebo JE, Moskowitz MA. Synthesis of cluster headache pathophysiology. *In* Olesen J, Tfelt-Hansen P, Welch KMA, eds. The Headaches. New York: Raven Press; 1993:574–575.

3

Taking a Headache History

Merle L. Diamond, M.D.

Glen D. Solomon, M.D.

Introduction

A detailed and relevant history geared to the headache patient is the most important factor in making correct diagnoses (Table 3–1). Through careful questioning and direction of the inquiry, a specific headache profile evolves that in many instances pinpoints the diagnosis because the majority of patients with headache have negative results on neurological and physical examinations. The essentials of a headache history should be set down in a short, concise manner so a pattern evolves and the clinician is able to identify the type of headache that is present.

Table 3–1 History of the Patient with Headache

Patient's name:
Date of initial visit:
Types:
Headache onset:
Location:
Frequency:
Severity:
Exertional aspects to headache:
Duration:
Aura:
Premonitory symptoms:
Associated symptoms:
Sleep pattern:
Family history:
Menses (if applicable):
Seasonal:
Emotional:
Tests:
Headache medications:
Other medications:
Surgical:
Medical:
Allergies (1) Drugs:
(2) Foods:
(3) Alcohol:
(4) Tobacco:
Neurological examination:
Physical examination:

Sample histories are presented at the end of the chapter. The headache history is begun by asking the patient for a precise description of headache; it is quite common for a patient to have two or three separate types of headache. The charting of the headache frequency by the patient for 1 or 2 months (the headache calendar) often provides clues to the type of headache present. Table 3–2 is a sample headache calendar kept by a patient with migraines; Table 3–3 depicts coexisting migraine and tension-type (mixed-headache syndrome) headaches.

Onset

The physician is interested in the specific time of life when the headaches began. Headaches that start in childhood, adolescence, and the second and third decades of life are often vascular, such as migraine. Headaches that occur later in life suggest an organic etiology, or they may be due to psychogenic illness, such as depression. The occurrence of a headache after a traumatic episode, such as the death of a loved one, a serious financial loss, and so forth, may be the key to an underlying depression. Headaches that occur because of high blood pressure are usually present on awakening and often disappear during the day. Migraine can awaken a patient at 3:00 or 4:00 AM, but more often, cluster headaches occur at night and frequently awaken the patient several hours after going to sleep. Sinus headache usually begins gradually in the morning and increases in severity during the day. Headache related to anxiety without an obvious depressive component often follows a specific stressful incident (e.g., a patient's headache starts with the death of a brother from a brain tumor).

Table 3–2 Headache Calendar

Patient's Name: ____________________

Date	Time (record hour and AM/PM) *Onset*	*Ending*	(*1) Severity of Headache	(*2) Psychic and Physical Factors	(*3) Food and Drink Excesses	Medication Taken and Dosage	(*4) Relief of Headache
12/1/96	12 noon	4 PM	8	12		Imitrex 50 mg × 2	3
12/2/96							
12/3/96							
12/4/96							
12/5/96							
12/6/96							
12/7/96	7 AM	3 PM	10	15		Imitrex 50 mg × 2	3
12/8/96	8 AM	6 PM	8	15		Anaprox 275 mg × 2	5
12/9/96	8 AM	12 noon	4	15		Midrin × 2	2
12/10/96							
12/11/96							
12/12/96							
12/13/96							
12/14/96	7 AM	12 AM	8		C, G, S	Imitrex 50 mg × 2	3
12/15/96							
12/16/96							

***1: Severity Scale**

1	*5*		*10*
None	Mild	Moderate	Severe

***4: Relief Scale**

1	*5*		*10*
COMPLETE	MODERATE	MILD	NO RELIEF

***2: Psychic and Physical Factors**

1: Emotional upset/family or friends
2: Emotional upset/occupation
3: Business/reversal
4: Business/success
5: Vacation days
6: Weekends
7: Strenuous exercise
8: Strenuous labor
9: High-altitude location
10: Anticipation anxiety
11: Crisis/serious
12: Postcrisis period
13: New job/position
14: New move
15: Menstrual days
16: Physical illness
17: Oversleeping
18: Weather
19: Fasting
20: Missing a meal
21: Other

***3: Food and Drink Excesses**

A: Ripened cheese (pizza)
B: Herring
C: Chocolate
D: Vinegar
E: Fermented foods *(pickled or marinated, sour cream/yogurt)*
F: Freshly baked yeast products
G: Nuts *(peanut butter)*
H: Monosodium glutamate *(MSG; Chinese food)*
I: Pods of broad beans
J: Onions
K: Canned figs
L: Citrus food
M: Bananas
N: Pork
O: Caffeinated beverage *(cola)*
P: Avocado
Q: Fermented sausage *(cured cold cuts)*
R: Chicken liver
S: Wine
T: Alcohol
U: Beer

(Patients on Nardil and/or Marplan should follow the original diet given them.)

Table 3–3 Headache Calendar

Patient's Name: ______________________________

Date	Time (record hour and AM/PM) *Onset*	*Ending*	(*1) Severity of Headache	(*2) Psychic and Physical Factors	(*3) Food and Drink Excesses	Medication Taken and Dosage	(*4) Relief of Headache
8/15/96	7 AM	11 AM	5	5		Advil X 4	4
	7 PM	10 PM	6	1		Fiorinal X 2	4
8/17/96	6 PM	12 AM	8	2	A	Fiorinal X 4	5
8/18/96	11 AM	3 PM	9	17		Imitrex 12 mg SQ	3
8/19/96	8 PM	1 AM	4	18	F	Advil X 2	4
8/20/96	6 AM	10 PM	10	15		Imitrex 12 mg SQ	7
						Fiorinal X 3 Thorazine 25 mg rectal supp	4 2
8/21/96	9 AM	12 noon	6	15		Aleve X 2	4
8/22/96	8 AM 6 PM	11 AM 9 PM	5	11		Advil X 2 Aleve X 1	3 4
8/23/96	1 PM	3 PM	3		H	Advil X 2	2
8/24/96	11 AM	4 PM	6	17		Excedrin X 2	4
8/25/96	7 AM	10 PM	10		A, S	Imitrex 12 mg SQ	6
8/26/96	9 AM	2 PM	6	20		Aleve X 2	4

***1: Severity Scale**

1	*5*		*10*
None	Mild	Moderate	Severe

***4: Relief Scale**

1	*5*		*10*
COMPLETE	MODERATE	MILD	NO RELIEF

***2: Psychic and Physical Factors**

1: Emotional upset/family or friends
2: Emotional upset/occupation
3: Business/reversal
4: Business/success
5: Vacation days
6: Weekends
7: Strenuous exercise
8: Strenuous labor
9: High-altitude location
10: Anticipation anxiety
11: Crisis/serious
12: Postcrisis period
13: New job/position
14: New move
15: Menstrual days
16: Physical illness
17: Oversleeping
18: Weather
19: Fasting
20: Missing a meal
21: Other

***3: Food and Drink Excesses**

A: Ripened cheese (pizza)
B: Herring
C: Chocolate
D: Vinegar
E: Fermented foods *(pickled or marinated, sour cream/yogurt)*
F: Freshly baked yeast products
G: Nuts *(peanut butter)*
H: Monosodium glutamate *(MSG; Chinese food)*
I: Pods of broad beans
J: Onions
K: Canned figs
L: Citrus food
M: Bananas
N: Pork
O: Caffeinated beverage *(cola)*
P: Avocado
Q: Fermented sausage *(cured cold cuts)*
R: Chicken liver
S: Wine
T: Alcohol
U: Beer

(Patients on Nardil and/or Marplan should follow the original diet given them.)

Under the general heading of *onset,* the physician also asks about the length of illness. Many migraine or depressive sufferers will give a 20-, 30-, or 40-year history of headache. The chronicity of their headache suggests that they do not have a progressive neurological lesion. Conversely, the sudden onset of severe headache and diagnostic neurological signs precludes a self-limited headache syndrome.

Location

It is important to know whether the cephalalgia is generalized over the entire head or localized on one side. It is also important to know whether the pain switches from one side of the head to the other; migraine headaches frequently act in this way. In the absence of increased intracranial pressure, generalized head pain may indicate psychogenic disease. Focal pain on one side of the head may be migraine, but it can also be due to organic disease. Pain localized to the eye alone should make the clinician suspicious of ocular disease or cluster headache. The "hatband" distribution of head pain indicates tension-type headache.

Frequency

Migraine may occur at sporadic intervals during a lifetime. By the time medical advice is sought, an identifiable pattern is often established. Usually, in females, there is an association with the menstrual cycle. Often, there is an absence of the headache pattern during vacations and after the third month of pregnancy, but some headaches appear only during periods of relaxation. Cluster headache may be seasonal, and the series often occur in the spring and autumn in cycles lasting from 1 to 2 weeks to 4 or 5 months. Some patients experience chronic cluster headache with remission periods lasting less than 14 days. Chronic tension-type headache is continuous and may last for years.

Duration

If the headache is due to organic causes, it is usually continuous and progressively increases in intensity. The headache due to migraine is episodic and lasts from 6 hours to 3 days or even longer. Cluster head pain can last from several minutes to less than 4 hours. As mentioned above, chronic tension-type headache is often persistent.

Severity

The severity of the pain in migraine is often described as intense. Characteristically, it is a pulsating or throbbing rather than constant pain. The pain of cluster headache is also throbbing, but it is frequently described as deep, boring, and very severe. Tic douloureux is a shock-like, transient, stabbing pain, typically neuritic in character. Pain of tension-type headache is often dull, nagging, and persistent, with occasional exacerbations of more severe pain.

Prodromata

The major types of migraine are differentiated by the presence of aura or prodromal symptoms occurring 30 to 60 minutes before the acute headache. The prodromata or warning signs of migraine with aura are usually limited to visual symptoms (Table 3–4). It is believed that both the positive and negative eye prodromes originate in the visual cortex portion of the occipital lobe. The metamorphopsias indicate a disturbance of function in the optic radiation of the posterior temporal zone. Other auras may take the form of paresthesias, defects in mobility, and, rarely, a disturbance of the sense of smell. Vague, premonitory symptoms may present in both types of migraine, starting 24 to 48 hours before the onset of an acute attack. These symptoms include hunger, fatigue, nervousness, or bursts of energy. Tumors and angiomas of the occipital lobe can also cause

Table 3–4 Ocular Prodromata of Migraine

Positive	Teichopsia (fortification spectra) Zigzags Flashing lights and colors
Negative	Scotomata Hemianopsia
Metamorphopsia	Illusions of distorted size, shape, and location of fixed objects

teichopsia, or fortification spectra, but it occurs more persistently than in migraine.

Associated Symptoms

The migraine attack may include a wide variety of symptoms occurring in association with the pain. Photophobia, nausea, vomiting, and urinary and focal neurological changes may be seen. With cluster headache, a modified Horner's syndrome may appear, including ptosis and constriction of the pupil. Lacrimation, flushing, or blanching of the face and a mucoid discharge from the nostril on the side ipsilateral to the headache may occur during a cluster attack. Overt glaucoma is characterized by a steamy cornea and difficulty in seeing. If subarachnoid hemorrhage has occurred, meningeal signs will appear rapidly. Sudden loss of power in the arms or legs with associated headache suggests a stroke, either thrombotic or hemorrhagic. Be alert to unilateral tinnitus or diplopia, which may be evidence of an intracranial mass. Associated epilepsy is usually an ominous sign.

Sleep Habits

The identification of sleep disturbances can be extremely important in determining the etiology of chronic tension-type headaches. Difficulty falling asleep is indicative of anxiety. The physician should consider an environmental stress syndrome or psychological factors that may be producing the problem. If the patient has frequent or early awakening, depression is suggested, and questioning should be directed toward a possible depressive component. Patients with migraine can be awakened by severe headache during the night but are usually helped by sleep. Patients with cluster headache are frequently awakened by their severe head pain, and the intensity of the pain forces them into ceaseless activity until the attack subsides.

Precipitating Factors

Among the multiple factors that precipitate migraine are fatigue, loss of sleep, stress, menstruation, bright sunlight, and foods and drugs containing tyramine and other vasoactive materials. Less common factors include alcohol, prolonged hunger, and high humidity. Cough headache, contrary to popular belief, is not always associated with an intracranial tumor, can often be benign, and may occur as part of a vascular headache syndrome.

Emotional Factors

The patient's relationship to his or her family, as well as the patient's occupation, social life, environmental stresses, and sexual habits should all be ascertained in detail by the interviewer. Such emotional factors as these have special relevance to headache. Careful questioning about other physical, emotional, and psychic symptoms may uncover an underlying psychological illness that has been masked by the cephalalgic patient. Overt depression should be obvious to the interviewer. It is possible to uncover a stressful situation with associated anxiety through a simple inventory of the factors mentioned above.

Relationship to Occupation

Emotional factors and stress on the job are common headache causatives. There are certain specific occupations, however, that have a built-in predisposition to head pain. Patients providing services to the public are particularly susceptible. Abattoir workers are subject to Q fever, with intense headache as one of the symptoms. The nitrites to which munitions workers are exposed cause vasodilation of the cerebral vessels that mimics vascular headaches. Mechanics and others can get headaches from carbon monoxide present in poorly ventilated work areas.

Family History

Migraine is a familial illness, whereas cluster headache is not. Depression also frequently occurs in families. Studies suggest a hereditary relationship of migraine. If both parents have experienced migraine, there is a 70% chance that the children will also have migraine; if only one parent has had migraine, the children's chances are reduced to about 45%. If neither parent has had migraine but there is a history of migraine in other family members, it will occur in about 25% of the children.

Seasonal Relationship

Cluster headaches are more common in the spring and autumn. Depression associated with chronic tension-type headaches often occurs during holiday seasons, at a time linked with family gatherings.

Menstrual and Obstetrical Factors

Approximately 70% of female migraineurs will report a relationship between their headaches and their menstrual cycle. The headaches often occur immediately before, during, or shortly after their period. Some patients will complain of headaches in midcycle, about the time of ovulation. Migraine tends to disappear by the third month of pregnancy, only to return after delivery. Remission of the migraine attacks typically occurs with onset of menopause. The administration of hormones in the postmenopausal period can prolong the headache syndrome. Conversely, migraine that reappears at the time of the menopause may be relieved by the ingestion of estrogens. The use of oral contraceptives is known to increase the severity, frequency, duration, and complications of migraine.

Owing to the increasing incidence of hyperprolactinemia, every female patient should be specifically asked about the presence of galactorrhea and amenorrhea.

Medical History

Questions should also be asked about recent or remote head trauma. Subdural hematomas may occur after trivial blows. A recent spinal tap performed for anesthesia or diagnosis may cause a self-limited headache. A low spinal fluid pressure syndrome has been described, which can be associated with a chronic subdural hematoma. A history of seizures, one-sided headache, and neck stiffness indicates the possibility of an aneurysm or angioma present with a slow leak.

Surgical History

If a person reports prior surgery on a mole or other tumor, the lesion may have metastasized to the brain, producing headache. A past history of tuberculosis may have significance regarding possible spread to the brain. Obviously, any previous cranial surgery should alert the physician to previous head trauma, tumor, aneurysm, or other significant brain disease. A prior history of spinal anesthesia may have triggered the headaches.

Systems Review

A complete careful review of the systems should be done in all headache workups. Disease of the eyes, ears, nose, throat, teeth, and neck should be emphasized because all can produce local head pain.

Allergy

The relationship of headache to seasonal allergy should be sought. Patients may experience increased headaches accompanying their hay fever or seasonal allergy symptoms as part of increased capacity for vasomotor activity. Researchers have not been able to show, however, that migraine or other forms of headache result from a specific antigen–antibody reaction.

Previous Tests for Headache

Physicians see countless patients who have had repeated, sophisticated workups. The age and adequacy of these studies, considered with the history and current physical findings, dictate whether these studies should be repeated. Headache may be associated with metabolic diseases, such as hypothyroidism, or with significant anemia, so there is no substitute for an adequate medical survey. However, if the patient has previously undergone an adequate workup and there are no neuro-

Table 3–5 New Patient Headache Treatment History

Previous consultations with physicians	
Names of physicians	***Date***
1.	
2.	
Previous hospitalization *(for headaches)*	
Place	***Date***
1.	
2.	
Previous emergency department visits *(due to headaches)*	
Place	***Date***
1.	
2.	

logical or historic reasons to order any further tests, it is prudent to avoid repeating expensive and potentially dangerous studies.

Past Treatments and Effectiveness

A history of previous treatments can be a key to the diagnosis, as well as to the selection of therapies (Table 3–5). If the patient has consulted various physicians and had multiple hospitalizations and emergency department visits, admission to a specialized inpatient headache unit may be considered. A review of previous medications should also be an essential part of the history (Table 3–6). For example, if one knows that ergotamine tartrate has previously helped a patient, one can assume that the patient probably has migraine. If the patient has had a trial on antidepressants with some success, the likelihood of a diagnosis of depression is increased. However, antidepressants are also used for their analgesic effects; therefore, a history of past medications and their successes and/or failures acts as both a diagnostic and therapeutic clue to management of the patient.

Table 3–6 Drug History

Name of Drug	Period Drug Taken	Response*	Reason for Discontinuation of Drug

*1, Definitely not helpful; 2, not helpful; 3, uncertain; 4, helpful; and 5, extremely helpful.

Present Medications and Effectiveness

One should review in detail the medications used by the patient. Are they contributing to headache? This is especially true with asthma drugs, which are sympathomimetic and may exacerbate headache. Has the patient recently started to use vasodilators, such as niacin, papaverine, or dipyridamole? As stated, migraine may be exacerbated by the use of oral contraceptives. Nitrates can activate migraine in certain susceptible people. Indomethacin is another drug that can on occasion cause chronic head pain. The physician should pursue with vigor the drug history of the patient.

Case Histories

Headache 1: Migraine

T.E. is a 19-year-old man who describes episodic headaches involving one side of his head. His maternal grandmother and his father's brother have similar problems. As a child, he easily became carsick, found it difficult to play twirling games, and had recurrent episodes of unexplained vomiting without diarrhea, which puzzled the family pediatrician. His headaches started at age 12 and have continued episodically. They appear perhaps four to six times a year and often begin in midmorning. Initially, he notes a slight loss of vision in part of his visual field, after which he sees twinkling lights and a series of jagged lines that he can sometimes draw on paper. These visual images appear in both eyes. Promptly thereafter, as the visual images cease, his headache begins. It is localized to one side of the head, usually frontal, but with different attacks it may shift sides. The pain is severe and pounding, increases with bending over or straining, and is not particularly relieved by lying down. Shortly after the pain begins, he experiences significant nausea and vomiting and may vomit repeatedly. Bright lights and sound bother him, and on occasion he has left school to return to the dormitory. In his bedroom, he pulls the blind and tries to sleep. If he can get to sleep, he may waken free of headache. After approximately 6 to 12 hours, the headache begins to wane and is usually gone by 24 hours; then he is left depleted, with a feeling of exhaustion. His physician has diagnosed his problem as migraine with aura. He has used sumatriptan and the ergot derivatives to abort the headache. If these medications are taken during the aura phase or early in the course of the headache, he can sometimes abort the episode.

T.E. is recognized by his professors and peers to be extremely competent and meticulous to a fault. He is compulsive about details and consistently rechecks work on examinations. His organizational skills have led him to several leadership positions in high school and now on his college campus. Although the headaches can limit activities during the acute episodes, T.E. refuses to let the migraine affect his schoolwork and social life.

Headache 1 Outline

Types:	One
Onset:	Age 12
Location:	Unilateral, usually frontal
Frequency:	One every 2 to 3 months
Duration:	6 to 12 hours
Severity:	Very severe, can be incapacitating
Aura:	Twinkling lights, jagged lines
Associated symptoms:	Nausea, vomiting, photophobia, phonophobia, pain that may be relieved by sleep or vomiting
Sleep pattern:	No sleep disturbance
Emotional status:	Perfectionist, compulsive, well organized
Family history:	Maternal grandmother and father's brother have migraine
Seasonal relationship:	None
Precipitating factors:	Chocolate and cheese can trigger a headache

Headache 2: Coexisting Migraine with Tension-Type Headaches Due to Depression

L.V. is a homemaker, age 37, who enjoys good health with the exception of incapacitating headaches. She started having one-sided headaches at age 16 that were diagnosed as migraine but were helped by the ingestion of sublingual ergotamine tablets given to her by the family physician. These migraine-type headaches occurred almost weekly and lasted 2 to 3 days. She noted that the headaches started about 2 days before her menstrual cycle. The migraine increased in frequency and severity since she started taking birth control pills. During her two pregnancies, the headaches disappeared after the first trimester.

Currently, the severe headaches occur not only at her period but also one to two times per week. When the headache is severe, L.V. also has nausea and vomiting and occasionally sees black spots before her eyes. About 2 days before the attack, she notes excessive energy, often completing major projects around the home before the pain strikes. She has a very neat house, with everything in its place. Chocolate and red wine will trigger a severe headache. She remembers that her grandmother had similar headaches.

Three years ago, L.V. started experiencing another type of headache that was present on both sides of her head and the neck. On questioning, the patient revealed that she and her husband have been having marital problems for the past 4 years. This second type of headache is always present on awakening. She rarely has problems falling asleep but is always awake early, usually by 4:30 or 5:00 AM. L.V. feels depressed owing to her headaches, and she is losing interest in her home and children. She tries to sleep to escape and usually feels fatigued. She states she cannot tolerate the pain much longer because it lasts all day and sometimes into the night.

L.V. was placed on long-acting propranolol (80 mg) every morning and amitriptyline (50 mg) at bedtime. The birth control pills were discontinued. For the acute headaches, she is using naproxen sodium (275 mg) PRN. After 3 weeks, she began to show some improvement and is being followed carefully in the outpatient headache clinic.

Headache 2 Outline

Types:	Two: A and B
Onset:	A: Age 16 B: 3 years ago
Location:	A: Usually behind left eye, radiates to entire left side B: Bilateral, including the neck
Frequency:	A: One to two weekly; always at menses B: Daily
Duration:	A: 2 to 3 days B: Continuous throughout day
Severity:	A: Severe, may be incapacitating B: Dull ache, mild to moderate
Aura:	None
Associated symptoms:	A: Nausea, vomiting, occasionally sees black spots B: None
Sleep pattern:	Early awakening at 4:00 to 5:00 AM, without alarm
Emotional status:	Depression for 3 to 4 years due to headaches and marital problems; perfectionist; compulsive
Family history:	Maternal grandmother had migraine headaches
Seasonal relationship:	None
Menstrual relationship:	Severe headache starting 2 days before menses
Medical and surgical history:	Noncontributory
Precipitating factors:	Chocolate and red wine trigger headaches

Headache 3: Tension-Type Headaches

J.B. is a 49-year-old accountant who has complained of headaches for 20 years. The headaches occur almost daily and are not well localized, but he often describes a band of pain about his forehead that waxes and wanes. Sometimes, he notes pain in the neck and lower part of the head. He consumes large amounts of over-the-counter medications, switching from one to another, seemingly dependent on the vagaries of the latest television headache commercials. By his own admission, he is an aspirin-popper.

He has consulted many physicians and has been subjected to examinations and testing, but no cause for these headaches has been found. In addition to headache, he described chronic fatigue that is not relieved by rest. He sleeps poorly, has problems getting to sleep, and often wakes early in the morning. He often has a vague sense of being unwell. He has withdrawn from many social activities and rarely plays golf, his favorite pastime; they tire him and "are too much trouble besides." He would rather stay at home now. He has lost his appetite for sex. He is irritable, has trouble concentrating, and has a "short fuse." He is more emotional than formerly, feeling at times that he might weep without reason.

He recently reported to his physician, and another unsuccessful neurological survey was done. His physician then wisely referred J.B. to a clinical psychologist, and psychological testing was performed. A significant masked depression was expressed, particularly as body complaints. After a period of antidepressant therapy and counseling, he is somewhat improved, although his headaches are not entirely relieved. He continues to regularly consume rather large amounts of aspirin.

Headache 3 Outline

Types:	One
Onset:	Age 29
Location:	Bilateral pain across forehead, occasional pain in occipital region and neck
Frequency:	Almost daily
Duration:	Continuous throughout day

Severity:	Moderate to severe
Aura:	None
Associated symptoms:	None
Emotional status:	Feels unwell, irritable, anxious, depressed, decreased libido, fatigue
Sleep pattern:	Difficulty falling asleep, often has early and frequent awakening
Family history:	None
Seasonal relationship:	No relationship
Precipitating factors:	None

Headache 4: Cluster Headaches

M.Z., age 45, is a successful contractor who has always enjoyed good health. He was a former college football player, but in recent years has exercised little and gained 30 pounds during the past decade. He smokes heavily and on occasion drinks to excess. About 2 years ago, he experienced a series of excruciating, usually nocturnal headaches. The series of headaches began suddenly, lasted 3 weeks, and then ceased spontaneously. His physician was contacted at that time but offered no explanation for these episodes.

One month ago, the nocturnal headaches restarted, often awakening him at 3:00 AM. The pain is localized to and above the left eye. The left eye waters copiously with the onset of the headache. The left side of the nose is initially congested and later has rhinorrhea. His left eye becomes very red, perhaps because he rubs it. The pain is steady and intense, severe enough to make this stolid man cry for help. The pain usually lasts 45 minutes and then rapidly clears. For the remainder of the day, he feels perfectly well. During a series, he has noticed that even small amounts of alcohol can reproduce this set of symptoms, so he has stopped drinking completely in the past month. His physician was contacted again and advised M.Z. that he was working too hard and was too tense. During a week's vacation, he rested and the headaches continued. He was concerned that he might have a brain tumor. In the past several days, however, the headaches have started to decrease and are no longer as intense. He has not responded to any of the pain medications provided by his physician.

Headache 4 Outline

Types:	One
Onset:	2 years ago
Location:	Above left eye, never switches sides
Frequency:	During this current series, the headaches occur nightly; the last series of headaches was 2 years ago
Duration:	Acute headaches last 45 minutes
Severity:	Very severe, excruciating
Aura:	None
Associated symptoms:	Left-sided lacrimation, ipsilateral congestion, rhinorrhea, reddened pupil
Sleep pattern:	Headache awakens him nightly
Emotional status:	Noncontributory
Family history:	None
Seasonal relationship:	Both series have occurred during the spring
Precipitating factors:	During a series of headaches, alcohol will trigger an acute attack

Headache 5: Subarachnoid Hemorrhage

J.S., a 29-year-old attorney, was in his usual state of good health. He maintained his weight at moderate levels and practiced abstemious habits. A recent complete physical examination had been within normal limits. He had never complained of headache. Two weeks ago, while jogging, he experienced a sudden and severe head pain involving his entire head; the pain did not wax and wane and was not relieved by rest. He became ill and vomited and found no relief from aspirin, codeine, or an ice pack applied to his head by his wife. Shortly thereafter, he became sleepy and was not easily roused. His wife recognized immediately that a serious illness had occurred and drove him to the closest emergency department, but he could not walk from the car to hospital entrance. On admission, he was restless and moaning in pain and could not provide an adequate history. One pupil had become dilated, but other signs of neurological damage were not prominent. He was not paralyzed, but he demonstrated slight stiffness of the neck. Computed tomography scan of the head demonstrated blood in the ventricular system. A lumbar puncture was performed within the hour, and the spinal fluid obtained was bloody. After consultation among several specialists, angiograms were done that showed a leaking aneurysm of one of the brain arteries. This was eventually clipped successfully by a neurosurgeon, and J.S. is rapidly recovering.

Headache 5 Outline

Types:	One
Onset:	2 weeks earlier
Location:	Entire head
Frequency:	Only one attack
Duration:	Constant and unrelenting
Severity:	Severe, progressive
Aura:	None
Associated symptoms:	Vomiting, gradually became drowsy and comatose, dilation of the pupil, slight neck stiffness
Sleep pattern:	Negative
Emotional status:	Noncontributory
Family history:	None
Seasonal relationship:	No relationship
Medical and surgical history:	Negative
Precipitating factors:	Headaches started while jogging

Headache 6: Brain Tumor

L.R., age 60, began to note difficulty with his vision. He stated that his vision to the right was impaired, and he found it difficult to read. He was bumping into objects on the right side of his environment. He saw an ophthalmologist, who observed a visual field defect, although the patient's cooperation was not optimal.

L.R. reported a long history of chronic frontal and temporal headache that he associates with hay fever and sinusitis. He says that these headaches have not increased, but during the course of the interview and examination, he later states that he has more pain in the left side of the head, which is relatively constant and now is not easily relieved by medications. He describes great turmoil recently associated with problems with the Internal Revenue Service. These business difficulties have been very trying, and he blames many of his current problems on these issues. He takes large amounts of medication, including a sleeping pill, a tranquilizer, and an antihistamine, and he uses cigarettes and alcohol liberally.

When examined, he had a significant loss of visual acuity with a definite visual field cut on the right. His recent memory was poor. His speech was slow and suggested sedation. There was minimal weakness of the right leg. The patient followed directions poorly and seemed confused. He was admitted to a hospital where appropriate studies were completed, and a mass lesion was identified in the left temporal and occipital areas of the brain. He was transferred to a neurosurgical facility, where a well-circumscribed and encapsulated tumor was removed. The patient has made an excellent recovery, is headache free, and is no longer confused. However, he still has a slight right visual field defect. He continues to complain of difficulties with the Internal Revenue Service.

Headache 6 Outline

Types:	One
Onset:	1 year
Location:	Frontal and temporal areas
Frequency:	Constant throughout day
Duration:	Continuous
Severity:	Moderate to severe
Aura:	None
Associated symptoms:	Impaired vision, speech difficulties, some confusion
Sleep pattern:	Difficulty falling asleep
Emotional status:	Irritability
Family history:	None
Seasonal relationship:	No relationship
Precipitating factors:	Stress (?)

Conclusions

There are a multitude of diagnostic studies for the investigation of the headache patient. It is difficult to give specific advice regarding the extent of a diagnostic workup for an individual patient. Much depends on the diagnostic acumen of the examiner. We believe that if headache is a major complaint, a computed tomography scan or, preferably, magnetic resonance imaging of the brain should be done. If the headache pattern changes appreciably or if new neurological signs or symptoms appear, the study should be repeated.

4

Physical and Neurological Examination of the Patient with Headache

Merle L. Diamond, M.D.

Glen D. Solomon, M.D.

Introduction

After taking an all-inclusive history, every patient with headache, deserves a complete physical and neurological examination. Often, there will be no significant findings, but this cannot be assumed, even if the medical history suggests a specific diagnosis. The careful evaluation of the patient with headache is essential to rule out possible life-threatening causes and to establish appropriate diagnosis to select the treatment regimen.[1] The examination should include the following:

- General survey and physical examination
- Mental state
- Head
- Dental/jaw evaluation[2]
- Cervical spine
- Cerebellar functions
- Cranial nerves
- Motor functions
- Sensory functions
- Pathological reflexes

General Survey and Physical Examination

The physical examination of all patients must include measurement of vital signs. For example, hypertensive encephalopathy is a constellation of symptoms such as headache, nausea, vomiting, visual disturbance, seizures, confusion, and coma. It is a result of malignant hypertension, with typical blood pressures of 250/150 mm Hg.[1] Fever is an essential manifestation of toxic vascular headaches.

The facial characteristics and overall actions of a patient with headache may provide clues to the diagnosis. Depressed patients frequently are easy to spot by the downturning of the corners of their mouths and their generally sad appearance. The patient with migraine may have his or her clothes neatly folded and often will fold the paper examination gown on completion of the examination. Meticulous attention to personal appearance is a clue to the migrainous subject. Preparation of lists of symptoms and medications and careful documentation of headache frequency are other characteristics of the patient with migraine.

The patient with cluster headache may, during an attack, exhibit a complete or partial Horner's syndrome with ptosis, a constricted pupil of the affected eye, and flushing of the face; eye and nasal lacrimation also may occur. Graham[3] has described the typical facial characteristics of a patient with cluster headaches: flushed appearance, square jaw, accentuated glabellar creases, thick chin, and well-chiseled lower lip. Careful examination of the skin reveals telangiectases, coarse cheek skin (peau d'orange), and accentuated skin folds (Figs. 4–1 and 4–2).

Patients with cluster headache are characterized by motor restlessness. Those with migraine, in contrast, often retire to bed, seek out a dark room, pull the blinds, and desire isolation rather than company.

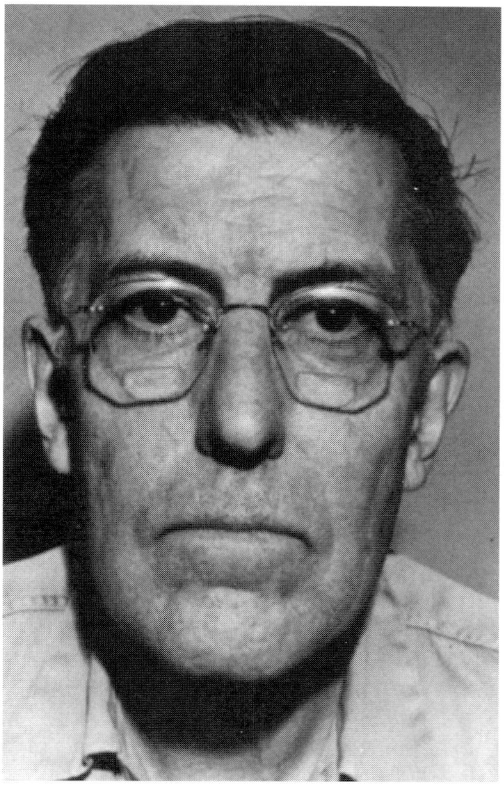

Figure 4–1 Patient exhibits typical facial characteristics of cluster headache.

Sometimes, the diagnosis of facial pain is obvious, such as in postherpetic neuralgia, where there are trophic changes in the skin related to the antecedent viral infection. Evidence of neurofibromatosis, with more than five accompanying brownish-disk lesions of the skin (*cafe-au-lait spots*), may indicate an increased predilection for intracranial tumors, particularly neuromas and meningiomas. Angiomata of the skin suggest intracranial angioma. External evidence of hypothyroidism, including puffy, dry skin; brittle hair; and loss of hair, can be associated with headache. We have seen several patients who had hypothyroidism and bizarre chronic headache of an uncertain type. Pituitary deficiency with smooth skin, lack of body hair, and testicular atrophy also is an infrequent cause of chronic headache if a pituitary tumor is present. Galactorrhea may be the sole manifestation of a prolactinoma.

One should question the headache patient carefully regarding surgical scars because they can be a clue to cerebral metastases, especially from such lesions as melanomas.

The general physical examination may reveal many disparate illnesses that can cause headache; hypertension, coarctation of the aorta, and abnormalities of the cervical spine are a few.

A distended bladder should be sought in the general physical examination of a patient with headache because this can be a cause of reflex "autonomic headache." Although headache caused by distended bladder is most common in paraplegic patients, it can occur in others.

Mental State

This subject can be assessed during the gathering of the history but can be further assessed during the physical examination. Examine the patient's orientation, memory, intelligence, and speech; obvious indications of either anxiety or depression may be present. Agitation and ceaseless activity may be evident. Failure to carry out the necessary tasks of the examination suggests inattention or dementia. Aphasia and other disorders of speech occurring in a right-handed person

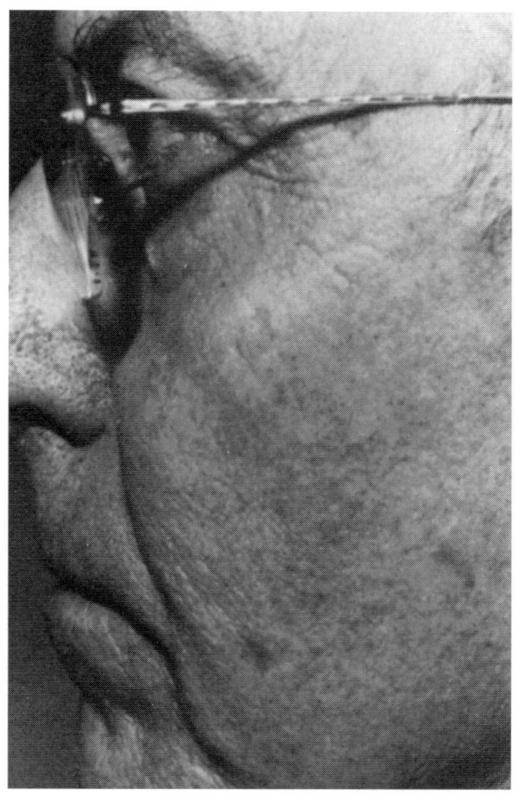

Figure 4–2 Closer examination of same patient reveals telangiectasis, peau d'orange, and accentuated skin folds.

indicate a lesion of the left hemisphere. Memory impairment for recent events and failure to remember relevant details discussed only a few minutes before should alert the examiner to early dementia that, if accompanied by chronic headache, will require intensive neurological investigation.

Head

A careful examination of the head is required for all patients with cephalalgic pain. Evidence of local infection, hardened temporal arteries (temporal arteritis), a trigger point (tic douloureux), dysfunction of the temporal mandibular joint with spasm of muscles of mastication and crepitus, and tenderness over one of the sinus areas should be carefully sought in all patients. The practitioner should perform auscultation of the head and neck, searching for bruits that may be a clue to a possible aneurysm, carotid stenosis, or angioma. Headache that occurs with coughing or with to-and-fro movements of the head may indicate a midline lesion, such as a cyst of the third ventricle.

Dental/Jaw Evaluation

Many persons with headache will present to a physician and report previous dental examinations and procedures without any benefit. The patient may have undergone evaluation and treatment for temporomandibular joint dysfunction or malocclusion. A simple examination may reveal abscess or dental caries that could affect the headache condition. The patient should also be questioned about previous dental surgeries and the use of dental appliances.

Cervical Spine

Muscle spasm, rigidity, and reduced range of motion of the cervical spine can be indicative of muscle or spinal disease of the neck that is a cause of chronic head and neck pain. Cervical spondylosis with headache is common in the elderly.

Cerebellar Functions

Cerebellar tumors (primary or metastatic), cerebellopontine angle tumors, and large acoustic neurinomas may produce dyscoordination and signs of truncal ataxia with associated difficulties in equilibrium and steady movement. A wide-based gait is a common early manifestation of cerebellar disease. Abnormal finger-to-nose or heel-to-knee tests often are indications of cerebellar dysfunction. Headache is relatively uncommon in cerebellar disorders unless increased intracranial pressure develops.

Cranial Nerves

Olfactory Nerve (I)

The loss of the sense of smell most often is due to local pathology in the nose and its accessory structures. A head injury or a tumor of the olfactory nerve in the olfactory groove may cause a unilateral disturbance of smell. If there is accompanying mental confusion, a frontotemporal tumor should be suspected.

Optic Nerve (II)

An eye examination is most important and must be included in the study of every patient with headache. Simple observation may reveal the "steamed cornea" so typical of overt glaucoma. Testing of the pressure with the fingers also can elicit a difference in pressure between the two eyes; this difference should be confirmed through tonometry. Gross examination of the visual fields should be performed, and if the examination is in any way abnormal, the visual fields should be plotted. Examination of the fundi is imperative because evidence of papilledema, optic atrophy, hemorrhages, or exudates may indicate an organic brain lesion, hypertension, or diabetes, among other diagnoses.

Oculomotor and Trochlear Nerves (III and IV)

A patient who complains of sudden pain behind the eye, with an accompanying third nerve palsy, should be evaluated for an expanding aneurysm. If the pupil on one side shows progressive enlargement, progressive compression of the oculomotor nerve is suggested. Herniation of the temporal lobe through the tentorium should be suspected (Table 4–1).

Table 4–1 Clinical Manifestations of Temporal Lobe Herniation

Compressed Structure	Clinical Manifestations
Third cranial nerve	Dilated pupil ipsilateral to herniation
Midbrain	
Physiological transection	Decerebrate rigidity
Reticular formation	Impairment of consciousness progressing to coma
Ipsilateral cerebral peduncle (direct compression)	Contralateral hemiparesis progressing to hemiplegia
Occlusion of aqueduct of Sylvius	Headache due to acute hydrocephalus
Contralateral cerebral peduncle (displaced against the sharp free edge of the tentorium)	Hemiparesis ipsilateral to herniation (false localizing sign)
Posterior cerebral artery as it crosses the tentorial edge to reach the occipital lobe (calcarine cortex)	Contralateral homonymous hemianopsia, false localizing sign

Abducens Nerve (VI)

Lesions, such as a lateral sinus thrombosis, may produce a unilateral sixth nerve paralysis. Bilateral sixth nerve paralysis may occur in acute hydrocephalus or cerebral edema.

Trigeminal Nerve (V)

The face and mucous membranes of the head should be examined for the trigger points of trigeminal neuralgia. Corneal testing should be performed with a wisp of cotton. Motor function of the trigeminal nerve is tested by opening the jaw against resistance.

Facial Nerve (VII)

This nerve is evaluated by testing the motor power of the facial muscles. Evidence of a residual stroke or facial palsy may be elicited.

Remember that the upper part of the face is bilaterally innervated and that the lower part of the face is contralaterally innervated. There are four possible levels of facial nerve dysfunction on a peripheral basis, from above downward:

1. A lesion at or proximal to the geniculate ganglion will lead to loss of tearing of the ipsilateral eye, hyperacusis, paralysis of the facial muscles, and loss of taste of the anterior two thirds of the tongue.

2. A lesion above the origin of the muscle to the stapedius gives rise to all of the findings mentioned, but loss of tearing of the ipsilateral eye will not be noted.

3. Involvement of the facial nerve in the facial canal above the origin of the chorda tympani gives rise to the lesions mentioned, excluding hyperacusis and loss of tearing of ipsilateral eye.

4. Involvement of the facial nerve at the stylomastoid foramen or below produces weakness of the facial muscles. Taste, hearing, and tearing are unaffected.

With a suprasegmental facial paresis, the lower part of the face is more profoundly affected than the brow because the brow is bilaterally innervated.

The face also may be affected in lesions of the basal ganglia as in parkinsonism. Here, lack of movement of the face is primarily noted.

Auditory Nerve (VIII)

Both cochlear and vestibular functions should be tested. Simple tests of hearing should be done. Such procedures as calorics and rotational tests may be necessary. Unilateral tinnitus and deafness should always be investigated to rule out an acoustic neuroma. Posterior fossa myelography and angiography may be necessary.

Glossopharyngeal, Vagus, Accessory, and Hypoglossal Nerves (IX, X, XI, and XII)

Most often, involvement of these structures is not associated with serious headache problems. Lingual pain may occur in cranial arteritis. Bilateral absence of the pharyngeal reflex may be a hysteric phenomenon, but disease of the brainstem also should be ruled out.

Motor Functions

Basically, there are three motor systems:

1. Lesions of the pyramidal or corticospinal system produce paralysis or weakness, spasticity, and hyperactive deep tendon reflexes.

2. Lesions of the extrapyramidal system produce instability of posture and disorders of muscle tone, as well as slowness of movement in nonparalyzed limbs.

3. The cerebellar system primarily in-

volves accuracy of movements of the trunk and limbs. The cerebellum can be divided into two basic functional parts. The vermis is related to movements of the trunk, whereas the hemispheres serve primarily coordination of the extremities, particularly the arms. It also is important to remember that the cerebellar tracts cross twice, so a lesion involving the right cerebellar hemisphere produces difficulty with the right arm and right leg.

Lower motor neuron disease is characterized by wasting, weakness, atrophy, and loss of deep tendon reflexes, depending on the extent of the lesion.

Sensory Functions

Central or peripheral lesions of the nervous system can be uncovered by careful sensory testing. Two-point discrimination is particularly important in assessment of cortical sensation. A disturbance of astereognosis, or failure to recognize the size or shape of objects, can be the only sign of a parietal lobe tumor.

The basic sensory pathway consists of a three-neuron pattern. The primary sensory neuron has its cell body outside the central nervous system, usually in the dorsal root ganglia. The second neuron must cross the midline. The third neuron has its cell body in the opposite thalamus and radiates to the cortex. A large proportion of the sensory cortex is taken up by sensation from the face, especially the mouth and tongue, and from the hand, especially the thumb and first finger. This may in part be responsible for the common complaints of abnormalities of head and neck sensation, especially head and neck pain.

The integrity of the parietal lobes is always responsible for normal perception of the body image. If there is loss of parietal function, extinction may occur. The patient will deny appreciation of sensation of the body subserved by the diseased parietal lobe when bilateral sensory testing is performed.

Reflexes

It is important to remember the concepts of upper motor neuron and lower motor neuron disease. The upper motor neuron system organizes groups of muscles to mediate movement of body parts. The lower neuron system organizes individual muscles.

Deep Tendon Reflexes and Superficial Reflexes

- Achilles reflex: <u>S-1</u> and S-2
- Quadriceps reflex: L-2, <u>L-3, and L-4</u>
- Low abdominal: T-11 and L-1
- Upper abdominal: T-6 and T-9
- Hoffman reflex: C-7, <u>C-8, and T1</u>
- Brachioradialis reflex: C-5 and <u>C-6</u>
- Biceps reflex: <u>C-5</u>, and C-6
- Triceps reflex: C-6, <u>C-7, and C-8</u>
- Jaw reflex: midpons

The underlined numbered segments indicate the dominant or main spinal segments involved. If present, pathological reflexes are a sign of organic brain or spinal cord disease.

By testing the deep tendon reflexes, as well as the superficial reflexes, one can sample the influences of both the upper and lower motor neurons on the reflex arcs. Beginning from the lower extremities and proceeding proximally, the plantar response depends on the intactness of the L-5, S-1, and S-2 segments. If the plantar response is extensor, it indicates that the corticospinal pathway serving the L-5, S-1, and S-2 segments has been disturbed.

Conclusion

An adequate history, a thorough physical examination, and a competent neurological examination usually enable the physician to make a correct headache diagnosis and do much toward reassuring the patient.

References

1. Perkins AT, Ondo W. When to worry about headache: Head pain as a clue to intracranial disease. Postgrad Med 1995;96:197–208.
2. Canales R, Ayachi S. Evaluating and treating the patient with a headache. Phys Asst 1998;16:26–44.
3. Graham JR. Cluster headache. Postgrad Med 1974;56:181–185.

5

Neurodiagnostic Imaging in the Investigation of Headache

Jordan M. Prager, M.D.

David Lewin, M.D.

Introduction

The number of Americans with headache who seek medical attention is staggering—there are about 18 million annual patient visits.[1] Previously, the relevant neuroimaging question when evaluating a patient with headache was whether to obtain a computed tomography (CT) scan. The question is now more complex and involves whether to image and whether to obtain a CT scan or to use magnetic resonance imaging (MRI).

Physicians who take care of patients with headache are well aware that most results of neurodiagnostic imaging examinations in this population are normal,[2–4] but unexpected findings include tumor, post-traumatic abnormalities, and vascular anomalies that account for a patient's headaches. At times, the neurological examination is highly predictive of these positive findings. Frequently, however, dramatic findings on neuroimaging studies are a surprise. Even patients with textbook migraine or tension-type (muscle contraction[1]) headaches can develop a meningioma or subarachnoid hemorrhage.[4] Given the number of patients with migraine and tension-type headache, it is not surprising that this occurs.

The specter of liability is also always present. Patients with a several-year history of typical migraine may develop new neurological signs; imaging obtained at the time of these signs can show underlying disease such as vascular malformation or tumor. Unfortunately, baseline diagnostic imaging may not have been obtained when the patients first presented with typical headache. These cases may result in a lawsuit and are settled with considerable time and expense. Because of these basic medical and socioeconomic factors, an argument may be made to obtain a baseline imaging study when a patient's headache becomes sufficiently severe that he or she seeks medical attention. In a more academic viewpoint, the American Academy of Neurology issued the following statement as a practice guideline: "In adult patients with recurrent headaches that have been defined as migraine—including those with visual aura—with no other focal neurologic signs or symptoms, the routine use of neuroimaging is not warranted. In patients with atypical headache patterns, a history of seizures, or focal neurologic signs or symptoms, CT or MRI may be indicated."[5]

Which neuroimaging examination is appropriate? With a few important exceptions, MRI is the preferred examination because it is distinctly more sensitive to subtle tumors, vascular malformations, and inflammatory disorders and provides superior assessment of lesions by virtue of imaging equally well in any anatomic plane. CT is superior in the emergency setting for patients with acute headache or trauma or when there is suspicion of subarachnoid hemorrhage. We document these conclusions with descriptions of MRI and CT and examples of typical findings seen in association with headaches.

Computed Tomography

CT was developed for clinical use in the early 1970s and became a common examination by 1980. CT links a computer and an x-ray source to produce a relatively simple set of images from a mountain of complex data. A highly focused x-ray beam, variably absorbed by tissues of differing density within the body, is rotated around the patient. X-rays incompletely absorbed by the patient's tissues pass through the imaged region and are measured by highly sensitive detectors. Hundreds of separate measurements of x-ray intensity are collected for each CT "slice." Mathematical algorithms are then used to create a gray-scale image from the data set.

Each point, or pixel, within a CT slice is assigned a numerical value, called a Hounsfield unit (HU); CT was pioneered by G. N. Hounsfield. The scale represents relative x-ray attenuation and ranges from −1000 to +1000, with water measuring 0. Air and fat are negative and thus dark; acute blood, soft tissues, and bone are positive and thus bright (Fig. 5–1).

As CT scanners have evolved, scan times have been drastically reduced while image quality has improved. Newer scanners use slip-ring technology so the examining table can move continuously during the scan. Scan times may be reduced to 1 second per slice, with slices as thin as 1 mm.

Different tissues may be highlighted manually after the CT image data are collected, aiding in the search for acute blood or bone lesions. The term *windowing* refers to this highlighting process; the range of HUs selected for gray-scale imaging, as well as the *zero point* (or window center), can be manually selected to answer specific diagnostic questions. Smaller window widths highlight subtle soft tissue differences, such as gray matter–white matter differentiation. The typical CT scan of the head selects a window and level to highlight differences between gray matter and white matter. This has a cost because there is blurring between the cortex and inner table of the skull. To better visualize this area for subdural hematomas, a "wider" window may be used. Contrast enhancement with iodinated materials is useful to detect breakdown in the blood-brain barrier, as occurs with tumor or infection.[6]

CT scanning is excellent for the detection of acute hemorrhage (Fig. 5–2) and bony abnormalities such as fracture. Patients may be easily monitored during scanning, and the examination can be performed quickly. CT is therefore an excellent modality for evaluation of the acutely injured patient and for the detection of subarachnoid hemorrhage. Additional uses of CT include the detection of sinus disease, calcific lesions, and calvarial and temporal bone abnormalities and when MRI is contraindicated (e.g., in patients with cardiac pacemakers, cochlear implants, some metallic surgical clips, or severe claustrophobia).

CT is very sensitive for the detection of acute subarachnoid hemorrhage, with the exception of severe anemia (with decreased hemoglobin levels, blood becomes "isodense" with cerebral parenchyma) and posterior fossa bleeds (bone artifact limits visualization).[7] When the CT scan is positive for acute subarachnoid blood in the nontraumatic setting, angiography is usually indicated to locate and define the site of bleeding, which most commonly is an aneurysm (Fig. 5–3). The location of the aneurysm may be suggested by the area of highest concentration of blood; however, all major cerebral vessels must be studied to rule out multiple aneurysms (20% incidence in patients with aneurysm).

CT is also very sensitive for the detection of parenchymal hemorrhage; however, in this case, it is not specific. Primary causes such as hypertension, drug abuse, or amyloid angiopathy are sometimes not easily distinguished from secondary causes such as underlying tumor or vascular malformation (Figs. 5–3 and 5–4). In these cases, MRI or angiography may help to define the cause of bleeding, provided the patient can tolerate the examination.[7]

Imaging of acute cranial trauma is first obtained in the CT scanner, which is sensitive for bony injuries, acute subdural or epidural hemorrhage, chronic subdural hematomas, and parenchymal volume loss (Fig. 5–5). Subacute subdural hematomas (1 to 4 weeks old) may transiently become "isodense" with brain parenchyma on CT; during this phase, MRI may be used to clearly show the pathology (Fig. 5–6).

CT is an effective tool in the diagnosis of acute sinus inflammatory disease and is superior to MRI in defining the bony anatomy of the paranasal region (Fig. 5–7). CT is also indispensable to the ear, nose, and throat surgeon in delineating the anatomy and pathology of the temporal bones and middle ear structures. It is complementary to MRI, which defines soft tissue involvement by tumor and infectious and inflammatory lesions in this region.

In the emergency setting, CT is usually sufficient to exclude conditions that require

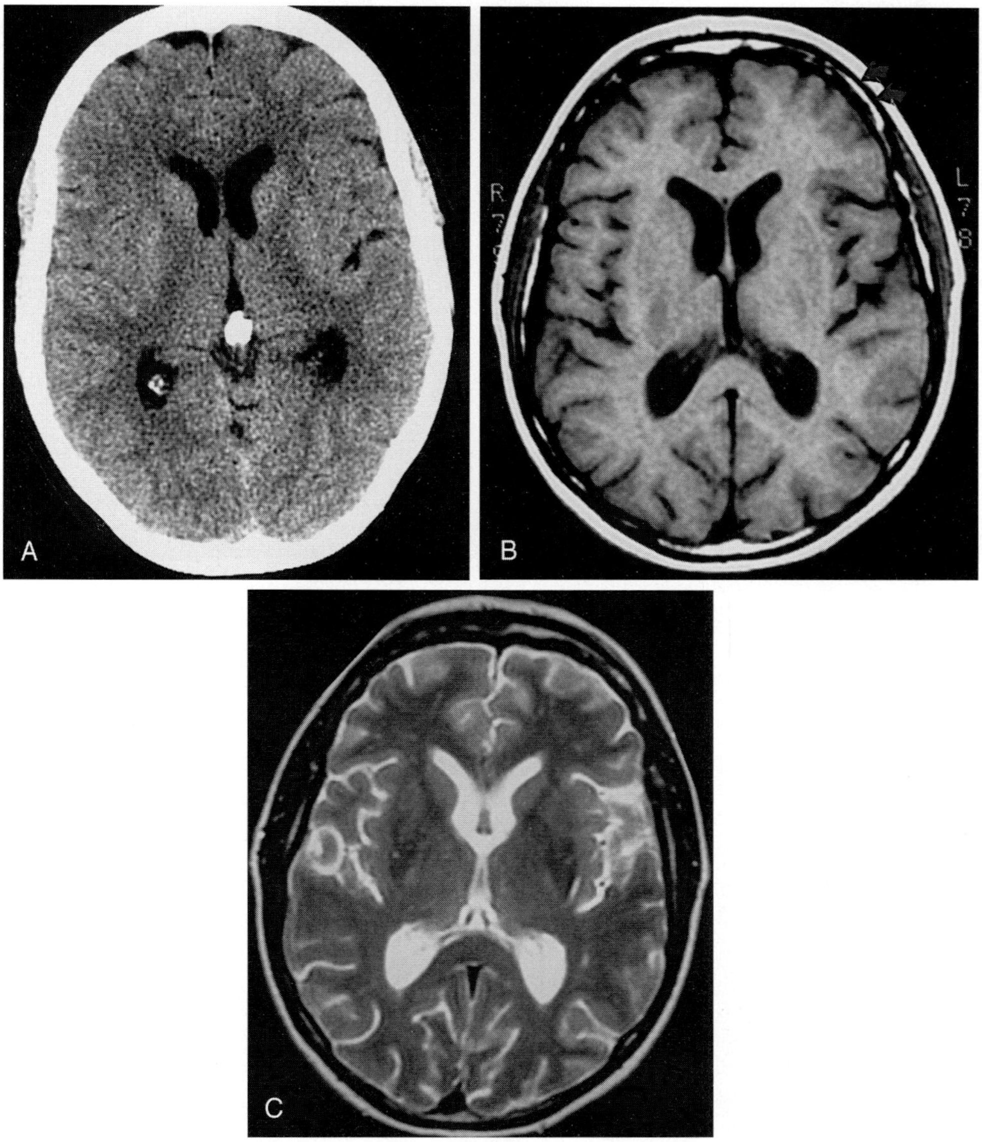

Figure 5–1 Normal CT scan and MRIs. *A,* CT scan. *B,* T1-weighted MR image. *C,* T2-weighted MR image. Note the superficial similarities between the CT scan and T1-weighted MRI. There is a bright peripheral rim on both images. On CT, this is referred to as increased density or attenuation (the more x-rays attenuated, the brighter is the resulting image). On MRI, brighter areas are referred to as increased signal intensity. MRI and CT "bright" areas, however, represent different anatomic structures. On the CT scan, the increased attenuation represents the bony calvarium. (Note the increased attenuation, calcified pineal gland.) On the T1-weighted image, this represents subgaleal fat overlying the bony calvarium. The bony calvarium on the T1-weighted image is represented by a thin black line for the outer table of the skull *(curved arrows* in *B),* variable increased signal from fat in the medullary cavity, and a thin black line centrally representing the inner table of the skull. Cerebrospinal fluid is dark on both CT scan and T1-weighted MR image. On the CT scan, gray matter is brighter than white matter, whereas the reverse is true on T1-weighted MR image. With the T2-weighted image, cerebrospinal fluid becomes bright, white matter becomes dark, and gray matter is intermediate. A general rule is that structural anatomy is better visualized with T1-weighted images, and physiology or functional disturbance is better visualized with T2-weighted images.

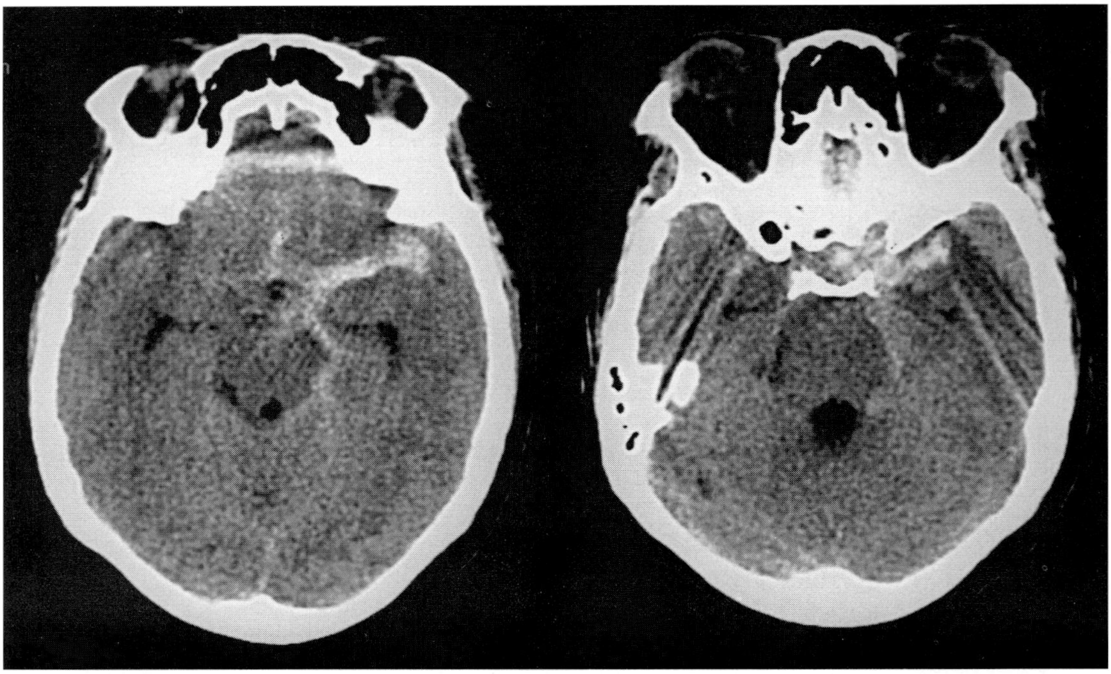

Figure 5–2 Subarachnoid hemorrhage. The CT scan views clearly demonstrate the increased attenuation (brighter) material in the basilar cisterns. This acute subarachnoid hemorrhage is in the suprasellar cistern, extending into the left medial sylvian fissure.

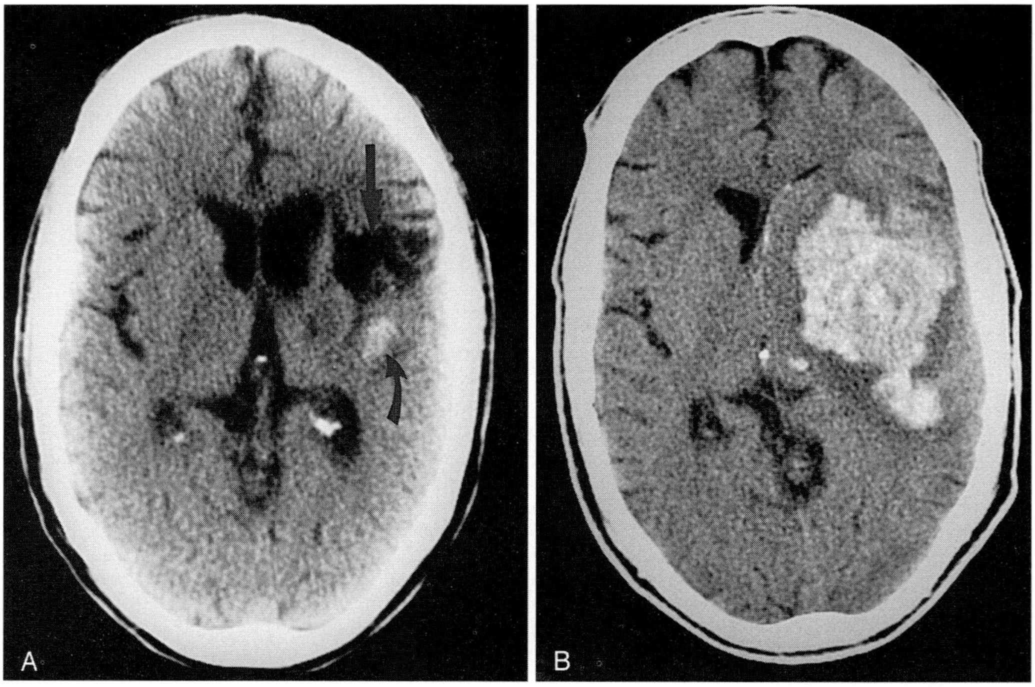

Figure 5–3 Aneurysm. *A,* The CT scan appears at first glance to be from an older patient with long-standing vascular disease. However, the patient is 42 years old and a chronic crack cocaine user. Note the old infarction in the left frontal cortex *(arrow),* as well as the generalized atrophy. The increased attenuation (bright) structure in the region of the left medial sylvian fissure is an unruptured aneurysm *(curved arrow).* The patient signed out against medical advice, complaining of a headache. He returned 2 days later with gross subarachnoid and intraparenchymal hemorrhage *(B).*

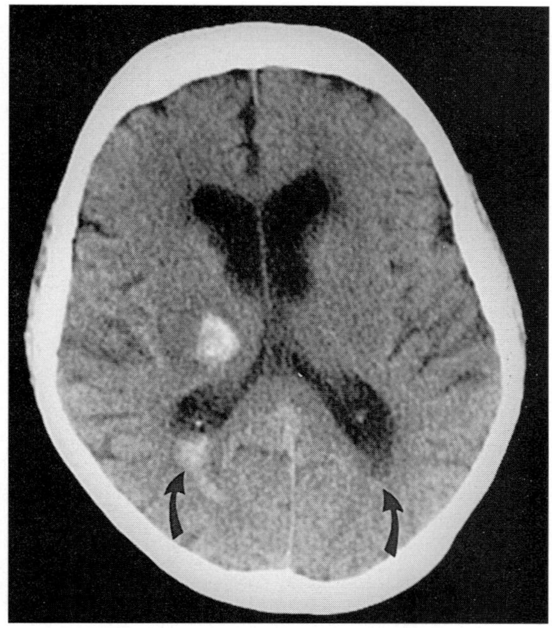

Figure 5–4 Hematoma. The CT scan shows increased attenuation in the region of the right thalamus; this is a typical location for hypertensive hemorrhage. Other typical locations include the putamen, pons, and central cerebellar hemispheres. It is unusual, although not exceedingly rare, to see lobar hemorrhage with hypertension. Note intraventricular blood layering in the occipital horns of the lateral ventricle *(curved arrows).*

immediate treatment. When inconclusive or negative findings are present and physical signs or symptoms continue to be concerning, MRI is indicated to narrow the list of differential possibilities. In the nonemergency setting, MRI is often the examination of choice.

Magnetic Resonance Imaging

Unlike CT, which uses the partial attenuation by the body of an x-ray beam, MRI measures the response of the body to a strong magnetic field. Magnetic field strength in clinical MRI is typically 0.5 to 1.5 T. A *tesla* (T) is a unit of magnetic field strength equal to 10,000 G (gauss); the magnetic field of the earth is about 0.5 G.

When biological tissue is placed in a strong magnetic field, the magnetic moments (axes) of the hydrogen protons in the tissue align in the direction of the magnetic field. A specialized antenna, or *coil,* directs a radiofrequency wave at the tissue (using the resonant frequency of the protons in the tissue), caus-

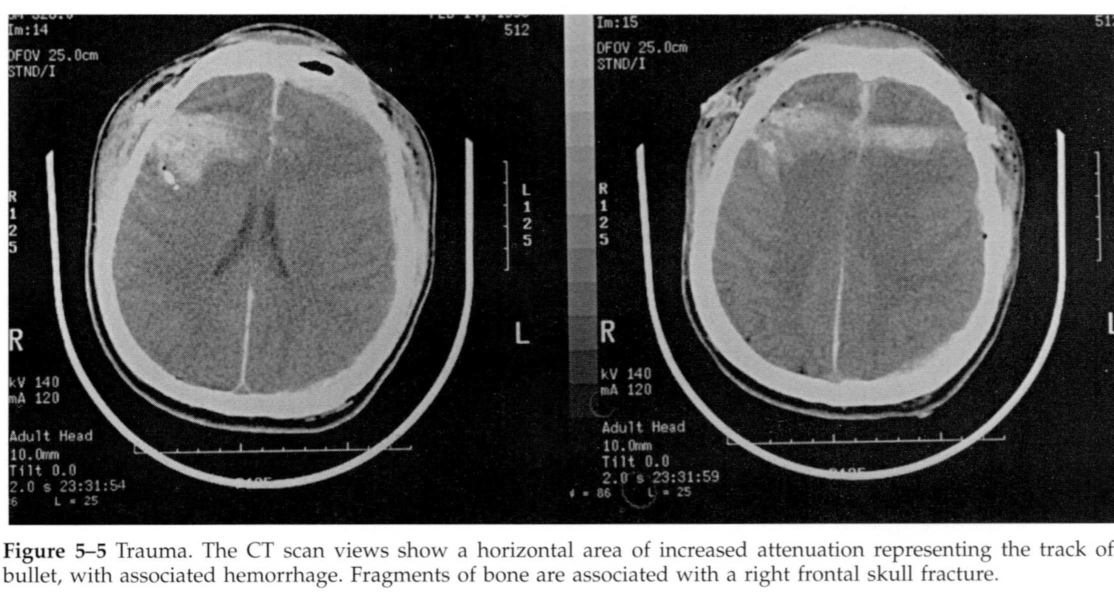

Figure 5–5 Trauma. The CT scan views show a horizontal area of increased attenuation representing the track of a bullet, with associated hemorrhage. Fragments of bone are associated with a right frontal skull fracture.

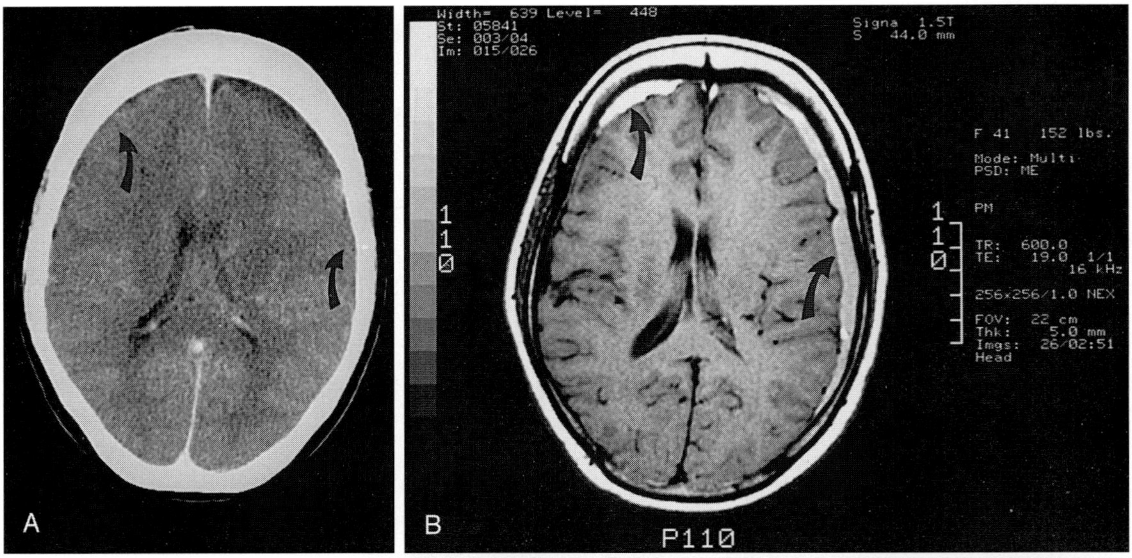

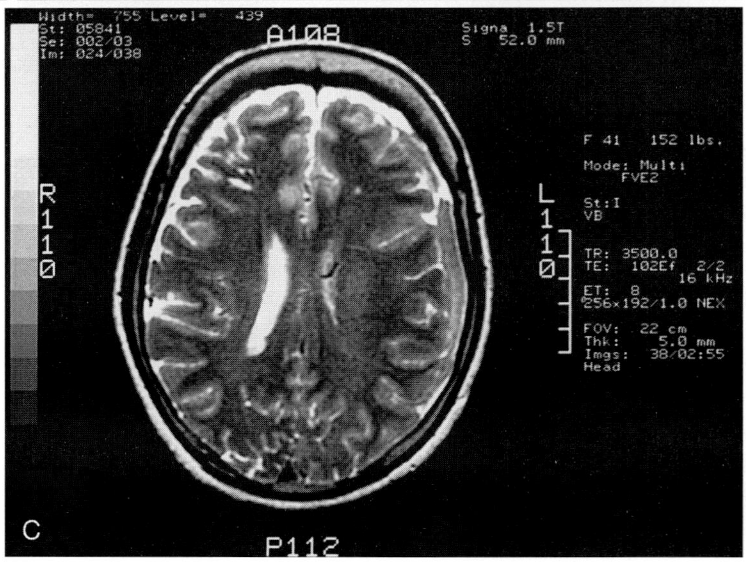

Figure 5–6 Subdural hematoma. *A,* CT scan. *B and C,* T1- and T2-weighted MR images. Subacute subdural hematomas occur when blood products degrade, generally 1 to 3 weeks after the initial hemorrhage. During this phase, the hematoma may have attenuation similar to parenchyma on CT scan. This is referred to as an isodense subdural hematoma *(curved arrows).* At the same time, however, the MR signal from subdural hematoma is bright on both T1- and T2-weighted images *(curved arrows)* and is quite obvious. The initial trauma may be somewhat trivial, especially in older patients; they may not even remember the initial trauma. Therefore, older patients with chronic headache should especially be considered for MRI instead of CT.

ing a significant number of protons to deflect out of alignment with the field and into phase with each other. The radiofrequency coil is then turned off, and the protons return to both their former alignment with the magnetic field and their random phase orientations. As they return to the *relaxed* state (the direction of the magnetic field), they give off radiofrequency waves, which are picked up by the same coil (now acting as a receiver) and converted to image data through a complex mathematical algorithm, the Fourier transformation. By altering the sequence of radiofrequency pulses and adjusting the magnetic field to vary along different axes, equally detailed images can be obtained in any imaging plane—typically axial, coronal, and sagittal.

T1-weighted images highlight tissues with protons that return quickly to alignment with the magnetic field (e.g., fat, subacute blood, and highly paramagnetic substances such as gadolinium, which we discuss). Tissues with rapid return to alignment are represented as high-intensity signal (bright areas) on T1-weighted images; this is referred to as *T1 shortening.* T2-weighted images highlight tissues with protons that remain in phase with each other for a relatively long time after the radiofrequency pulse is turned off. Water is the prototypical *bright* signal on T2, and relative brightness on T2 is referred to as *T2 lengthening.*

Gadolinium is a paramagnetic intravenous contrast agent that causes enhancing structures to appear bright on T1-weighted

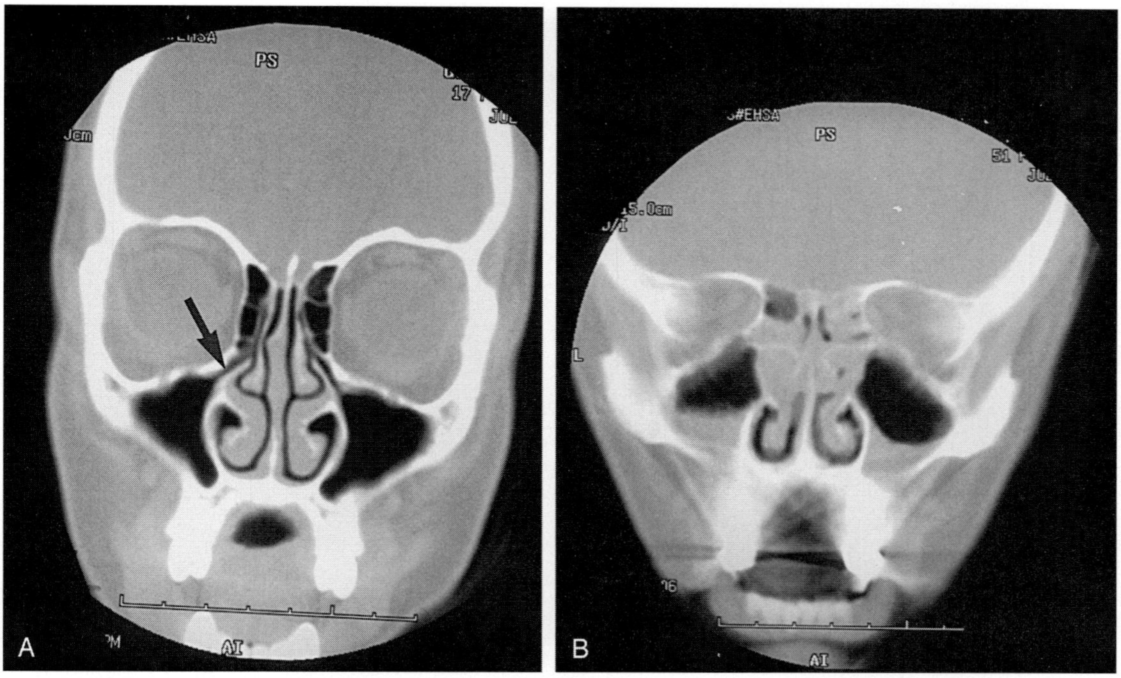

Figure 5–7 Sinus CT scan. *A,* This normal study demonstrates the paranasal sinus anatomy, including the outlet (infundibulum), from the maxillary antrum *(arrow).* This also is a space for outflow from the ethmoid and frontal sinuses. *B,* Marked sinusitis. There are air-fluid levels in the paranasal sinuses. There also is polypoid soft tissue in the nasal cavity.

MR images. Gadolinium enhancement is analogous to the enhancement seen on contrast-enhanced CT in which there has been breakdown in the blood-brain barrier. It is useful in imaging tumor, acute infarction, infectious and inflammatory conditions, and vascular anomalies. Gadolinium enhancement effects are most prominent on T1-weighted images, with a much smaller effect on T2-weighted images.[6]

Field strength is directly related to the signal-to-noise (SNR) ratio. Higher field strength results in higher SNR; however, higher field strength magnets require a more narrow aperture and confinement for the patient. Lower field strength scanners are advertised for the use of heavier or claustrophobic patients. These patients also find it more difficult to hold still during the examination. The combination of lower field strength and increased movement considerably limits the quality of the low field examination. If there is a question of a subtle abnormality on a low field examination or if low field examination fails to detect an abnormality in a patient with very suggestive history and physical examination, further attempts to obtain a high field examination may be valuable.

Chronic headache is best evaluated with MRI because of its superiority in imaging tumor, infection, and vascular pathology (Figs. 5–8 to 5–10), as well as clearly demonstrating white matter disease and pathological changes in the posterior fossa, a prominent "blind spot" for CT. MRI may be used to detect typical abnormalities in patients with migraine that are invisible on CT (Fig. 5–11),[8] and it is highly sensitive in the imaging of subtle post-traumatic abnormalities, as well as other entities associated with headache, such as TMJ dysfunction (Fig. 5–12), trigeminal neuropathy, venous sinus thrombosis, and Chiari's malformation (Fig. 5–13).

MRI and CT are both highly sensitive for hydrocephalus, which may be a cause of acute headache arising after trauma or infection (Fig. 5–14). Obstructive hydrocephalus can often be diagnosed with CT, which may reveal a mass obstructing the ventricular system (Fig. 5–15). MRI is frequently required to further define the anatomic position of the lesion in several imaging planes before surgery. In addition, MRI may be used to detect abnormal enhancement of the meninges in patients with meningitis (Fig. 5–16).

Patients with migraine may demonstrate abnormal areas of high signal in the cerebral white matter called *white matter foci.* This

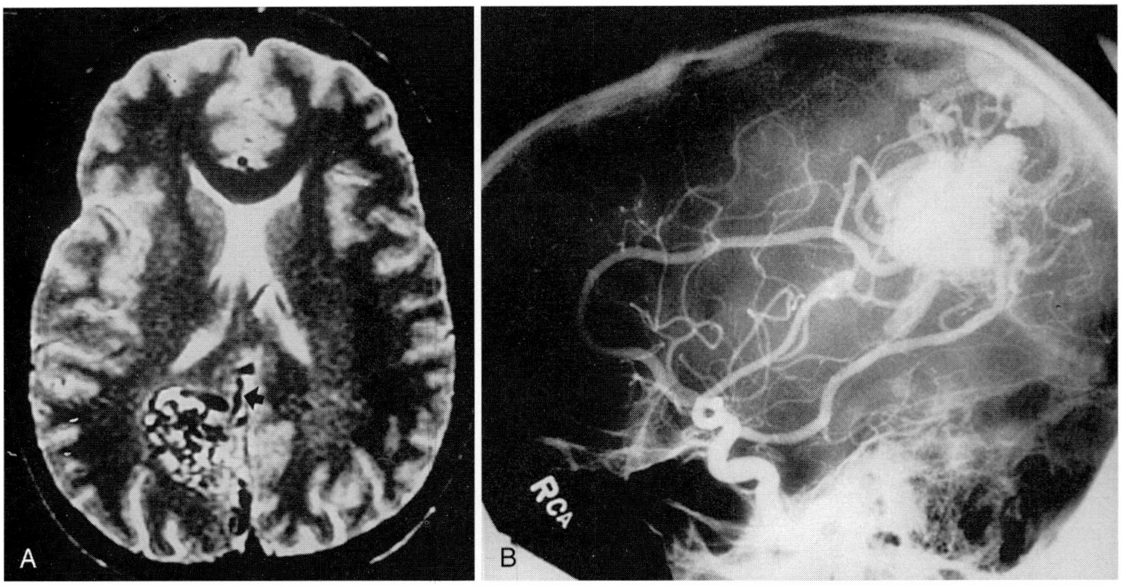

Figure 5–8 Arteriovenous malformation (AVM). *A,* T2-weighted MR image. *B,* Angiogram. AVM may have a nonspecific appearance on CT, with local atrophy, calcification, and, at times, visualization of prominent vessels. On MRI there is a more characteristic appearance, with serpiginous areas of increased and decreased signal representing various manifestations of flow and hemorrhage. Flow void from draining vein *(arrowhead)* is demonstrated on this T2-weighted MR image. Angiogram shows abnormal vessels, as well as feeding arteries and draining veins.

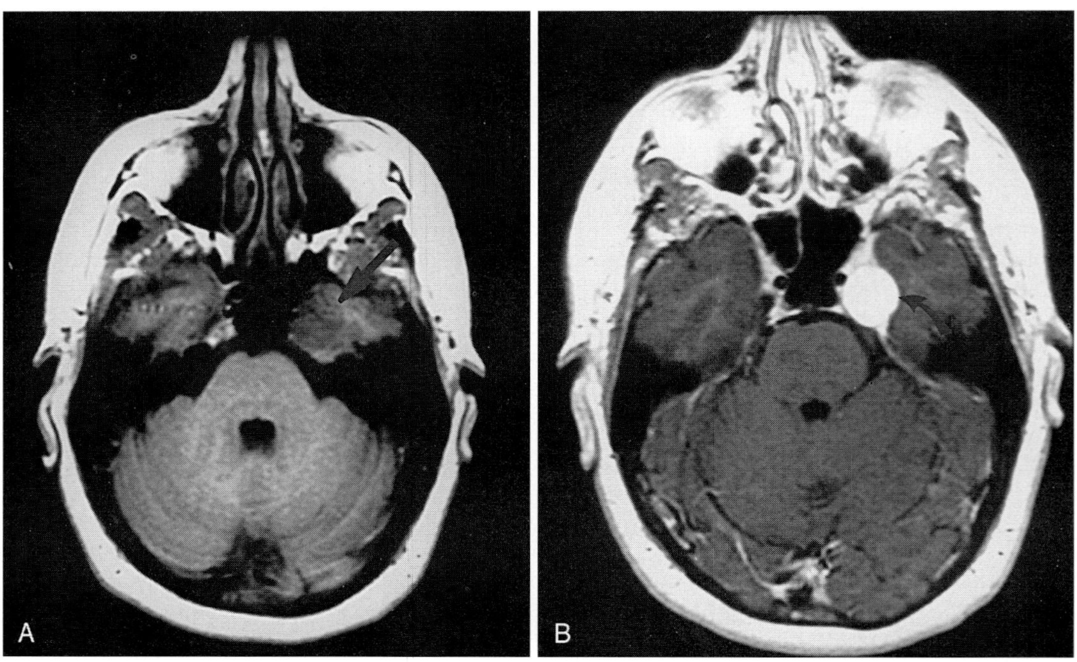

Figure 5–9 Meningioma. *A,* T1-weighted image. *B,* T1-weighted image with gadolinium. Meningioma may be difficult to diagnose without intravenous contrast material. It may appear similar to underlying parenchyma on both CT and MRI *(arrow).* Intravenous contrast enhancement *(curved arrow)* is extremely helpful in the diagnosis. These neoplasms are most often superficial, exerting a mass effect on adjacent parenchyma, and may present in association with headaches.

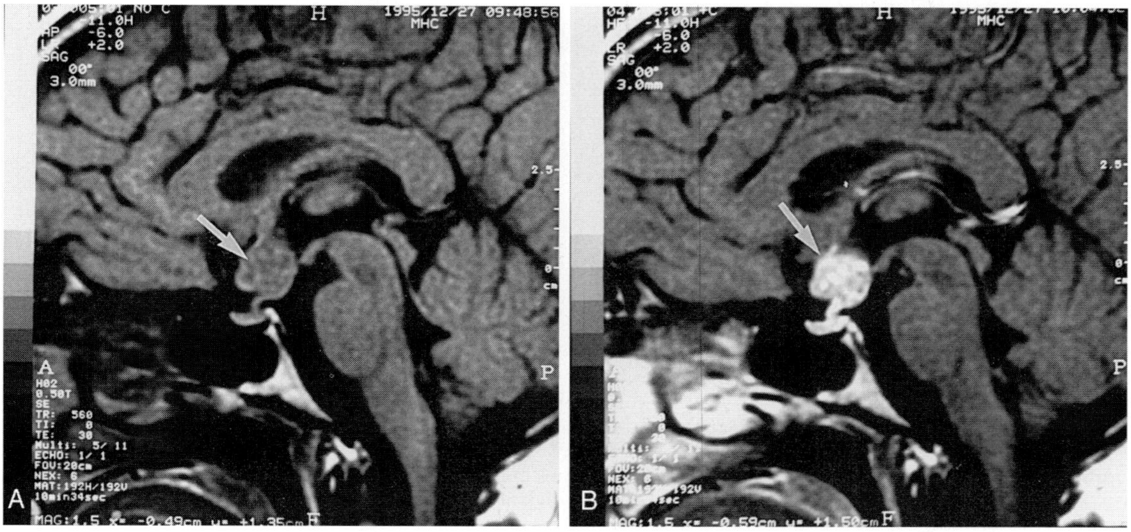

Figure 5–10 Germinoma. *A,* T1-weighted image. *B,* T1-weighted image with gadolinium. This patient is a young woman seen by psychiatry and internal medicine consults for continuing headaches and a "myriad of soft complaints." She finally had an MRI study that showed a prominent suprasellar lesion with characteristics most suggestive of germinoma *(arrow),* which was confirmed through surgical pathologic examination.

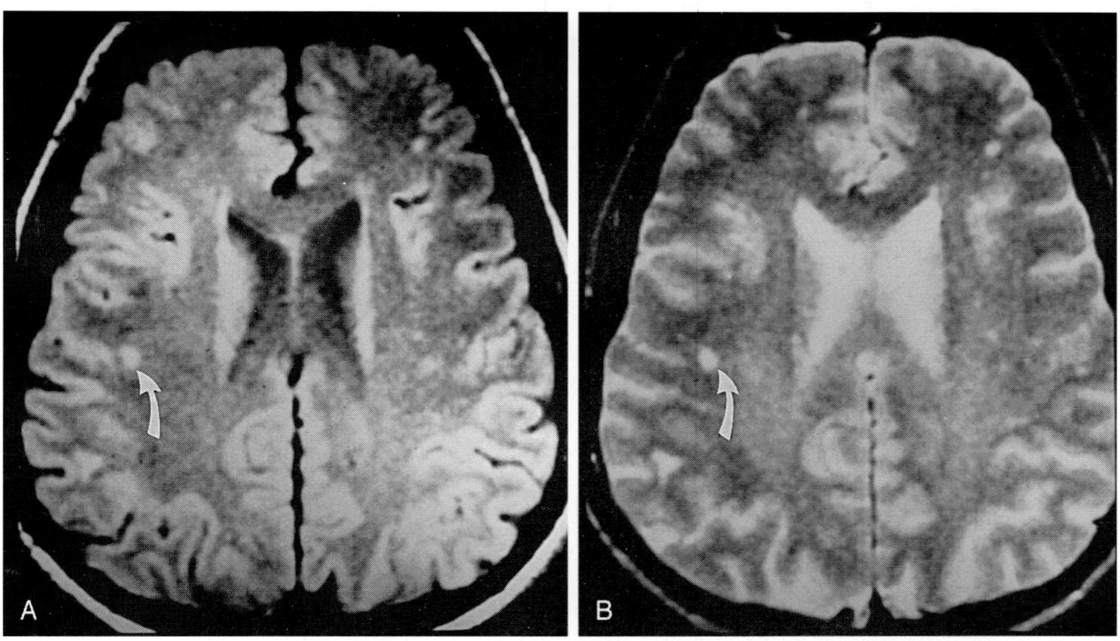

Figure 5–11 Migraine. *A,* Intermediate. *B,* T2-weighted image. On MRI, there frequently are small foci *(curved arrows)* of increased signal on T2-weighted images, usually subcortical in location. These must be differentiated from the white matter foci of multiple sclerosis, which are typically periventricular and more oval in configuration. Bright T2 foci are also seen with hypertension, and in the elderly population in general. These foci are also more generally periventricular and are smaller than those seen in migraine. Many more rare conditions may also present with bright T2 foci.

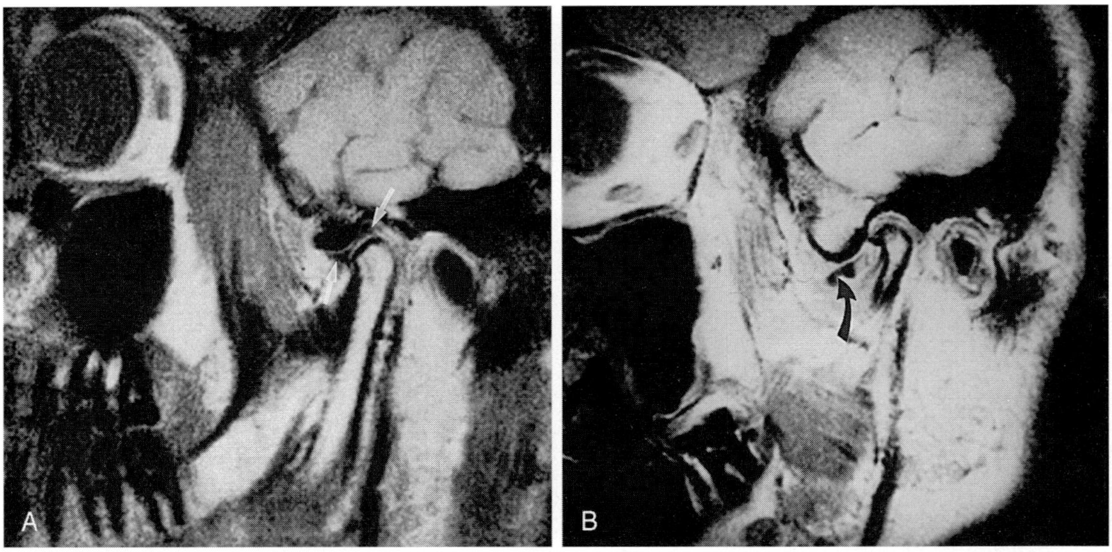

Figure 5–12 Normal and abnormal views of the temporomandibular joint (TMJ). *A,* Bow tie–shaped low signal in the joint represents normally placed TMJ disk *(arrows). B,* This disk is displaced anteriorly *(curved arrow).*

finding is seen more often in patients with migraine (25% to 68%) than in controls (6%) but is not specific for migraine. It may be related to the inherent vascular instability of these patients, and it is seen at a younger age in patients with migraine than in asymptomatic controls. The current flurry of research in "functional" MRI, which seeks to characterize areas of relative high and low perfusion within the brain, may yield more sensitive images of migraine.[8]

Angiography and Magnetic Resonance Angiography

Cerebral angiography is an invasive vascular study usually performed via a femoral artery

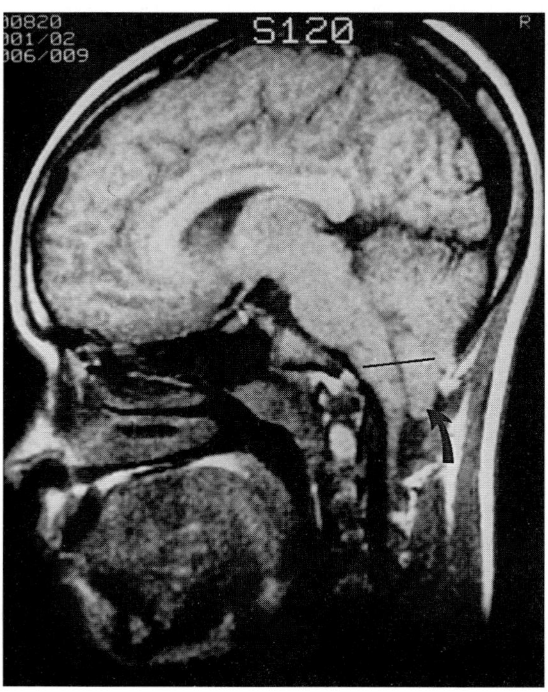

Figure 5–13 Chiari I malformation. Sagittal T1-weighted view of the head demonstrates another reason for the superiority of MRI in the evaluation of chronic headache. The considerable artifact from the skull base seen on CT is not a problem with MRI. This particular examination clearly shows the cerebellar tonsils *(curved arrow)* descending below the level of the foramen magnum *(black line).*

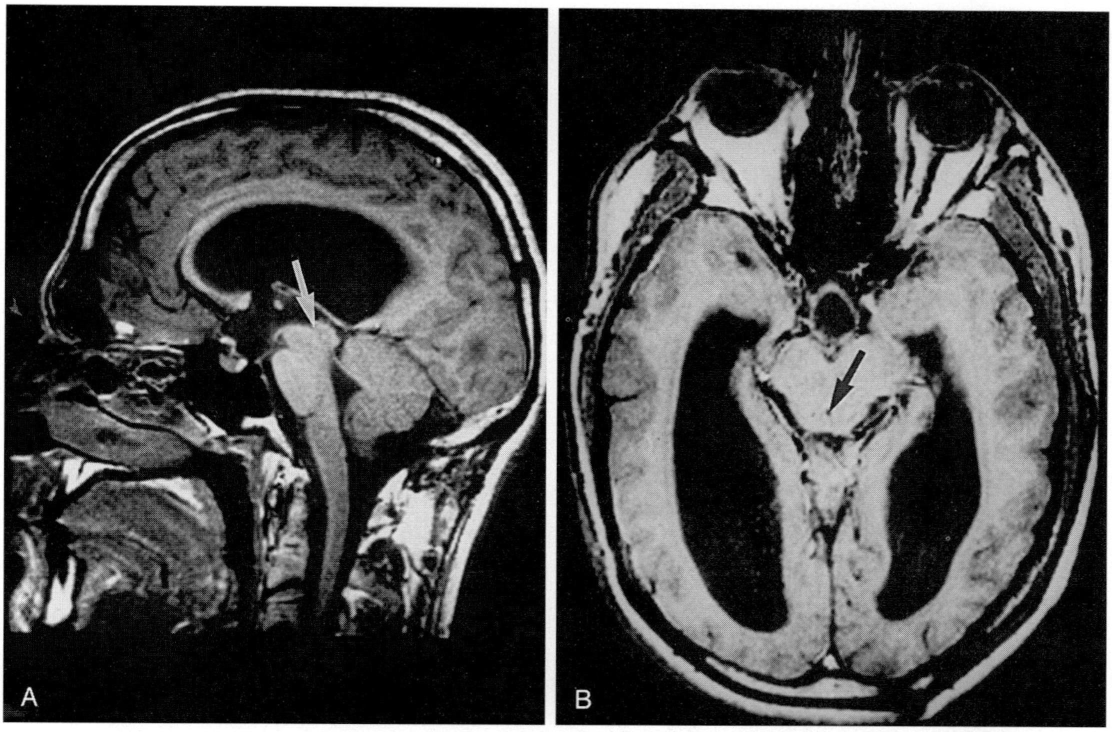

Figure 5–14 Hydrocephalus. Sagittal *(A)* and axial *(B)* T1-weighted images demonstrate marked enlargement of the third ventricle and lateral ventricles. The small size of the aqueduct *(arrow)*, with a normal fourth ventricle, is indicative of aqueductal insufficiency. These patients may present with acute hydrocephalus after trivial trauma or infection.

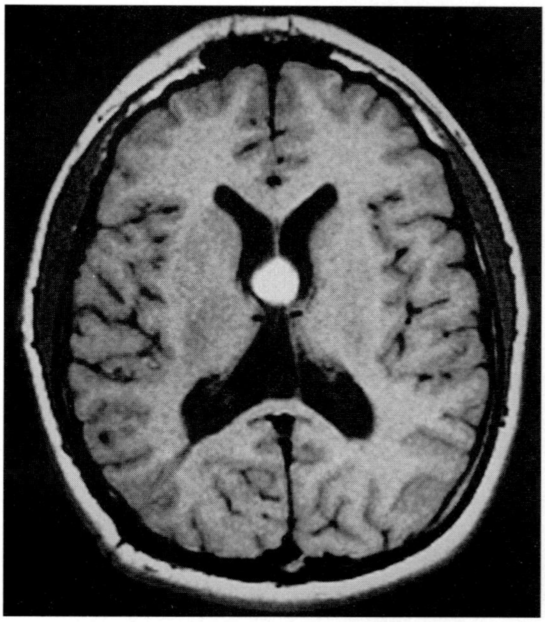

Figure 5–15 Colloid cyst. MR image of a colloid cyst shows typical increased signal in the superior/anterior aspect of the third ventricle. Colloid cyst headaches may be positional. Typically, while bending forward, the colloid cyst acts as a ball-valve joint in the third ventricle, obstructing outflow from the lateral ventricles and causing headache.

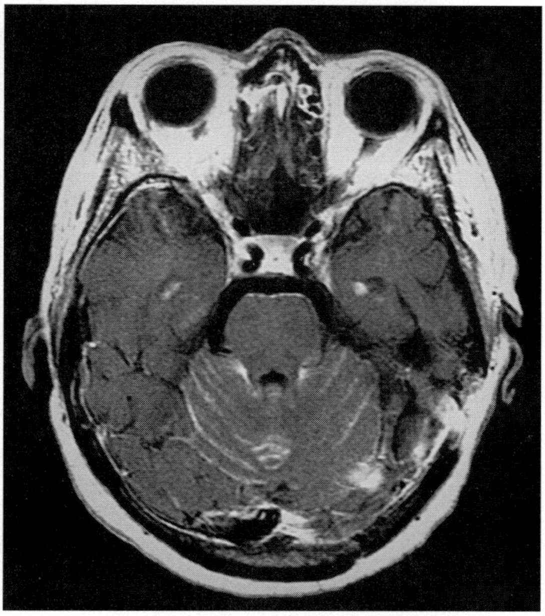

Figure 5–16 Meningitis. T1-weighted MR image with gadolinium. Pial enhancement, especially in the cerebellum, is prominently noted in this patient with carcinomatous meningitis. Enhancement also coats the pons anteriorly and is present in the temporal horns.

puncture to place a long, flexible catheter into the aorta. With a wire for guidance, the catheter may be selectively placed in the carotid artery or branch vessel, as well as the vertebral artery. Studies are typically done with digital subtraction, a process in which nonvascular background anatomy is electronically subtracted from the final image. With digital subtraction, smaller amounts of contrast may be used, and greater detail can be visualized.

Cut film angiograms are rarely used. Sometimes cut film is used to evaluate small vessel vasculitis or, less often, aneurysm description. In centers experienced in the use of catheter angiography, morbidity is between 0.5% and 1.0%.[9–11] Morbidity may be somewhat greater in patients with active vascular pathology at the time of the angiogram, such as stroke in evolution.

Magnetic resonance angiography (MRA) is a noninvasive technique that exploits MR signal intensity differences between flowing blood and stationary tissue. Through suppression of stationary background tissue and highlighting of flowing blood, vascular structures can be imaged (Fig. 5–17). The data can be acquired in a three-dimensional volume,

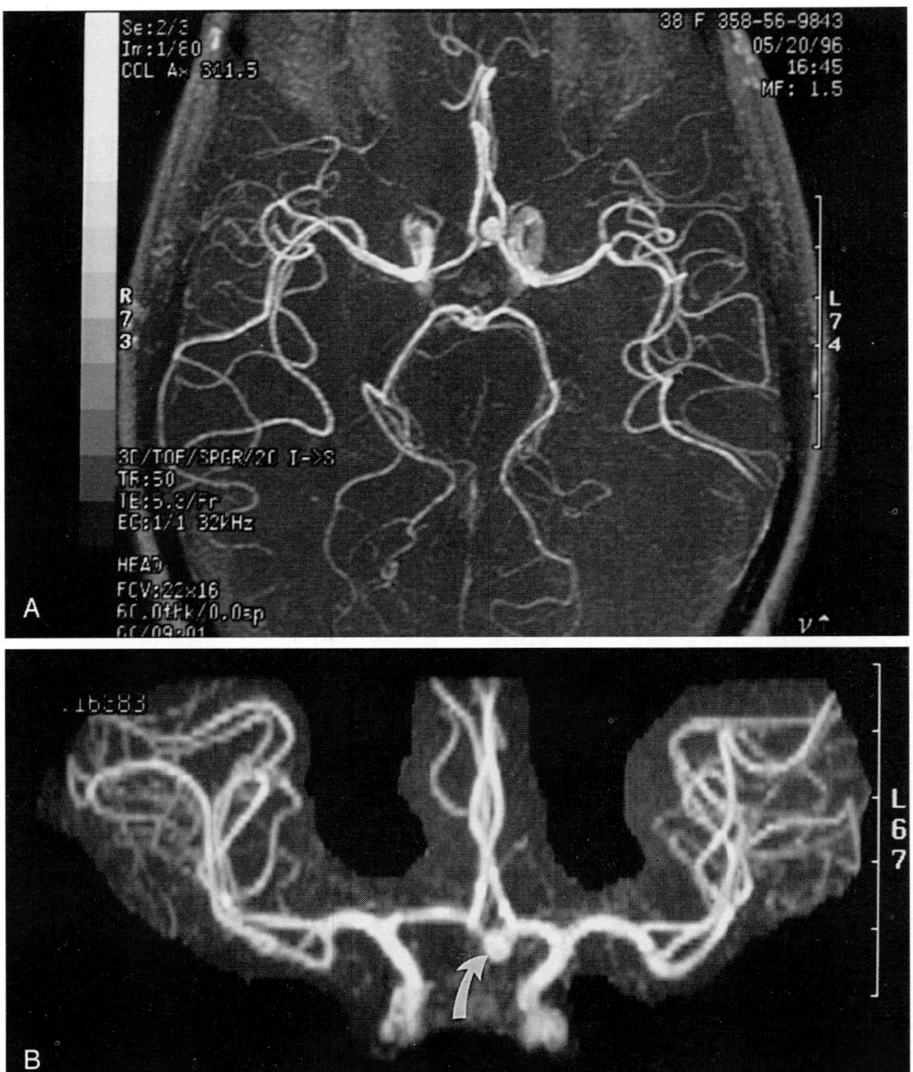

Figure 5–17 MRA takes advantage of two principles: stationary tissue may be saturated or subtracted from an image, whereas structures moving into a region of tissue, such as flowing blood, may be enhanced. Both of these principles serve to highlight flowing blood. On the examples shown, the distal internal carotid arteries are distinguished, as well as the proximal anterior and middle cerebral arteries. Distal branches appear fairly symmetric. This is not an example of a normal MRA. An anterior communicating artery aneurysm originating from the left side is shown *(B, curved arrow).*

resulting in vascular images that can be projected from different perspectives.

MRA is regularly used to visualize aneurysms of more than 5 mm. Aneurysms smaller than this are less reliably imaged.[12, 13] The debate about the use of MRA for aneurysm detection is quite complex, and many technical issues remain to be examined. MRA techniques are still developing. The current wisdom appears to be that for patients with relatively mild suspicion for aneurysm (i.e., unusual headaches or family history of aneurysm), MRA is probably adequate. If, however, there is strong suspicion of aneurysm due to symptoms and physical findings, catheter angiography is indicated; it remains the gold standard.

Catheter angiography remains the examination of choice when considering the diagnosis of vasculitis, which may be strongly suggested by MR findings. Acute venous sinus thrombosis may be definitively diagnosed via MRI; however, catheter angiography also offers the possibility of treatment via administration of thrombolytic agents.

It is also possible to obtain a CT angiogram (CTA). This technique is performed using *spiral* imaging (the examination table moves continuously through a rotating x-ray tube, which describes a "spiral" around the patient). With this technique, an intravenous bolus of contrast material is delivered, and rapid axial CT images are obtained in a volume of tissue. The initial two-dimensional source images are very helpful in the evaluation of vascular anatomy and its relationship to neighboring bony structures. Three-dimensional vascular anatomy may be reconstructed by "stacking" the two-dimensional images with the use of a computer. Both CT angiography and MRA are well suited for evaluation of the cervical portion of the carotid arteries.

Myelography

The use of myelography, which involves intrathecal contrast injected via lumbar puncture, has diminished significantly because of the highly accurate images of the spine provided by MRI for evaluation of back pain; it is still used when MRI fails to disclose an abnormality in a patient with significant physical findings or for preoperative surgical planning. The most common and significant complication of myelography is a spinal headache resulting from the lumbar puncture. Multiple studies have documented a lower incidence of spinal headache when smaller-gauge needles and when pencil-point needles (as opposed to beveled needles) are used.[14]

References

1. Caesar T. Acute headache management. The challenge of deciphering etiologies to guide assessment and treatment. Emerg Med Rep 1995;16:117–128.
2. Frishberg BM. The utility of neuroimaging in the evaluation of headache in patients with normal neurologic examinations. Neurology 1994;44:1191–1197.
3. Mitchell CS, Osborn RE, Grosskreutz SR. Computed tomography in the headache patient: Is routine evaluation really necessary? Headache 1993;33:82–86.
4. Weingarten S, Kleinman M, Elperin L, et al. The effectiveness of cerebral imaging in the diagnosis of chronic headache. Arch Gen Intern Med 1992;152:2457–2462.
5. Practice parameter: The utility of neuroimaging in the evaluation of headache in patients with normal neurologic examinations (summary statement): Report of the Quality Standards Subcommittee of the American Academy of Neurology. Neurology 1994;44:1353–1354.
6. Grossman RI, Yousem DM. Neuroradiology: The requisites. *In* Techniques in Neuroimaging. St. Louis, MO: Mosby; 1994;2–14.
7. Prager JM, Mikulis DJ. The radiology of headache. Med Clin North Am 1991;75:525–544.
8. Prager JM. Neurodiagnostic imaging in migraine. *In* Rose FC, ed. New Advances in Headache Research, 3d ed. London: Smith-Gordon; 1994.
9. Heiserman JE, Dean BL, Hodak JA, et al. Neurologic complication of cerebral angiography. AJNR Am J Neuroradiol 1994;15:1401–1407.
10. Ramadan NM, Gilkey SJ, Mitchell M, et al. Postangiography headache. Headache 1995;35:21–24.
11. Waugh JR, Sacharias N. Arteriographic complications in the DSA era. Radiology 1992;182:243–246.
12. Huston J 3rd, Nichols DA, Luetmer PH, et al. Blinded prospective evaluation of sensitivity of MR angiography to known intracranial aneurysms: Importance of aneurysm size. AJNR Am J Neuroradiol 1994;15:1607–1614.
13. Winn HR. Intracranial aneurysms and MR angiography: Questions and answers. AJNR Am J Neuroradiol 1994;15:1617.
14. Prager JM, Roychowdhury S, Gorey MT, et al: Spinal headaches after myeolograms: Comparison of needle types. AJR 1996;167:1289–1292.

6

Migraine Headache

Seymour Diamond, M.D.

Introduction

It has been estimated that in the United States, 18 million women and 5.6 million men have severe migraine headaches.[1] According to a study that used the International Headache Society classification, estimates of lifetime prevalence were 25% for women and 8% for men.[2] The term *migraine* comes from the French and is derived from the Greek word *hemicrania*, which means *half a head*.

It would perhaps be helpful to define migraine as it is currently understood clinically (Fig. 6–1). The outstanding feature of the migraine syndrome is periodic headache, which usually is unilateral in onset but may become generalized. The headaches are associated with irritability and nausea and often with photophobia, vomiting, constipation, and diarrhea. Not infrequently, the attacks are ushered in by scotomata, hemianopsia, unilateral paresthesia, and speech disorders. The pain commonly is limited to the head, but it may include the face and even the neck. Often, other members of the patient's family have similar headaches. Cranial artery dilation occurs during the attack, but permanent structural damage is rare. Other body accompaniments are abdominal distention, cold cyanosed extremities, vertigo, tremors, pallor, dryness of the mouth, excessive sweating, and chilliness. Many patients have noticed, either just before or during the migraine headache attack, that rings on the fingers are difficult to remove. Others describe and call attention to the "thickness of the skin," which appears and feels edematous. Pale urine or low specific gravity also indicates a widespread disturbance in water metabolism as an accompaniment of the headache.

Some clinicians prefer to limit the use of the word "migraine" to headaches that are always strictly unilateral throughout the attack. There is no objection to such a precise use of the term except that it results in profitless subdivisions of overlapping headache syndromes. Many persons with strictly unilateral periodic headaches also have, from time to time, attacks that become bilateral or are bilateral from the start. It seems justifiable to include such kindred headaches in one general class called *migraine* or *migraine variants*, of which the members have vascular mechanisms in common.

Classification of Migraine

The classification of headache by the Ad Hoc Committee of the National Institutes of Health has served as a foundation on which other headache classifications have developed.[3] The International Headache Society published a hierarchically constructed classification and operational diagnostic criteria for all headache disorders.[4] The document is primarily a research tool but will, in time, undoubtedly influence the diagnosis and classification of headache. The enduring and much simpler classification that divides migraine into common, classical, hemiplegic, and ophthalmoplegic will enable the practitioner to arrive at the diagnosis and will help in selecting the appropriate therapy. Common to all these types is a tendency for vascular dilatation to occur, which represents the headache phase of the migraine attack.

In migraine with aura (classic migraine), the patient experiences an aura of focal neurological symptoms that localize to the cerebral cortex or brainstem and initiate or accompany the headache phase. The aura represents ini-

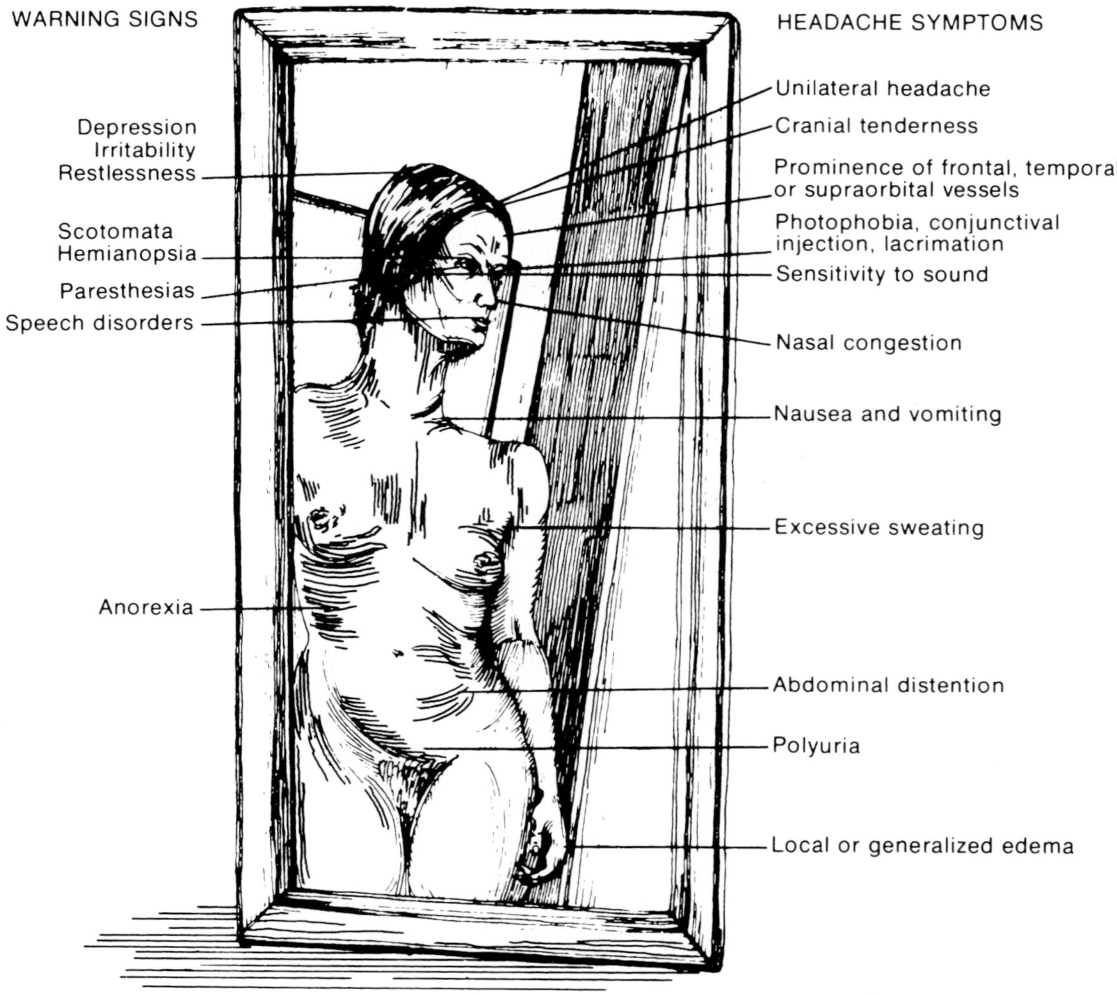

Figure 6–1 Clinical features of migraine.

tial vasoconstriction that gradually develops over 5 to 20 minutes and usually lasts less than 1 hour. In migraine without aura (nonclassic or common migraine), the headache phase is not preceded by an aura. Migraine without aura is believed to occur more frequently; however, the two types of migraine are not mutually exclusive. Many patients experience a mixture of headaches with or without auras.

For simplicity, if any headache in the patient's history was preceded by focal neurological signs, the classification of migraine with aura is applied, although the majority of headaches may be aura free.

Hemiplegic and ophthalmoplegic migraines are considered more severe forms of migraine with aura. If recurrent migraine becomes associated with permanent neurological residual damage to the nervous system, the term *complicated migraine* is used. In these patients, one or more of the aura symptoms continues for longer than 1 hour but less than 1 week.

Neuroimaging results are usually normal. If the symptoms persist for longer than 1 week or if ischemic infarction is demonstrated on neuroimaging, then a *migrainous infarction* has occurred.[2]

Sex Distribution

Migraine is more common in women than in men. Estimates have varied, but most experts agree that 60% of patients with migraine are women.

Family History

Migraine patients will frequently relate a history of their disorder in a close blood relative. Most twin studies of migraine have suggested that genetic factors account for a significant degree of the variance of the trait. Increases of twofold to sevenfold in monozygotic versus dizygotic concordance rates have been reported.[5–7] In a 1993 study, a genetic link was identified for familial hemiplegic migraine in a DNA region on human chromosome 19.[8] Whether the problem is hereditary or familial is conjecture, but a positive family history is obtained in as many as 70% of affected individuals.

Age Distribution

Migraine may appear in childhood. In one epidemiological investigation, the report noted that among those aged 12 to 29 years old, within 1 month before the interview, 3.0% of males and 7.4% of females had had a migraine headache.[9] Usually, migraine begins before the age of 40—most commonly in the second and third decades of life. Occasionally, the first symptoms present in the fifth and sixth decades. Migraine tends to decrease with advancing age. In many older patients, the prodromal preheadache symptoms persist after the headaches disappear.

Factors Influencing Attacks

Stress and Fatigue

In my experience, many but not all patients with migraine are obsessive, compulsive, and rigid. They keep long lists documenting their attacks, treatment, and medications. The stress situations of life, such as menopause, puberty, and change of school or job, seem to paralyze their adapting mechanisms. This inability to adapt creates anger and resentment and has been described as the repressed hostility of the migraine patient. Physicians who deal with headache need to emphasize that a patient's migrainous attacks may not represent the essence of the problem at hand. Consider the remark of a woman who said angrily, "Doctor, will you stop talking about my headache and discuss my other symptoms: my tendency to fatigue, my inability to keep up with my husband, and the social and work tasks I set up for myself?" Attacks occur more frequently when the patient is excessively tired. Migraine patients as a whole tend to build for themselves lives with too many environmental demands. They are extremely sensitive to overload. They may suffer situational anxieties in addition to those caused by deeper subconscious conflicts.

Many migraine sufferers will relate that their initial attacks occurred in close proximity to extended periods of emotional distress, such as loss and bereavement or physical illness.[10] In many patients, the emotional triggers may not precipitate for a considerable time, but in other migraineurs, the acute migraine attack may occur on the same day as the stressful event.[11]

Blau[12] conducted a study of 50 migraine patients to review previous observations that the migraine attack is often resolved by sleep. Fourteen of his subjects stated that they were able to decrease the duration of the migraine attack by sleeping for an average of 2.5 hours. These migraineurs used various methods of falling asleep, such as retiring to a dimly lit or darkened room and closing the door to ensure quiet. One important observation in this study was discussed: the need for the migraine patient to be cognizant of the various methods to abort the acute attack and the need to individualize these methods.

In addition to sleep, biofeedback is a useful nonpharmacological method of treating migraine. The mechanism for its success is probably twofold. First, pain and relaxation are dichotomous, and if one can relax, then pain must decrease (Table 6–1). Second, Dalessio and his associates[13] at Scripps Clinic in La Jolla, California, described an *adaptation-relaxation* reflex that is characterized by dilation of blood vessels in the hand and arm and then reduction in blood flow in the arteries of the temporal lobe of the brain. The reflex is learned through biofeedback training and is essential to successful conditioning of hand temperature. The long-term effects of training in relaxation and stress-coping in patients with migraine were shown to be clearly effi-

Table 6–1 Electromyographic Feedback Exercises: Relaxation of Facial Area with Neck, Shoulders, and Upper Back

Let all your muscles go loose and heavy. Just settle back quietly and comfortable. Wrinkle up your forehead now; wrinkle and smooth it out. Picture the entire forehead and scalp becoming smoother as the relaxation increases . . . now frown and crease your brows and study the tension . . . let go of the tension again. Smooth out the forehead once more . . . now, close your eyes tighter and tighter. Feel the tension . . . and relax your eyes. Keep your eyes closed, gently, comfortably, and notice the relaxation . . . now clench your jaw, bite your teeth together; study the tension throughout the jaw. . . . Relax your jaw now. Let your lips part slightly . . . appreciate the relaxation . . . now press your tongue hard against the roof of your mouth. Look for the tension. All right, let your tongue return to a comfortable and relaxed position . . . now purse your lips, press your lips together tighter and tighter . . . relax the lips. Note the contrast between tension and relaxation. Feel the relaxation all over your face, all over your forehead and scalp, eyes, jaws, lips, tongue, and your neck muscles. Press your head back as far as it can go and feel the tension in the neck; roll it to the right and feel the tension shift; now roll it to the left. Straighten your head and bring it forward and press your chin against your chest. Let your head return to a comfortable position, and study the relaxation. Let the relaxation develop . . . shrug your shoulders right up. Hold the tension . . . drop your shoulders and feel the relaxation. Neck and shoulders relaxed . . . shrug your shoulders again and move them around. Bring your shoulders up and forward and back. Feel the tension in your shoulders up and forward and back. Drop your shoulders once more and relax. Let the relaxation spread deep into the shoulders, right into your back muscles; relax your neck and throat, and your jaws and other facial areas as the pure relaxation takes over and grows deeper . . . deeper . . . ever deeper.

cacious and were maintained at 3 years of follow-up.[14]

Psychological Patterns in Migraine Patients

For centuries, the personality profile of the migraine sufferer has been a point of discussion and disagreement. As early as 1743, the physician D. Junkerius wrote that the primary cause of migraine is anger, especially when it is tacit and suppressed. The role of suppressed anger as a precipitant to migraine attacks has long been accepted. Fromm-Reichman[15] concluded that migraine sufferers "could not stand to be aware of their hostility against beloved persons; therefore, they unconsciously tried to keep this hostility repressed, and finally expressed it by the physical symptoms of migraine."

In the late 1930s, Wolff conducted a comprehensive study of the personalities of migraine patients.[16] He concluded that various "pernicious, emotional reactions," not necessarily anger, were precipitants of migraine attacks. In subjects predisposed to migraine, attacks often occur during such reactions; hence, the personality functions of these persons become important. Wolff's accounts of the childhood of the migraineur revealed that more than half were "delicate," shy, withdrawn, and extremely obedient. These traits coexisted, however, with an unusual stubbornness or inflexibility. These contrasting qualities were often a prominent feature of the child's personality.

Courteous, gracious, polite behavior was associated in the same person with obstinancy, defiance, or even rebellion. Temper tantrums occasionally resulted from frustration. Characteristically, these children were sensitive, trustworthy, and energetic. Generally respected and admired by parents and teachers, they eventually were given responsibility at an early age.

During adolescence and later, these children were more than usually preoccupied with moralistic and ethical problems, particularly concerning sex. In adults, these preoccupations took more definite form and were sometimes accentuated to an exceptional degree. Ninety percent of the migrainous subjects were ambitious and preoccupied with achievement and success. Many said they lost their ability to feel tired. They were conscientious, persistent, and exacting and attempted to arrange or bring order wherever possible. They were frequently described as meticulous, well dressed, hard workers, and perfectionists. They were also unforgiving and inflexible, with many experiencing difficulty in sexual adjustment.

Bille[17] described children with migraine as fearful, tense, sensitive, and easily frustrated. These findings were quite consistent with Wolff's original work. Jonckheere[18] described the migraine sufferer as obsessive and/or aggressive. Henryk-Gutt and Rees[19] said these people had greater neuroticism, hostility, and anxiety than control groups. Rogado's group[20] also depicted the migraineur as an obsessive-compulsive personality with a greater incidence of hysteria and hypochondriasis than normal subjects. Philips[21] reviewed the studies of Howarth,[22] Maxwell,[23] and Henryk-Gutt and Rees[19] and concluded that there was only support for the view that migraine sufferers were more neurotic than age-matched control subjects. Rorschach records of migraine sufferers reviewed by Ross and McNaughton[24] showed these patients had a tendency toward rigidity, persistence toward success, difficulty in sexual adjustment, perfectionism, conventionality, intolerance, and obsessive-compulsive features. In contrast, the majority of the research reported in the 1980s showed that migraine sufferers in general have normal personality profiles.[25–27]

In general, the psychological studies and interviews with migraine patients do not support the widely held view that the migraine patient is likely to be compulsive, inhibited in the expression of anger, prone to neurotic defenses, and dependent. It is probable that selection biases prevent clinicians from observing a representative sample of patients with migraine. Certainly, the possibility of experiencing the sudden, sometimes disabling pain of migraine attacks could generate responses of irritability, anxiety, or dependency in any person. Because studies show that only 50% of migraine sufferers consult physicians, it therefore is possible that the traits considered to be causes or predispositions to migraine may simply be characteristics that correlate highly with persons seeking medical attention. The debate continues with reputable neurologists and headache specialists supporting both sides of the question.

Dietary Migraine

No clinical problem is more perplexing to the practicing physician than the relationship of foods and beverages to the production of migraine. A great deal of folklore surrounds the subject, and little scientific work has been done to clarify the issue. Furthermore, various misconceptions about diet and migraine are given credence by articles in the popular press. Thus, the physician may encounter patients who have constructed elaborate diets in the hope of escaping recurrent migraine attacks. Occasionally, these diets assume ridiculous extremes; for example, one may find that a patient is living primarily on scallions, bananas, or onions. The purpose of this section is to make some sense out of a confusing clinical dilemma and, at the least, to stress those facts that seem conclusive.

Alcohol

Unquestionably, some ingested substances provoke vascular headaches in susceptible individuals. Alcohol, for example, produces a vascular headache in migraine patients, particularly if they are in a migraine phase. Alcoholic beverages are the most cited triggers of migraine attacks by migraineurs.[28] Patients with cluster headache are notoriously sensitive to even small amounts of alcohol, and they learn to avoid alcohol during the period of cluster headache recurrence. Alcohol is a nonspecific vasodilator, which probably accounts for its precipitation of the vascular headache process. The vasodilation is assumed to be the result of depression or alteration of the central vasomotor centers because the direct action of alcohol on blood vessels is insignificant. Moderate amounts of alcohol do not affect cerebral blood flow, but severe intoxication causes a significant increase in cerebral blood flow, with diminished cerebrovascular resistance.

Some patients with migraine claim that red wine, but not alcohol in general, could provoke a headache. Red wine has been suggested to contain a migraine-provoking agent that is neither alcohol nor tyramine.[29] The complex phenol compounds (flavanoid phenols) are found in much higher concentrations in red wine than in white wines.

Tyramine

Foods that contain tyramine, a vasoactive amine, may precipitate headache, particularly in patients who are treated with monoamine oxidase inhibitors (MAOIs). Tyramine-rich foods include strong or aged cheeses, pickled herring, chicken livers, canned figs, and the pods of broad beans (Table 6–2). Tyramine acts as a sympathomimetic amine, both directly and through the release of norepinephrine. It is theorized that the release of norepinephrine from tissues results in selective cerebral vasoconstriction; when tissue stores of norepinephrine are exhausted, rebound dilation of the extracranial vessels occurs, producing headache. Patients with migraine appear to metabolize tyramine in a manner different from that of normal control subjects; in a study conducted by English investigators, dietary migraine patients excreted less conjugated tyramine, both before and after an oral load of that substrate, than did normal subjects.[30]

However, in a controlled study of exclusion of dietary vasoactive amines in children with migraine, the investigators found a significant decrease in the number of headaches when vasoactive amines were eliminated from the diet.[31] The study demonstrated that dietary manipulation improved migraine; all children who were on the high-fiber diet reported a decrease in headaches. Further investigation of dietary factors is warranted.

Aspartame

Aspartame (NutraSweet), an artificial sweetener, was approved for use in carbonated beverages in July 1983. As of July 1991, more than 5000 aspartame-related complaints were received by the Food and Drug Administration,[32] with neurological and behavioral symptoms, including headache, being the most common complaint.[33] Controlled studies have been equivocal in their findings about aspartame's effects on migraine.[34]

Cured Meats

Sensitivity to sodium nitrite has been reported in a patient who noted the onset of moderately severe headaches after the ingestion of cured meat products, such as hot dogs, bacon, ham, and salami.[35] This type of vascular headache is usually bitemporal or bifrontal and is described as throbbing and occasionally accompanied by facial flushing.

Elimination Diets

My approach to this problem has been to eliminate foods and beverages that contain vasoactive substances from the diets of patients with migraine. I then have the patient gradually reintroduce the foods as a trial to determine whether a headache will be triggered. Thus, patients receive recommendations that include avoidance of alcohol, particularly some wines that contain large amounts of histamine; aged or strong cheese; pickled herring; chicken livers; chocolate; and canned figs. The patients are not advised to avoid milk products. Large amounts of monosodium glutamate (MSG) may produce a generalized vasomotor reaction that may include headache *(Chinese restaurant syndrome)*. Use of excessive amounts of MSG is unwise.[36]

If patients persist in their contention that a specific substance is provoking headaches, I suggest that they participate in an experiment that is performed in the laboratory. An appropriate amount of the suspected substance is prepared in powdered form and put into capsules so that ingestion of this substance can be compared, in a double-blind study, with consumption of a similar amount of lactose. After a control period of about 1 week, the experiment is set into motion. The patients ingest the capsules for 2 weeks, and then the code is broken. Invariably, it is demonstrated that headaches occur from lactose ingestion as often as from the "offending" substance.

Hypoglycemia

The quality and quantity of food consumed by the patient with migraine are important. Hypoglycemia exerts a profound effect on the tone of the cranial blood vessels. If the sugar content of the blood is reduced by insulin or other means, conspicuous cerebral vasodilation occurs. For example, headache is a prominent symptom of insulin shock. Furthermore, in patients with migraine, the relative hypoglycemia produced by fasting may evoke typical vascular headaches. Reactive hypoglycemia occurring after ingestion of an excessive carbohydrate load may also precipitate vascular headache in a susceptible person. Because of these factors, patients with migraine are advised to eat three well-balanced meals a day and avoid an overabundance of carbohydrates at any single meal. Avoidance of oversleeping on weekends is also recommended. Excessive sleep may alter the body's normal blood sugar level and thus precipitate headaches when a rigid schedule of awakening is not maintained.

Miscellaneous

Substances such as chocolate and glutamate are triggers of migraine. These substances contain little or no tyramine. β-Phenylethylamine, a potent vasoactive amine, has been identified as the agent in chocolate as respon-

Table 6–2 Headache Diet

Each day, eat three meals with a snack at night or six small meals spread throughout the day.
All food, especially high-protein foods, should be prepared and eaten fresh. Do not eat leftovers held for more than 1 day.
The foods listed in the "caution" column have smaller amounts of tyramine or other vasoactive compounds. (Caffeinated beverages may be used in allowed amounts.)
Each person may have different sensitivities to a certain level of tyramine or other vasoactive compounds in foods; use restricted foods in limited amounts.

Allowed	Use with Caution	Avoid
Beverages		
Decaffeinated coffee Fruit juices Club soda and sparkling waters Caffeine-free carbonated beverages	Limit caffeinated beverages to no more than two servings per day Limit alcoholic beverages to one serving: wine, vodka, or scotch	All alcoholic beverages not specified in caution column
Meat, fish, poultry, eggs		
Freshly purchased and prepared meats Fish and poultry Eggs Tuna fish, tuna salad (with allowed ingredients)	Bacon Sausage Hot dogs Corned beef Ham Any luncheon meats with nitrites added (may not be high in tyramine) Meat with tenderizer (e.g., MSG) added Caviar	Products that are: Aged Dried Fermented Smoked Pickled Pepperoni Salami Liverwurst Nonfresh meat or liver Pickled herring
Dairy		
Milk Processed cheese	Parmesan or romano as a garnish (2 tsp) or minor ingredient Yogurt Buttermilk Sour cream	Aged cheese
Breads, cereals, pasta		
Commercially prepared yeast products Products leavened with baking powder All hot and dry cereals All pasta	Homemade yeast breads and coffee cake Sourdough breads	Any with restricted ingredients
Vegetables		
Any vegetables not on avoidance list	Raw onion	Fava or broad beans Sauerkraut Fermented soy products like miso and pickles

Table 6–2 Headache Diet *Continued*

Allowed	Use with Caution	Avoid
Fruits		
All fruits not on restricted list	Limit intake to ½ cup per day from each group: citrus, avocados, bananas, figs, raisins, papaya, passion fruit, red plums	
Nuts, seeds		
		All nuts: peanuts, peanut butter, pumpkin seeds, sesame seeds, walnuts, pecans, etc.
Soups		
Soups made from allowed ingredients Homemade broths	Canned soups with: Yeast Meat extracts Monosodium glutamate (MSG)	
Desserts, sweets		
Any made with allowed foods and ingredients	Chocolate-based products	Mincemeat pie
Ingredients listed on food labels		
Any not listed in the restricted section		MSG* (in large amounts) Nitrites (found in processed meats) Yeast, yeast extracts, brewers yeast Meat extracts Meat tenderizers (papain, bromelin) Seasoned salts (containing MSG) Soy sauce Teriyaki sauce
Fats, oils, miscellaneous		
All cooking oils and fats White vinegar Commercial salad dressing with allowed ingredients in small amounts All spices not listed in restricted ingredients	Fermented vinegars (wine, apple, etc.)	Mixed dishes made with restricted ingredients: macaroni and cheese, beef stroganoff, cheese blintzes, oriental foods, pizza Frozen dinners: read labels to check for restricted ingredients

*MSG and nitrites do not have the same effect as tyramine-containing foods but can cause headache in many people.

sible for triggering migraine attacks.[37] The headache caused by chocolate may not develop for up to 24 hours after ingestion.[38]

Hormonal Changes

Approximately 70% of female migraineurs note a relationship between their headaches and their menstrual cycle. The influence of hormonal changes and the role of oral contraceptives and hormone replacement therapy on headaches are described in Chapter 8.

Allergy, Epilepsy, and Migraine

I do not believe that there is any relationship between migraine and allergy or epilepsy. Migraine patients may note an increase in headache during or after an allergic episode, related to increased vasomotor activity. In addition, the vasoconstrictive phase of migraine presumably can set off seizure activity in one predisposed to seizures, but this series of events must be rare. Electroencephalographic changes have been reported in migraine patients, but their importance is conjectural. An occasional migraine patient with a significant dysrhythmia may respond to anticonvulsants.

In an earlier report, I presented studies on migraine and atopy.[39] Serum IgE levels were evaluated in 116 patients with headache by the radioimmunoassay technique. A second group consisted of 504 patients who were seen at a headache clinic during a period of 2 months. Elevation of the serum IgE was noted in 5.7% of the migraine population in both groups, which was approximately the same incidence of elevated serum IgE in the normal population. This incidence is far below that seen in atopic disorders. In the second group of 504 patients, the prevalence of atopic disorders in migraine patients and their relatives was approximately the same as the prevalence in patients with chronic tension-type headaches. The numbers are close to the prevalence of atopy in the normal population or their relatives and are not statistically significant. There is, therefore, no increase in the prevalence of atopy in the relatives of patients with migraine headaches. This study casts further doubt on any supposed relationship among atopy, allergy, elevation of the serum IgE, and migraine. It now seems evident, from this and other careful studies, that migraine is not an allergic phenomenon and is not related to the atopic disease.

Other Vascular Conditions and Migraine

Various conditions are triggered by vasospasm of selected arteries.[40] In one series, migraine with aura and Raynaud's phenomenon were studied in patients with variant angina. It was observed that these two conditions occur concomitantly with variant angina on a more frequent basis than in the control groups. This observation suggests the possibility of an underlying defect or mechanism that may partially account for all three conditions. A possible diagnosis could then be made of generalized arterial vasospasm, a single clinical syndrome that could be treated with a single agent. Another suggestion of this study is that attacks occurring in various arterial beds usually occur at different times and are triggered by a variety of mechanisms. This finding would then indicate that local factors may participate in the pathogenesis of these disorders.

Raynaud's Phenomenon

In one study, it was reported that Raynaud's phenomenon occurred more frequently in migraine patients.[41] Of special note, it was observed that drugs usually used in migraine therapy, such as the ergots and β-blockers, did not necessarily precipitate Raynaud's phenomenon. Cigarette smoking also did not precipitate the symptoms of Raynaud's phenomenon. In the general population, Raynaud's phenomenon occurs five times more frequently in females than in males. However, in studying migraineurs, it was noted that Raynaud's phenomenon was more prevalent in males. This finding has been attributed to the generalized tendency of vasospasm in cases of migraine.

Raynaud's phenomenon occurs very commonly in scleroderma and primary Sjögren's syndrome. One study evaluated 191 subjects with various connective tissue disorders and diagnosed migraine in 46% of patients with primary Sjögren's syndrome, 32%

of patients with scleroderma, and 11% of normal control subjects.[42]

Systemic Lupus Erythematosus

The possible relationship of migraine to systemic lupus erythematosus (SLE) has been reviewed.[43] Migraine with aura was found to be more prevalent in patients with SLE than in control groups. However, there were no statistically significant data about the prevalence of migraine without aura for the two groups. None of the case subjects were on concomitant oral contraceptives.

Recently, researchers have been investigating the association of the lupus anticoagulant and migraine.[44, 45] Further expanded studies are needed to support this association.

Mitral Valve Prolapse

Numerous reports have linked migraine with mitral valve prolapse.[46, 47] Mitral valve prolapse was observed in 15 of 100 migraineurs and in 7 of 100 control patients.[48] Pfaffenrath's group[49] studied 43 patients with migraine (with and without aura) and 19 migraineurs with hemiplegic migraine and determined that migraine with aura is not associated with mitral valve prolapse more frequently than other forms of migraine.

Due to the common incidence of these conditions, a study with a larger population should be conducted to allow for a definitive correlation. The physician should rule out mitral valve prolapse in younger patients with complicated migraine or stroke symptoms.

Multiple Sclerosis

A review of the records of 1113 patients with multiple sclerosis found 44 cases whose initial attack or subsequent exacerbations were heralded by a migraine-type headache.[50] The majority of the patients had no history of headache.

Site and Character of Headache

The most frequent history obtained is that of a dull ache that progressively worsens and finally develops into throbbing or pulsating pain. As it becomes stabilized, the headache may again become constant and nonthrobbing. About 70% of migraine is unilateral and frequently affects the frontal and temporal regions, but it may settle behind the eye. The pain can radiate across the head and to other regions of the face and neck surrounding the primary pain site.

Number, Duration, and Onset of Attacks

The number of attacks varies; in severe cases, attacks may occur every few days, whereas in moderate cases, attacks may occur only once or twice a year. Most frequently, patients report two to four attacks monthly. Most migraine episodes last longer than 4 hours, usually for 1 or 2 days. A severe attack can last up to 6 days. The onset can occur at any time and may be precipitated by various factors. It is not uncommon for a migraine patient to awaken with a headache.

Occasionally, pain in other areas, such as the temple, bregma, occiput, mastoid, or tongue, occurs concomitantly with substernal chest pain as a manifestation of myocardial ischemia. Cardiac pain has been observed in some cases of migraine that sometimes present during an acute attack of angina.[51, 52] The exact mechanism of this pain has not been determined.

The Attack

In the initial phase of migraine, the *prodromal phase*, vasoconstriction occurs, followed by vasodilation during which the headache manifests. In about 35% of cases, the patient has the typical migraine with aura as described. The patient notes an aura (most often visual) that may precede the attack by 10 to 20 minutes. Then, the typical one-sided, pulsating headache occurs with its associated symptoms. Migraine without aura does not have preheadache prodromes; however, premonitory symptoms occur in both forms of migraine. These symptoms, which are often vague, included mood changes, increased appetite, and excessive yawning, which may precede the "headache" by as long as 24 hours.

Prodromes in Order of Frequency

The prodromes in order of frequency are:

1. Scotomata, or blind spots
2. Teichopsia, or fortification spectra—a zigzag pattern resembling a fort (Fig. 6–2)
3. Photopsia, or flashing of lights and colors
4. Paresthesias
5. Visual and auditory hallucinations; Alice in Wonderland syndrome described by Lewis Carroll, who experienced migraine, who saw the distorted figures of "Alice" as part of his migraine attack

Other Rare Prodromes

Diplopia, ataxia, vertigo, syncope, and hyperosmia may occur. The prodromes usually resolve before each attack, but on occasion can remain permanent. As a person with migraine grows older, he or she may note only the prodrome without the subsequent headache.

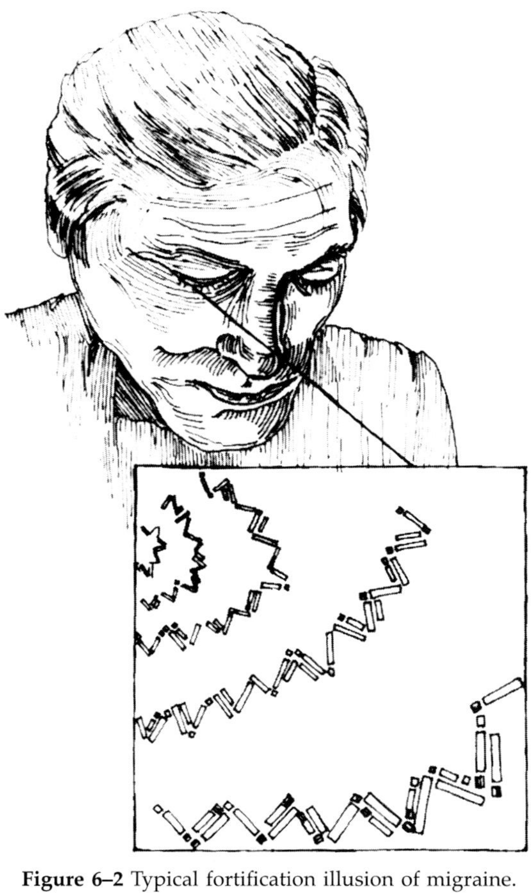

Figure 6–2 Typical fortification illusion of migraine.

Symptoms Accompanying Migraine Attacks

- Photophobia—Undue sensitivity to light, preferring darkened room. Noise can also increase discomfort.
- Nausea and emesis—Occurs in 90% of migraines. Rarely, diarrhea ensues. Dehydration may occur if recurrent emesis persists.
- Arteries (vascular changes)—Cold hands and feet, tenderness over the superficial vessels over the part of the head where the headache occurs, and pale skin of the face often are noted.
- Other body changes—During attack, there most often is an increase in weight, with sodium retention and an oliguria. As the patient improves, diuresis often occurs. Hyperesthesia of the scalp is a frequent complaint of the patient with migraine.

Special Types of Migraine

An occasional patient with migraine will note neurological manifestations that persist beyond the immediate headache period. Such complications include hemiparesis, hemisensory defects, occlusion of the retinal artery, and ophthalmoplegia. I assume that these complications are related to the prolonged vasoconstriction or vasodilation occurring as part of the migraine process. If the brain becomes sufficiently ischemic during these vasoactive changes, permanent damage related to cerebral infarction may ensue. This situation is termed *complicated migraine*.[53, 54]

The incidence of complicated migraine is uncertain, but the most widely accepted studies suggest that less than 1% to 2% of patients with migraine experience episodes that could be characterized as complicated migraine. With the advent of computed tomography, it has been realized that cerebral infarction, edema, and atrophy may be consequences of migrainous attacks.[55, 56] The significance of these findings remains to be determined. It should be remembered that computed tomography (CT) scans may be normal for some patients with lifelong migraine. Likewise, no obvious association between abnormalities has been discovered by CT scanning and persistent treatment with ergot derivatives.

Ophthalmic migraine is associated with a third nerve or other ocular nerve palsy. It is usually transient but may become permanent.

The occurrence and recurrence of this problem suggest the diagnosis, as opposed to an intracranial aneurysm, producing a third nerve palsy.[57]

Hemiplegic migraine is associated with motor (and sensory) changes of hemiplegia.[58] It may persist for days or weeks. This is a rare form of migraine that is commonly familial.[59]

Migraine Therapy

Migraine has been described by some as a self-limited neurogenic sterile inflammation. Its aura pattern has been described as a *spreading oligemia* or spreading depression associated with a decrease in cerebral cortical blood flow. For years, the investigational pendulum has swung back and forth between findings that support an arterial process and findings that support a cerntral nervous system process as the basis for migraine pathogenesis. Unfortunately, however, neither the details nor the cause of migraine has truly come to light.

Pharmacologically, it appears that managing the migraine patient involves the use of drugs that block stimulation of the platelets, trigeminovascular system, substance P release, or neurogenic inflammation. For abortive purposes, agents that prevent substance P and calcitonin gene-related peptide (CGRP) release (e.g., ergotamine or the triptans) or stop neurogenic inflammation (e.g., such as the nonsteroidal anti-inflammatory agents [NSAIDs]) have been found to be useful. For prophylactic purposes, agents that inhibit trigeminovascular stimulation appear to have the most efficacy; these include such drugs as β-blockers, calcium channel blockers, antidepressants, methysergide, divalproex sodium, and NSAIDs.

Managing the patient with migraine revolves around three interrelated objectives:

- Minimizing symptomatology
- Reducing disability
- Improving quality of life

In an effort to achieve these objectives with the greatest degree of safety, pharmacological therapy must be selected on a case-by-case basis after a thorough evaluation of a patient's history and physical examination (Table 6–3).

Table 6–3 Data Necessary to Individualize Therapy Selections

1. What are the patient's age, weight, and gender?
2. Does the patient have other physical and/or psychiatric comorbidities?
3. What is the patient's reproductive status? Is the patient concerned about compromising libido or fertility? Is the patient pregnant?
4. Does the patient have known drug sensitivities?
5. What time of day do headache attacks occur?
6. Does the headache develop slowly, begin abruptly, or awaken the patient from sleep?
7. Are headache attacks associated with menses or ovulation?
8. Where is the patient during the attacks?
9. Does each attack create the same level of disability?
10. Does the patient work? If so, does the work involve the operation of dangerous machinery? Does the patient drive?
11. Does the patient have childcare responsibilities?
12. Is the patient an athlete, or does he or she participate in recreational activities that involve strenuous physical exercise or the use of dangerous equipment?

For example, all things being approximately equal, it is possible that any two patients may respond equally well to the prophylactic use of a β-blocker. If, however, one of those individuals is a professional athlete, the issue of possible adverse effects on athletic performance would likely preclude this choice from the physician's repertoire. Similarly, the use of a narcotic, muscle relaxant, or other central nervous system depressant might be considered a poor choice for a patient who is traveling all day or is at home throughout the day caring for three toddlers.

Depending on a patient's individual presentation and circumstances, selections may be made from any or all of the following categories of medication:

- Abortive
- Symptomatic (pain relief)
- Prophylactic

Both physician and patient should be aware that making the appropriate selection or selections can be a prolonged process that may require frequent office visits and many thoughtful, interactive discussions. It also is important for patients to be appraised of the fact that migraine is a disorder whose symptoms may wax and wane throughout the course of a lifetime. Therapeutic selections chosen within the framework of one set of circumstances or one stage of life may be ineffective, inappropriate, or both in the framework of another. Thus, although pharmacological therapy can greatly reduce pain and suffering, it is not likely to render the patient completely headache free, given the complex variables involved.

Equipped with the knowledge that breakthrough headaches can occur, patients are more likely to focus on an overall pattern of improvement than on intermittent or isolated events. Given the diverse arsenal of available agents, however, the vast majority of patients with migraine can expect to gain some degree of control over their migraine attacks.

Abortive Therapy

Ideally, abortive agents should be started as early as possible in the attack or during the aura. The agents of choice in migraine abortive therapy include the triptans, NSAIDS, ergotamine preparations, and phenothiazines (Table 6–4).

Triptans

During the past three decades, there have been tremendous gains in our knowledge of migraine pathogenesis, with investigations into the relationship between serotonin and migraine.[60] Some researchers suggested that the release of serotonin from the platelets triggers migraine. The release of serotonin from perivascular terminals of putative serotonergic nerve fibers has been identified as the initiator of an acute migraine attack. Systemic metabolic changes in serotonin metabolism have also been suggested as migraine causative factors. Serotonergic drugs, such as reserpine, are recognized as migraine provocateurs.

Serotonin (5-HT) agonists, such as the triptans (sumatriptan, naratriptan, zolmitriptan, rizatriptan, eletriptan, and frovatriptan), ergotamine, and dihydroergotamine, have demonstrated efficacy in aborting migraine attacks and have variable affinity for the 5-HT_{1A}, 5-HT_{1B}, 5-HT_{1D}, and 5-HT_{1F} receptors. Their antimigraine effect is exerted via a receptor-mediated neural pathway in both the central nervous system and the trigeminal nerve, at which point neurogenic inflammation is blocked.[61]

As a serotonin receptor agonist that inhibits release of 5-HT, norepinephrine, acetylcholine, and substance P, sumatriptan is highly effective in blocking inflammation and producing vasoconstriction in dilated cranial arteries. As the first triptan to be approved for migraine abortive therapy, sumatriptan has gained universal acceptance for first-line treatment of an acute migraine attack.[62]

When first introduced, sumatriptan was available only for subcutaneous administration. At a subcutaneous dose of 6 mg, the terminal half-life of sumatriptan is reported as approximately 2 hours. This agent also is available in oral preparations and a nasal spray. The 100-mg oral dose of sumatriptan reportedly provides improvement within 4 hours in approximately 75% of patients. The 50-mg dose (oral) is commonly prescribed. The intranasal preparation, which received approval in 1998, is available in a 20-mg dose, and 75% of patients have reported relief within 120 minutes after inhalation.[63]

Sumatriptan is generally well tolerated, with minor and transient side effects, including flushing, throat discomfort, neck and chest tightness or pain, tingling, and nausea. If the autoinjectable preparation is used for subcutaneous administration, the patient may experience local irritation at the injection site.

Sumatriptan use has been limited due to the occurrence of chest symptoms, although their presentation does not necessarily indicate cardiac ischemia due to the constriction of coronary arteries. The patient may complain of headache recurrence within 24 hours after initial successful treatment of an attack. In a few patients who do not maintain the dosing limitations, rebound phenomena have been observed.

If the first dose of sumatriptan is not effective or provides only partial relief, a second dose may be repeated after 1 hour or anytime within the next 24 hours. However, a 5-day hiatus should be maintained between treatment days.

Because sumatriptan can potentially cause coronary vasospasm, it should never be administered intravenously. This agent should never be used concomitantly with the ergotamine preparations or MAOIs.[64] Sumatriptan is contraindicated in patients with ischemic heart disease (or those presenting with symptoms or signs consistent with ischemic heart disease), prior history of myocardial infarction, documented silent ischemia, Prinzmetal's angina, uncontrolled hypertension, hemiplegic or basilar artery migraine,

Table 6–4 Migraine Abortive Therapy

Agent	Route	Dosage
Sumatriptan	SC	6 mg at onset; may repeat after 1 hour; up to 12 mg/24 hr
Sumatriptan	PO	Start with 25 to 50 mg at onset. If ineffective, dose can be repeated in 1 hour, up to 100 mg.
Sumatriptan	Nasal spray	20 mg, 1 spray in one nostril at onset, may repeat within 2 to 24 hours, limited to 2 sprays per day
Naratriptan	PO	1 mg or 2.5 mg; may repeat in 4 hours; only 2 per 24 hours; 4- to 5-day hiatus between treatment days.
Rizatriptan	PO—oral tablets or dissolvable tablets	5 mg or 10 mg at onset; may repeat in 2 hours; only 2 per 24 hours; 4- to 5-day hiatus between treatment days.
Zolmitriptan	PO	2.5 mg or 5 mg at onset; may repeat in 2 hours; only 2 per 24 hours; 4- to 5-day hiatus between treatment days.
Ergotamine tartrate	SL	2 mg under tongue at onset, may repeat every 30 minutes, up to 3 tablets per day, 5 tablets per week. Maintain 5-day hiatus between treatment days.
Ergotamine tartrate with caffeine	PO	Two 1-mg tablets at onset, may repeat 1 tablet every 30 minutes, up to 6 tablets per day; 10 tablets per week. Maintain 5-day hiatus between treatment days.
Ergotamine tartrate with caffeine	Rectal	One suppository at onset, may repeat at 1 hour, up to 2 per day, 5 per week; may begin with ½ suppository at onset, repeat by ½ within 1 hour. Maintain 5-day hiatus between treatment days.
Dihydroergotamine	IM, SC	1 mg at onset, may repeat at hourly intervals, up to 3 injections per day. Maintain 5-day hiatus between treatment days.
Dihydroergotamine	Nasal spray	2 mg, 1 spray in each nostril; repeat in 15 minutes, up to 3 mg per day
Isometheptene mucate with dichloralphenazone and acetaminophen	PO	Two capsules at onset, may be repeated 1 tablet every hour, up to 5 capsules per day, 15 per week.
Aspirin, acetaminophen, and caffeine	PO	Two tablets at onset, may repeat in 4 hours. If headache persists, professional consult should be sought.
Naproxen sodium	PO	825 mg initially, 550 mg after 1 hour
Flurbiprofen	PO	50–100 mg at onset; repeat every 6 hours
Etodolac	PO	300 mg TID
Mefenamic acid	PO	500 mg at onset
Diclofenac sodium	PO	50–75 mg BID or QID
Chlorpromazine	IM	50–100 mg
Prochlorperazine	IM	10–25 mg
Lidocaine	Intranasal	15 drops of 4% solution to the nostril ipsilateral to the pain. May be repeated in 5 minutes, up to 4 times per day.

pregnancy, or hypersensitivity to sumatriptan.

In the past year, three other triptans (zolmitriptan, naratriptan, rizatriptan) have received approval for migraine abortive therapy. Zolmitriptan and rizatriptan are selective $5\text{-HT}_{1B/1D}$ receptor agonists. Naratriptan is a second-generation 5-HT_{1D} receptor agonist.

Studies of zolmitriptan have demontrated that this agent is absorbed rapidly. Long-term studies showed relief of attacks within 2 hours in 81% of 2058 patients who used zolmitriptan for moderate to severe migraine attacks. Zolmitriptan was effective in relieving associated symptoms of migraine such as nausea, photophobia, phonophobia, and reduced activity impairment.[64a] Side effects were similar to those experienced with sumatriptan. The most frequently reported adverse effects were nausea, dizziness, prickling or tingling of the skin, drowsiness, warm or cold sensations, and tightness of the neck or throat, or jaw pain. This agent is available for oral administration in doses of 2.5 mg and 5.0 mg.

Naratriptan has a half-life of 6 hours, which is longer than that of other triptans and which can affect the recurrence rates. In a parallel group study, headache relief was reported 4 hours after dosing in 60% of patients receiving naratriptan, 2.5 mg.[64b] This study also noted a low incidence of side effects, with nausea and vomiting as the most frequently reported symptoms. It is available in 1.0-mg and 2.5-mg oral tablets.

Rizatriptan is also absorbed rapidly after oral administration. In a multicenter study,[64c] onset of effect was observed as early as 30 minutes after administration of the 10-mg dose. In general, rizatriptan is well tolerated, with the most commonly reported side effects being bitter taste, dizziness, somnolence, asthenia/fatigue, and nausea. These symptoms were dose-related. Rizatriptan is available in 5-mg and 10-mg doses as standard oral tablets or in disks for oral disintegration, which can be taken without water. Two other triptans (eletriptan, frovatriptan) are awaiting approval.

Ergotamine and Derivatives

Until the introduction of sumatriptan, ergotamine was the first-line choice in the abortive treatment of migraine headaches for more than 50 years. Ergotamine preparations are still prescribed. Ergotamine is an α-adrenergic–blocking agent with a direct stimulating effect on the smooth muscle of peripheral and cranial blood vessels, and it produces depression of central vasomotor centers. It also has properties of serotonin antagonism.

Ergotamine is available for oral, sublingual, and rectal administration. Absorption of ergotamine and its derivatives is quite variable. In the United States, caffeine has been added to the oral and rectal preparations to enhance the absorption of the active ingredient. The route of administration should be dependent on what is most acceptable to the individual patient. Sublingual preparations should be considered if the oral route is too slow or is not well-tolerated. Rectal suppositories are the best absorbed of the nonparenteral preparations and are especially helpful for those patients experiencing associated gastrointestinal symptoms. However, rectal administration would not be appropriate in patients who find them awkward to use or in those with associated diarrhea. Doses should be increased to a single effective dose, administered as early as possible in subsequent attacks. Patients experiencing migraine with aura should be instructed to use the drug during the prodromal phase. To prevent rebound headache, a 5-day hiatus must be maintained between treatment days.

Side effects of ergotamine administration include nausea, vomiting, diarrhea, cramping, dizziness, transient paresthesias, stroke, hypertension, myocardial ischemia/infarction, and peripheral vasospasm. Ergotamine preparations are generally contraindicated in the elderly and/or in patients with peripheral vascular disease, thrombophlebitis, severe hypertension, coronary ischemia, angina, renal or hepatic disease, or recent infection. Excessive consumption of the ergotamine agent may lead to symptoms of vasoconstriction and ultimately to ergotism. Ergotamine should never be used in pregnancy; it should be used cautiously in patients with peptic ulcer and recent infection.

Dihydroergotamine

An effective ergot derivative, dihydroergotamine (DHE), has recently been "rediscovered" as a 5-HT_1 receptor agonist. DHE also is potent at a number of other biogenic amine receptors. This agent differs from ergotamine in having less association with nausea and increased venoconstrictor effects.

DHE has long been available for parenteral administration, and a nasal spray form has been approved.[65] The route of administration is significant in obtaining relief because it influences the speed of action. Parenteral administration provides the patient with the quickest action, but self-injection techniques may not be tolerable for many patients. Waiting to receive an injection at the physician's office or at the local emergency department may delay the immediate action required. The nasal spray form of DHE may be more acceptable to the patient and can provide quick relief of the headache symptoms.[66] For parenteral administration (intramuscular, subcutaneous, intravenous), DHE is available in 1 mg/1 mL ampules. The nasal spray is administered in 2-mg doses.

DHE is contraindicated in patients with peripheral arterial disease, ischemic heart disease, uncontrolled hypertension, Prinzmetal's angina, hemiplegic or basilar artery migraine, impaired hepatic or renal function, sepsis, pregnancy, or hypersensitivity to ergot alkaloids. A 5-day hiatus between days of use must be maintained to prevent rebound phenomena, and it should never be used concomitantly with the triptans or other ergotamine derivatives.

Isometheptene

In patients who cannot tolerate ergotamine or its derivatives or the triptans, a mild vasoconstrictor, isometheptene, may be indicated. Isometheptene is a sympathomimetic amine that acts by constricting dilated cranial and cerebral arterioles. It is available in combination with dichloralphenazone (a mild sedative) and acetaminophen. It is especially helpful in patients with mild to moderately severe migraine if taken early in the attack. Isometheptene can also be used on the second or third day of a migraine attack, when the patient is prevented from repeating a dose of an ergotamine or its derivatives. Isometheptene has minimal side effects. It is contraindicated in patients with uncontrolled hypertension or severe cases of renal or hepatic disease, hypertension, or organic heart disease. Isometheptene should never be used concomitantly in patients receiving an MAOI.

Nonsteroidal Anti-inflammatory Drugs

For patients with mild to moderately severe migraine attacks, the NSAIDs are excellent alternatives for migraine abortive therapy. A possible explanation for their efficacy involves their ability to inhibit prostaglandin synthesis and thus prevent neurogenically mediated inflammation in the trigeminovascular system. The NSAIDs may also interfere with serotonin neurotransmission and modulate vasoconstriction. The side effects associated with short-term NSAID therapy are usually minor and can include nausea, abdominal distress, dyspepsia, diarrhea, dizziness, and tinnitus. Because of their capacity to induce gastrointestinal bleeding, the NSAIDs should be avoided in patients with peptic ulcer disease. The NSAIDs are also contraindicated in patients with renal dysfunction.

Phenothiazines

The phenothiazines chlorpromazine and prochlorperazine have demonstrated efficacy in migraine abortive therapy in the emergency department setting.[67] The success of these agents in migraine abortive treatment is related to their dopaminergic and adrenergic effects. Their sedative and antinauseant actions are beneficial for the associated symptoms of an acute migraine attack.

Lidocaine

The use of intranasal lidocaine has been suggested as an alternative agent for migraine abortive therapy.[68] However, relapse is common and occurs early after treatment.

Pain Relief Measures

Although the patient may have used abortive agents appropriately, the symptoms associated with migraine may persist (Table 6–5). Narcotic analgesics may be used to control the pain of infrequent attacks but should be avoided in patients who experience chronic migraine. If not contraindicated, the NSAIDs are an excellent alternative. Among the NSAIDs that have been used successfully for symptomatic relief of migraine are aspirin, ibuprofen, naproxen sodium, and ketoprofen. Ketorolac is available for intramuscular administration and can be used effectively for self-administration as well as in the emergency department and outpatient clinic.[69]

Aspirin, Acetaminophen, and Caffeine

A combination analgesic of aspirin, acetaminophen, and caffeine (Excedrin Migraine) is the first over-the-counter agent to be approved for migraine relief. It is recommended for the acute treatment of mild to moderate migraine headache without associated vomiting and disability. This agent certainly provides easy and cost-effective treatment of acute migraine headaches.

Opioids

For some patients, the use of simple analgesics is not effective or may be contraindicated.

Table 6–5 Symptomatic Agents in Migraine

Agent	Route	Dosage
Analgesics		
Aspirin	PO	500 mg BID
Ketoprofen	PO	12.5–25 mg BID
Naproxen sodium	PO	275–550 mg BID
Ibuprofen	PO	200–400 mg every 4 hours
Ketorolac	PO	10 mg QID
Ketorolac	IM	60 mg BID
Butorphanol	Intranasal	1 mg in one nostril; if pain persists, an additional 1 mg dose may be used within 60–90 minutes; the two-dose sequence may be repeated every 3–4 hours
Antinauseants		
Metoclopramide	PO	10–20 mg at onset; may repeat every 6–8 hours
Metoclopramide	IM	10–20 mg at onset; may repeat every 6–8 hours
Metoclopramide	IV	10 mg at onset; may repeat in 6 hours
Chlorpromazine HCl	PO	25–50 mg; may be repeated at 6-hour intervals
Chlorpromazine HCl	Rectal	100 mg suppository; may repeat at 6-hour intervals
Chlorpromazine HCl	IM	25–50 mg; may repeat at 6-hour intervals
Chlorpromazine HCl	IV	0.1 mg/kg via slow IV push; may repeat at 6-hour intervals
Prochlorperazine	PO	25–50 mg; may repeat at 6-hour intervals
Prochlorperazine	Rectal	25-mg suppository; may repeat at 6-hour intervals
Prochlorperazine	IM	10 mg; may be repeated at 6-hour intervals

The opioid analgesics can provide effective pain relief but cannot be used for frequent headaches because of the risk of habituation.

Transnasal Butorphanol

Butorphanol, originally provided for parenteral injection, is available for transnasal administration.[70] The exact mechanism of butorphanol is unknown. Its analgesic benefit is related to its agonist activity at the κ receptor and its partial agonist (mixed agonist-antagonist) activity at the μ receptor, in contrast to the morphine-like analgesics that are full agonists at both the μ and κ receptors. Also, butorphanol is associated with less respiratory depression and euphoria than the morphine-like analgesics.

The nasal mucosa are highly vascular, thus facilitating the rapid intake and absorption of transnasal butorphanol, which has a lipophilic nature. The most common reported side effects of butorphanol are somnolence, dizziness, and nausea and vomiting. Of course, somnolence may be a desired effect in some migraine sufferers. Dysphoria and hallucinations have been reported in rare cases. Transnasal butorphanol is contraindicated in patients with a hypersensitivity to butorphanol or benzethonium chloride, as well as patients dependent on narcotics or those who have recently received repetitive doses of an opioid. Acute opiate withdrawal symptoms have been observed in patients after repeated doses of opioids or in patients who experience decreased efficacy of other opioids. The abrupt discontinuation of transnasal butorphanol after prolonged use of higher doses can pose a potential risk for withdrawal symptoms.

Dependency and abuse problems have been reported in patients treated with transnasal butorphanol. Transnasal butorphanol is not indicated in patients with frequent headaches or in patients with prior histories of medication abuse. Dose and prescription limits should be maintained on all analgesic agents.[71]

Antiemetics

The associated gastrointestinal symptoms of migraine—nausea and vomiting—are often relieved with the use of the phenothiazines such as chlorpromazine and prochlorperazine. Again, their sedative effects may not be acceptable to many patients. Metoclopramide, which has minimal sedative actions, may be preferred by patients who want to return to normal activities after an acute attack.[72] This drug has been effective in the treatment of prolonged migraine attacks and status migraine because of its possible action in enhancing the absorption of oral agents and intravenous DHE.

Cold Packs

For many years, migraine sufferers have found relief by applying ice and other cold treatments to the affected site.[73] Commercial preparations, such as cold packs, are easy-to-use remedies for headache.

Prophylactic Therapy

Prophylactic therapy should be considered in patients who experience two or more migraine attacks per month, whose attacks are sufficiently severe to greatly affect their quality of life and ability to function, for whom abortive therapies have been unsuccessful, and for whom abortive therapies are contraindicated. Several prophylactic trials are reasonable as long as the provider is sufficiently comfortable and familiar with *both* the diagnosis *and* subsequent selections. With significant potential for reducing frequency, duration, and intensity of attacks, these therapies can be instrumental in the functional restoration of patients with chronic migraine (Table 6–6).

Table 6–6 Prophylactic Agents for Migraine

Agent	Route	Dosage
β-Blockers		
Propranolol	PO	80–240 mg daily in divided doses; long-acting preparation—60–160 mg in once-daily dosing
Timolol maleate	PO	5–30 mg daily
Nadolol	PO	40–80 mg daily
Atenolol	PO	50–100 mg BID
Metoprolol	PO	50–100 mg BID
Calcium channel blockers		
Verapamil	PO	240–360 mg daily in divided doses
Nimodipine	PO	30–60 mg daily
Nicardipine	PO	20–30 mg BID or TID
Neuroleptics		
Divalproex sodium	PO	250 mg BID, up to 1250 mg daily
Antidepressants		
Amitriptyline	PO	50–100 mg QHS
Protriptyline	PO	5–10 mg TID
Doxepin	PO	10–150 mg daily
Nortriptyline	PO	10–150 mg daily
Imipramine	PO	10–150 mg daily
Fluoxetine	PO	10–80 mg daily
Sertraline	PO	50–200 mg daily
Paroxetine	PO	20–60 mg daily
Trazodone	PO	15–60 mg daily
Bupropion	PO	200–300 mg daily
Venlafaxine	PO	37.5–75 mg BID
Phenelzine	PO	15–60 mg daily
NSAIDs		
Aspirin	PO	81 mg daily
Ketoprofen	PO	50–75 mg BID or TID
Naproxen	PO	250–750 mg daily
Naproxen sodium	PO	250–750 mg daily
Fenoprofen calcium	PO	600 mg TID
Flurbiprofen	PO	50–100 mg BID
Indomethacin	PO	25–50 mg TID
Piroxicam	PO	20 mg QAM
Nabumetone	PO	500–750 mg BID
Diclofenac sodium	PO	50–100 mg daily
Other agents		
Methysergide	PO	2 mg TID
Clonidine	PO	0.1 mg TID
Cyproheptadine	PO	4–16 mg daily
Ergotamine tartrate with phenobarbital and bellafoline	PO	One tablet TID

Once administration has begun, trials should be long enough (if sufficiently tolerated) to ensure the therapeutic levels have been achieved, yet short enough to avoid prolonged courses of nonproductive therapies. A time frame for trials of approximately 4 to 6 weeks is reasonable but may differ according to the medicine chosen and the individual response time of the patient. Beyond this period, if patients do not report improvement, evaluation for a different prophylactic choice may be warranted.

At this time, only a few medications have received approval from the Food and Drug Administration for migraine prophylaxis: propranolol, timolol, methysergide, and divalproex sodium.

β-Blockers

Propranolol, a nonselective β-adrenergic receptor–blocking agent, is considered to be the drug of choice in migraine prophylaxis.[74] The capacity of this drug to produce a blockade of β-adrenergic receptors that results in inhibition of arterial dilation and its ability to induce blockade of catecholamine-induced platelet aggregation are among the mechanisms of action that may account for its effectiveness.

Propranolol is especially beneficial for migraineurs with concomitant hypertension, angina pectoris, or thyrotoxicosis. The most common side effects include fatigue, gastrointestinal distrubances, insomnia, nightmares, hypotension, cold extremities, decreased resting heart rate, and sexual dysfunction. The drug is contraindicated in patients with asthma, chronic obstructive lung disease, congestive heart failure, or atrioventricular conduction distrubances and in patients receiving treatment with insulin, oral hypoglycemic drugs, or MAOIs. Abrupt withdrawal in patients with coronary heart disease may exacerbate coronary ischemia and lead to unstable angina or myocardial infarction.

If propranolol is contraindicated, treatment with another β-blocker may be considered. Both timolol and nadolol have demonstrated successful prophylaxis in many patients. For asthmatics or those with bronchial disorders, a cardioselective β-blocker, such as metoprolol or atenolol, may be substituted.

Methysergide

Closely related to the naturally occurring ergot alkaloids, methysergide is a semisynthetic lysergic acid derivative that lacks intrinsic vasocontractive properties. Its effectiveness in migraine prevention may be related to several mechanisms of action, including (1) peripheral serotonin antagonist effects on vascular receptors, (2) inhibition of serotonin release from platelets; and (3) central serotonin agonist effects.

Although methysergide is one of the most effective agents for migraine prophylaxis, it is generally reserved for use in patients with frequent, severe, disabling migraine that does not respond to less toxic agents. Adverse effects include nausea, vomiting, abdominal pain, ataxia, insomnia, drowsiness, leg cramps, paresthesias, edema, weight gain, hair loss, and hypotension. The long-term use of methysergide has been associated with retroperitoneal fibrosis, pleuropulmonary fibrosis, and fibrotic thickening of the cardiac valves. Therefore, patients on methysergide therapy should be evaluated at regular intervals to rule out pulmonary, coronary, or retroperitoneal fibrosis, as well as peripheral vascular disease. Patients should not be kept on methysergide therapy for longer than 4 to 6 months consecutively and should be given a 4- to 6-week drug hiatus. If the patient has been maintained on this agent for 6 consecutive months, an intravenous pyelogram should be performed to rule out retroperitoneal fibrosis. Methysergide is contraindicated in patients with a history of collagen diseases or fibrotic disorders, as well as peripheral vascular, coronary artery disease, severe hypertension, and thrombophlebitis.

Divalproex Sodium

Divalproex sodium is the most recent agent approved for migraine prophylaxis. It had been used since 1983 as an anticonvulsant agent, as well as for the indication of bipolar disorder. Its efficacy is linked to its capacity to increase synaptic levels of γ-aminobutyric acid (GABA). It has been helpful in some instances in which other prophylactic therapies are contraindicated. This agent may be of particular use in migraineurs with concomitant convulsive disorders.

The use of divalproex sodium has been limited by its side effect profile, which includes nausea, gastrointestinal distress, sedation, and hepatoxicity. Baseline complete blood count and liver function tests should be obtained before therapy and followed up on a timely basis. This agent should be avoided in any patient with a history of hepatitis or abnormal liver function. It has been effectively combined with tricyclic antidepressants in patients with chronic recurrent migraine.

Most investigations into the use of divalproex sodium in headache have involved migraine therapy, starting in 1988.[75] Long-term studies have examined its usefulness and safety for periods of 35 months and 5 years.[76, 77] In the latter study, 64% of the subjects with migraine experienced a favorable outcome on divalproex sodium at doses of 1000 to 1200 mg/day. The safe use of this agent was maintained for up to 63 months of therapy.

Nonsteroidal Anti-inflammatory Drugs

The NSAIDs have a unique place in the treatment of migraine in that their anti-inflammatory and analgesic properties make them appropriate choices for abortive, symptomatic, and prophylactic therapy. As platelet antagonists with the potential to affect abnormalities of platelet aggregation, and thus levels of serotonin, NSAIDs are of particular interest in the preventive treatment of those who have chronic migraine. Data collected from the U.S. Physicians' Health Study raise the possibility that the regular use of aspirin or other platelet-active drugs in this category might reduce the recurrence of migraine by approximately 20%.[78]

Gastrointestinal toxicity is the adverse side effect seen most often within this category of drugs. The risk of gastrointestinal toxicity escalates with increased dose (thus the lowest possible dose should be used), chronic use, alcohol ingestion, and smoking and in patients with a history of peptic ulcer disease. Patients should be monitored for gastrointestinal bleeding and for evidence of liver and/or kidney disease, both of which have been associated with chronic NSAID use.

Calcium Channel Blockers

The effectiveness of calcium channel blockers in migraine prophylaxis appears to be related to their ability to block the influx of calcium ions across the cell membrane of vascular smooth muscle and thereby inhibit arterial vasospasm, as well as to block platelet serotonin release and aggregation. Their effects on cerebral blood flow, neurotransmission, and neuroreceptor blockade may also enhance their efficacy. As with other agents that depend on down-regulation of serotonin receptors, their full effects may not be realized for 2 to 4 weeks after the initiation of treatment.

Verapamil is a papaverine-derived calcium-entry blocker with antiplatelet effects.[79] The drug is orally active and has long-term effects that promote its usefulness as a migraine preventive. Constipation is among the most common side effects of therapy, but as with any of the calcium blockers, flushing, lightheadedness, hypotension, rash, and nausea may also occur.

Nimodipine[80] has the highest marked selectivity for cerebral vasculature, but it has also been associated with more behavior changes, sedation, and other central nervous system effects than other calcium blockers. Muscle pains have also been reported.

In some parts of the world, flunarizine is used for migraine prevention. Nicardipine has also demonstrated some prophylactic benefits. Two other calcium channel blockers, nifedipine and diltiazem, have not been shown to be particularly useful for this purpose.

Patients using calcium channel blockers should be monitored carefully for adverse symptoms related to postural hypotension. This is especially important in patients who are concurrently taking other antihypertensive agents, including β-blockers. Due to their negative inotropic effects, calcium channel blockers should be used with caution in patients with concomitant congestive heart failure. Abrupt withdrawal of these agents should be avoided because of their potential to induce chest pain, rebound angina, or exacerbation of symptoms.

Antidepressants

The antimigraine effect of the antidepressant agents is believed to be relatively independent of their antidepressant effect, although the exact relationship remains uncertain. Tricyclic antidepressants (TCAs) are known to block the reabsorption of serotonin and, to a lesser degree, norepinephrine at nerve endings. They also exhibit anticholinergic and antihistaminic activity, which may contribute to their efficacy. With chronic TCA administration, the initial reabsorption effects are followed by slower, adaptive changes at the serotonin and norepinephrine receptor levels. The net effect is a re-regulation of abnormal receptors and consequent stabilization of the neurotransmitter relationship. Clinically, this down-regulation results in relief of symptoms and may explain the 2- to 3-week lag time that generally occurs between the initiation of treatment and the appearance of therapeutic effects.

TCAs are not considered to be a first-line migraine preventive but may be useful in some patients, particularly those with coexisting migraine and tension-type headache. Amitriptyline, one of the oldest antidepressants used in migraine therapy,[81] along with doxepin, nortriptyline, and imipramine, tends to be more sedating than protriptyline or desipramine. These agents may also cause constipation, dry mouth, weight gain, blurred vision, tachycardia, orthostatic hypotension, sexual dysfunction, and urinary retention and are not recommended in patients with narrow-angle glaucoma, prostatic hypertrophy, or cardiac conduction disturbances.

Some of the newer antidepressants, including the selective serotonin reuptake inhibitors (SSRIs) and others, appear to operate more specifically at the serotonin receptors and have a different side effect profile. As with the TCAs, however, a lag time of 2 to 3 weeks may occur before therapeutic effects are evident. Among the SSRIs, fluoxetine,[82] sertraline, and paroxetine have been beneficial, although nausea, insomnia, agitation, weight loss, and sexual dysfunction may be associated with their use. Among the other antidepressants, bupropion and trazodone have demonstrated some efficacy in migraine prophylaxis. Bupropion, however, has been known to produce agitation, anxiety, insomnia, and seizures and therefore is contraindicated for use in patients with a history of seizures or in those who are prone to electrolyte disturbances (e.g., bulimics). Trazodone has been associated with priapism and should be avoided in male migraineurs.

One of the MAOIs, phenelzine, has been found to be helpful in the preventive treatment of migraine.[83] It is not a first-line antidepressant agent, but it may be considered for use in refractory cases. MAO is the enzyme system responsible for the metabolic decomposition of biogenic amines throughout the body. Inhibition of MAO results in an increase in the concentration of endogenous epinephrine, norepinephrine, and serotonin in storage sites throughout the nervous system. Drugs that inhibit MAO activity have a wide range of clinical effects and must be monitored with extreme caution due to their potential interaction with several foods and drugs.

Adverse effects reported with MAOIs include dizziness, insomnia, hypomania, orthostatic hypotension, dry mouth, blurred vision, urinary retention, impotence, peripheral edema, and weight gain. Patients should be warned to avoid alcoholic beverages, tyramine-containing foods, and sympathomimetic drugs. When the body's MAO is inhibited, ingestion of large amounts of tryamine may result in a hypertensive crisis of sufficient severity to cause myocardial infarction or cerebrovascular accident. Due to the residual effects, a 2-week washout period is necessary before tyramine-containing foods or interactive drugs can be ingested.

Patients must be cautioned to not take any other medications without advice, including Contac, Dristan, Sinutabs, and nose drops or other drugs containing pressor agents. Tranquilizers may be used concomitantly with MAOIs. Narcotics, especially meperidine (Demerol), are known to produce hypotensive episodes when given in association with MAOIs and should be avoided.

Clonidine

Clonidine is a centrally acting α-adrenergic agonist whose efficacy in migraine prophylaxis is not comparable to that of the β-blockers. Clonidine has been found to be particularly helpful, however, in patients who experience food-related attacks.[84] Its mechanism of action may be related to its ability to block vasomotor reflexes and subsequently decrease vascular reactivity. Side effects associated with clonidine include drowsiness, dry mouth, constipation, disturbances of ejaculation, orthostatic hypotension, and depression.

Clonidine is given orally, beginning with a dosage of 0.1 mg twice a day and slowly increasing to a maximum of 2.4 mg daily. This drug should not be discontinued abruptly because of the danger of causing severe hypertensive crisis. Such hypertensive crises are due to a marked increase in the secretion of catecholamines from the adrenal medulla and may be fatal. If clonidine has to be discontinued, the dosage should be reduced gradually over 2 to 4 days.

Cyproheptadine

Cyproheptadine has been used successfully in the treatment of childhood migraine. Its antiserotonergic and antihistaminic effects have suggested its use for treatment of migraine in adults, although results in this category have been marginal. Sedation and excessive weight gain also limit its usefulness. The usual oral dosage is 4 mg four times a day, although this may be increased as required to a maximum divided daily dose of 32 mg. No fibrosis has been reported after the use of this drug, but the patient may experience dry mouth (xerostomia), drowsiness, and appetite stimulation.

Pizotifen

Although pizotifen is not available in the United States, it has been used extensively for migraine prophylaxis in other countries, demonstrating a high degree of success in reducing both the severity and frequency of attacks. It is structurally similar to cyproheptadine. Krakowski and Engisch[85] observed that pizotifen was an effective drug and compared favorably with other drugs used in the prophylaxis of migraine. Its effectiveness was enhanced by its minimal side effects and apparent antidepressant quality. These results were confirmed in another double-blind study by Lawrence and associates.[86] The side effect profile for this agent, which exhibits antiserotonergic, antihistaminic, and anticholinergic activity, includes increased appetite, weight gain, fluid retention, and muscle pain.

Status Migraine

When a migraine headache continues over 24 hours, there frequently is a sterile inflammation surrounding the enlarged vessel. The use of a corticosteroid, such as long-acting dexamethasone, 16 mg or methylprednisolone, 80 mg (intramuscular) will sometimes resolve a prolonged migraine.[87]

Raskin and Raskin[88] reported the results of a nonblind study comparing intravenous dihydroergotamine and metoclopramide administered every 8 hours for status migraine. A parallel group received intravenous diazepam with parenteral meperidine as needed. The results in the dihydroergotamine group were promising, with 49 of 55 patients becoming headache free within 48 hours.

Cyclic Migraine

Certain patients with migraine may experience a "clustering" of their attacks, followed by a relatively long remission.[89] The intermittent use of prophylactic agents, such as β-blockers, calcium channel blockers, NSAIDs, and methysergide, can be used to treat this cyclic type of migraine. Lithium carbonate has also been used successfully in patients with this migraine pattern.

References

1. Stewart WF, Liptpn RB, Celentano DD, Reed ML. Prevalence of migraine headache in the United States. JAMA 1992;267:64–69.
2. Rasmussen BK, Jensen R, Schroll M, Olesen J. Epidemiology of headache in a general population—A prevalence study. J Clin Epidemiol 1991;44:1147–1157.
3. Ad Hoc Committee on Classification of Headache. Classification of headache. JAMA 1962;179:717–718.
4. International Headache Society. Classification and diagnostic criteria of headache disorders, cranial neuralgias and facial pain. Cephalalgia 1988;8(suppl 7):4–96.
5. Harvald B, Hauge M. A catamnestic investigation of Danish twins. Dan Med Bull 1956;3:150–158.
6. Ziegler DK, Hassanein RS, Harris D. Headache in a non-clinic twin population. Headache 1975;14:213–218.
7. Lucas RN. Migraine in twins. J Psychosom Res 1977;21:147–156.
8. Joutel A, Bousser M, Biousse V, et al. A gene for familial hemiplegic migraine maps to chromosome 19. Nat Genet 1993;5:40–45.
9. Linet MS, Stewart WF, Celentano DD, Ziegler D, Sprecher M. An epidemiologic study of headache among adolescents and young adults. JAMA 1989;261:2211–2216.
10. DeBenedittis G, Lorenzetti A, Pieri A. The role of stressful life events in the onset of chronic primary headache. Pain 1990;40:65–75.
11. Köhler T, Haimerl C. Daily stress as a trigger of migraine attacks: Results of thirteen single-subject studies. J Consult Clin Psychol 1990;58:870–872.
12. Blau JN. Resolution of migraine attacks: Sleep and the recovery phase. J Neurol Neurosurg Psychiatr 1982;45:223–226.

13. Dalessio DJ, Kunzel M, Sternbach R, et al. Conditioned adaptation-relaxation reflex in migraine therapy. JAMA 1979;242:2102–2104.
14. Sorbi M, et al. Long term effects of training in relaxation and stress coping in patients with migraine: A 3-year follow up. Headache 1989;29:111–121.
15. Fromm-Reichman F. Contribution to the psychogenesis of migraine. Psychoanal Rev 1937;24:26–33.
16. Wolff HG. Personality features and reactions of subjects with migraine. Arch Neurol Psych 1937;37:895.
17. Bille B. Migraine in school children. Acta Paediatr 1964;64:499–508.
18. Jonckheere P. The chronic headache patient. Psychother Psychosom 1971;19:53–61.
19. Henryk-Gutt R, Rees WL. Psychological aspects of migraine. J Psychosom Res 1973;17:141–153.
20. Rogado AZ, Harrison RH, Graham JH. Personality profiles in cluster, migraine, and normal controls. Arch Neurol 1974;37:227–241.
21. Philips C. Headaches and personality. J Psychiatr Res 1976;20:535–542.
22. Howarth E. Headache, personality and stress. Br J Psychiatry 1965;119:1193.
23. Maxwell H. Migraine: Background and Treatment. Briston, PA: J. Wright; 1966.
24. Ross WD, McNaughton FL. Objective personality studies in migraine by means of the Rorschach method. Psychosom Med 1945;2:23.
25. Kudrow L, Sutkus BJ. MMPI pattern specificity in primary headache disorders. Headache 1979;19:18–24.
26. Sternbach R, Dalessio DJ, Kunzel M, Bowman G. MMPI patterns in common headache disorders. Headache 1980;20:311–315.
27. Cuypers J, Alternkirch H, Bunge S. Personality profiles in cluster headaches and migraine. Headache 1981;21:21.
28. Davidoff RA. Migraine: Manifestations, Pathogenesis and Management. Philadelphia: F. A. Davis; 1995;23.
29. Littlewood JT, Gibb C, Glover V, Sandler M, Davies PTG, Rose FC. Red wine as a cause of migraine. Lancet 1988;1:558–559.
30. Smith I, Kellow AH, Hanington E. A clinical and biochemical correlation between tyramine and migraine headache. Headache 1970;10:43.
31. Salfield SWA, et al. Controlled study of exclusion of dietary vasoactive amines in migraine. Arch Disease Child 1987;62:458–460.
32. Tollefson L, Barnard RJ. An analysis of FDA passive surveillance reports of seizures associated with consumption of aspartame. J Am Diet Assoc 1992;92:598–601.
33. Johns DR. Migraine provoked by aspartame. N Engl J Med 1986;315:456.
34. Van Den Eeden SK, Koepsell TD, Longstreth WT, et al. Aspartame ingestion and headaches: A randomized crossover trial. Neurology 1994;44:1787–1793.
35. Henderson WR, Raskin NH. Hot dog headache: Individual susceptibility to nitrite. Lancet 1972;2:1162.
36. Scopp AL. MSG and hydrolyzed vegetable protein induced headache: Review and case studies. Headache 1991;31:107–110.
37. Schweitzer JW, Friedhoff AJ, Schwartz R. Chocolate, β-phenylethylamine and migraine reexamined. Nature 1975;257:256.
38. Gibb CM, Davies PTG, Glover V, et al. Chocolate is a migraine-provoking agent. Cephalalgia 1991;11:93–95.
39. Diamond S, Medina JL. Double-blind study of propranolol for migraine prophylaxis. Headache 1976;16:24–27.
40. Miller D, Waters DD, Warnica W, et al. Is variant angina the coronary manifestation of a generalized vasospastic disorder? N Engl J Med 1981;304:763–766.
41. Zahavi I, Chagnac A, Hering R, et al. Prevalence of Raynaud's phenomenon in patients with migraine. Arch Int Med 1984;144:742–744.
42. Pal B, Gibson C, Passmore J, et al. A study of headaches and migraine in Sjögren's Syndrome and other rheumatic disorders. Ann Rheum Dis 1989;48:312–316.
43. Isenberg DA, Meyrick-Thomas D, Snaith ML, et al. A study of migraine in systemic lupus erythematosus. Ann Rheum Dis 1982;41:30–32.
44. Levine SR, Joseph R. Migraine and the lupus anticoagulant. Case reports and review of the literature. Cephalalgia 1987;7:93–99.
45. Hogen MJ. Lupus anticoagulant, anti-phospholipid antibodies and migraine. Can J Neurol Sci 1988;15:420–425.
46. Litman GI, Friedman HM. Migraine and the mitral valve prolapse syndrome. Am Heart J 1978;96:610–614.
47. Gamberini G. Further evidence on the association of mitral valve prolapse and migraine. Headache 1984;24:39–40.
48. Spence JD, Wong DG, Melendez LJ, et al. Increased prevalence of mitral valve prolapse in patients with migraine. Can Med Assoc J 1984;131:1457–1460.
49. Pfaffenrath V, Pöllmann W, Autenreith G, Rosmanith U. Mitral valve prolapse and platelet aggregation in patients with hemiplegic and non-hemiplegic migraine. Acta Neurol Scand 1987;75:253–257.
50. Freedman MS, Gray TA. Vascular headache: A presenting symptom of multiple sclerosis. Can J Neurol Sci 1989;16:63–66.
51. Samson JJ, Chietlin J. Pathophysiology of differential diagnosis of cardiac pain. Prog Cardiovasc Dis 1971;13:507–531.
52. Lefkowitz D, Biller J. Bregmatic headache as a manifestation of myocardial ischemia. Arch Neurol 1982;39:130.
53. Connor RCR. Complicated migraine: A study of permanent neurological and visual defects caused by migraine. Lancet 1962;2:1072.
54. Kallendovsky Z, Austin JH. Complicated mi-

graine: Its association with increased platelet aggregability and abnormal coagulation factors. Headache 1975;15:18–35.
55. Hungerford GD, du Boulay Gh, Zilkha KJ. Computerized axial tomography in patients with severe migraine: A preliminary report. J Neurol Neurosurg Psychiatry 1976;39:990–994.
56. Mathew NT, Meyer JS, Welch KMA, Neblett CR. Abnormal CT scans in migraine. Headache 1977;17:272.
57. Friedman AP, Harter J, Merritt HH. Ophthalmoplegic migraine. Trans Am Neurol Assoc 1961;86:169.
58. Bradshaw P, Parsons M. Hemiplegic migraine: A clinical study. Q J Med 1965;34:65.
59. Whitty CWM. Familial hemiplegic migraine. J Neurol Neurosurg Psychiatry 1953;16:172.
60. Fozard JR. 5-HT in migraine: Evidence from 5-HT receptor antagonists for a neuronal etiology. In: Sandler M, Collins GM (eds). Migraine: A Spectrum of Ideas. Oxford: Oxford University Press; 1990;128–141.
61. Peroutka SJ. Developments in 5-hydroxytryptamine receptor pharmacology in migraine. Neurol Clin 1990;8:829–838.
62. Plosker GL, McTavish D. Sumatriptan: A reappraisal of its pharmacology and therapeutic efficacy in the acute treatment of migraine and cluster headache. Drugs 1994;47:622–651.
63. Salonen R, Ashford E, Dahlof C, et al. Intranasal sumatriptan for the acute treatment of migraine. International Intranasal Sumatriptan Study Group. J Neurol 1994;241:463–469.
64. Freitag FG, Diamond S, Diamond ML, Urban GJ, Pepper B. Subcutaneous sumatriptan in patients treated with monoamine oxidase inhibitors and other prophylactic agents. Headache Q 1998;9:165–172.
64a. Rapoport AM, Ramadan NM, Adelman JU, et al. Optimizing the dose of zolmitriptan (Zomig,* 311C90) for the acute treatment of migraine. A multicenter, double-blind, placebo-controlled, dose range-finding study. Neurology 1997;49:1210–1218.
64b. Klassen A, Elkind A, Asgharnejad M, et al. Naratriptan is effective and well tolerated in the acute treatment of migraine. Results of a double-blind, placebo-controlled, parallel-group study. Headache 1997;37:640–645.
64c. Teall J, Tuchman M, Cutler N, et al. Rizatriptan (MAXALT) for the acute treatment of migraine and migraine recurrence. A placebo-controlled, outpatient study. Headache 1998;38:281–287.
65. Ziegler D, Ford R, Kriegler J, et al. Dihydroergotamine nasal spray for the acute treatment of migraine. Neurology 1994;44:447–453.
66. Gallagher RM. Acute treatment of migraine with dihydroergotamine nasal spray. Dihydroergotamine Working Group. Arch Neurol 1996;53:1285–1291.
67. Jones J, Pack S, Chun E. Intramuscular prochlorperazine versus metoclopramide as single-agent therapy for the treatment of acute migraine. Am J Emerg Med 1996;14:262–264.
68. Maizels M, Scott B, Cohen W, Chen W. Intranasal lidocaine for treatment of migraine: A randomized, double-blind, controlled trial. JAMA 1996;276:319–321.
69. Frederick RC. Parenteral NSAIDs in the treatment of migraine cephalalgia. Headache Q 1997;8:219–223.
70. Diamond S, Freitag FG, Diamond ML, Urban GJ. Transnasal butorphanol in the treatment of migraine headache pain. Headache Q 1992; 2:164–171.
71. Diamond S. Answering the challenge. Headache Q 1998;9:39–44.
72. Cameron JD, Lane PL, Speechley M. Intravenous chlorpromazine vs intravenous metoclopramide in acute migraine headache. Acad Emerg Med 1995;2:596–602.
73. Diamond S, Freitag FG. Cold as adjunctive therapy for headache. Postgrad Med 1986; 79:305–309.
74. Diamond S, Kudrow L, Stevens J, Shapiro DB. Long-term study of propranolol in the treatment of migraine. Headache 1982;22:268–271.
75. Sorenson KV. Valproate: A new drug in migraine prophylaxis. Acta Neurol Scand 1988; 78:345–348.
76. Thomas JR. The long term safety of divalproex sodium in the prophylactic treatment of patients with migraine. Cephalalgia 1995; 15(suppl 14):266. (Abstract)
77. Diamond S, Freitag FG, Diamond ML, Urban GJ, Pepper BJ, Bhambhavani D. Open-label long-term use of divalproex sodium in headache. Headache Q 1997;8:42–46.
78. Buring JE, Peto R, Hannekens CH. Low-dose aspirin for migraine prophylaxis. JAMA. 1990;264:1711–1713.
79. Solomon GD, Diamond S, Freitag FG. Verapamil in migraine prophylaxis: Comparison of dosages. Clin Pharmacol Ther 1987;41:202–207.
80. Formisano R, Falaschi P, Cerbo R, et al. Nimodipine in migraine: Clinical efficacy and endocrinological effects. Eur J Clin Pharmacol 1991;41:69–71.
81. Couch JR, Ziegler DK, Hassanein RS. Amitriptyline in the prophylaxis of migraine. Neurology 1976;26:121–127.
82. Bittman B, Emanuele S. Fluoxetine: Side effects and efficacy in a headache population. Headache Q 1992;3:82–85.
83. Anthony M, Lance JW. Monoamine oxidase inhibition in the treatment of migraine. Arch Neurol 1969;21:263–268.
84. Wilkinson M, et al. Clonidine in the treatment of migraine at the City Migraine Clinic in patients selected with tyramine. In: Dalessio DJ, et al (eds). Proceedings of the International Headache Symposium. Basel: Sandoz; 1971;219–221.

85. Krakowski AJ, Engisch R. A new agent for chemotherapy of migraine headaches: A controlled study. Psychosomatics 1973;14:302–308.
86. Lawrence ER, Hossain M, Littlestone W. Sanomigran for migraine prophylaxis; controlled multicenter trial in general practice. Headache 1977;17:109–112.
87. Edmeads J. Emergency management of headache. Headache 1988;28:675–679.
88. Raskin NH, Raskin KE. Repetitive intravenous dihydroergotamine for the treatment of intractable migraine. Neurology 1984;34(suppl 1):245.
89. Medina JL, Diamond S. Cyclical migraine. Arch Neurol 1981;38:343–344.

7

Cluster Headache

Todd Lewis, D.O.

Glen D. Solomon, M.D.

Introduction

The syndrome known as *cluster headache* had been considered a migraine variant.[1] The complete recognition of its periodic features led directly to the renaming of this fascinating, although punishing, condition in 1952.[2]

Cluster headache is the most uncommon of the primary headache syndromes,[3] with a prevalence of about 1:1000 persons. Some characteristics ascribed to the cluster sufferer are legendary, such as the leonine facies and hazel eye color.[4] The occurrence of the condition in men who use tobacco (and often alcohol) has been documented.[5] There is a relationship to the human biological clock that deserves further evaluation. The seasonal occurrence of cluster (i.e., spring and fall) is generally accepted, although the literature is confusing in this regard.[3] An association with arterial hypoxemia is interesting and perhaps of clinical importance.[6] The unusual nature of the symptoms and the frequent presence of certain physical findings are additional features that distinguish cluster headache from the more common primary headache syndromes.[7]

There is a general agreement among those who care for patients with headache that cluster headache is an "easy" diagnosis. Although its distinct features support this contention, the typical patient with cluster headache has spent many years with numerous consultations before an appropriate diagnosis has been made.[8] Sjaastad has summarized the clinical presentation of cluster headache by referring to five "pillars" upon which the diagnosis is based.[9, 9a]

- The headache is always unilateral. Except for rare exceptions, the most severe pain occurs within the distribution of the first and second divisions of the trigeminal nerve on either the left or right side. Other areas in which pain may be experienced include the occiput, neck, back, chest, and shoulder.[10]
- The headache is of excruciating severity. The duration of such pain is generally brief by comparison with the other primary headache disorders, lasting from 15 minutes to 2 hours.
- The headache is accompanied by certain autonomic phenomena, such as conjunctival injection, lacrimation, rhinorrhea, miosis, ptosis, and nasal congestion.
- Cluster headache is much more common in men. The accepted male-to-female ratio is estimated at 5:1.[11]
- The headache occurs with a striking periodicity. The term "cluster," coined by Kunkle et al,[2] refers to the rhythm that is characteristic of episodic cluster. The designation "chronic cluster" is an oxymoron because it refers to the absence of remissions and therefore to the absence of "clusters."[7] Although the nature of the attacks is not different between episodic and chronic cluster headaches, the patient with chronic cluster tends to respond less well to medical therapy.[3, 5, 12] Fortunately, only about 10% to 20% of patients meeting the criteria for cluster headache have chronic cluster headache.[3]

Etiology and Pathogenesis

The interaction of cerebral vascular elements and the trigeminal nerve has been implicated in the pathogenesis of both migraine and cluster headache.[13] Moskowitz[14] described an attractive model for cluster in the "pathophysiologic focus in the superior pericarotid cavernous sinus plexus." The neurochemical mediators and phenomena potentially involved include disordered vasomotor adrenoceptors,[15] oxygen desaturation,[6] erythrocyte choline concentrations,[16] central opiate activity,[17] substance P,[4, 17a] circadian rhythms,[7] and male hormones.[18]

Epidemiology

The prevalence of cluster headache has been estimated at 1:1000 adults[13] to 900:100,000 adults.[9] Approximately 85% of cluster sufferers are men.[9–11] Cluster headache usually occurs for the first time between the second and fourth decades, although it can begin at any age.[8, 9]

Clinical Features

"The syndrome is a very distinctive one, and its affinities to other forms of migraine have appeared questionable to some observers. There is usually an extremely acute onset of pain referred to the temple and the eye on one side; less frequently, pain may be felt in or behind the ear, or in the cheek and nose. The intensity of the pain may be overwhelming (one patient described it to me as an 'orgasm of pain'), and may drive patients into a frenzy. Whereas the majority of migraine patients sit or lie down, or wish to do so, the sufferer from migrainous neuralgia tends to pace up and down in a fury, clutching the affected eye and groaning. I have even seen patients beat their heads against the wall during the attack. The pain tends to be accompanied (and, on occasion, preceded) by a number of striking local symptoms and signs. The affected eye becomes bloodshot and waters, and there is a blockage or catarrh of the nostril on the same side. Sometimes the attack is accompanied or heralded by a flow of thick saliva, rarely by recurrent coughing. There may be a partial or complete Horner's syndrome on the affected side, and this may occasionally persist as a permanent neurological residue. The duration of the attacks may be as little as two minutes, and is rarely more than two hours. A majority of the attacks are nocturnal and wake the patient from deep sleep; some come on within a few minutes of waking in the morning, before the fogs of sleep have lifted. . . ."[1]

The International Headache Society (IHS) has formulated fairly strict criteria for the diagnosis of the primary headache disorders.[12] Although the list of features for cluster headache are much less poetic than the elegant description of Dr. Sacks, the IHS criteria (summarized in Table 7–1) is a valuable tool for dealing with the content of the headache history. Although the limited headache history can describe the essential requirements for an accurate diagnosis, a complete clinical evaluation is crucial to the optimal care of the patient.

A variety of diseases have been reported that present with cluster headache–like features (Table 7–2); neuroimaging, other special testing, or both therefore may be appropriate in the initial evaluation of such a patient. It should be recognized, however, that such cases of "symptomatic" cluster typically fail to fulfill IHS criteria or present unusual features that suggest their organicity.[19–26]

A thorough evaluation of the headache sufferer also serves to elucidate comorbidities, drug sensitivities, or other issues that may complicate or contraindicate certain otherwise appropriate therapies. Such an appraisal is particularly pertinent to the care of the cluster patient. This individual is more apt to have coronary artery disease or its

Table 7–1 Diagnostic Criteria

Cluster Headache (all of the following must be present)
At least 10 attacks of unilateral orbital or supraorbital pain or both
Severe or very severe pain
Untreated attacks lasting from 15 to 180 minutes
At least one of the following signs, on the same side as the headache
Conjunctival injection
Lacrimation
Nasal congestion
Rhinorrhea
Forehead and facial sweating
Miosis
Ptosis
Frequency of attacks from one every other day to eight per day
Attacks recurring on same side of head during an individual cluster period
One of the following
Typical history and normal examination
Suspected organic lesions on examination but normal neuroimaging results
Chronic Cluster Headache
Criteria for cluster headache (above)
Absence of remission for 1 year or longer, or remissions lasting less than 14 days

From the Headache Classification Committee of the International Headache Society. Classification and diagnostic criteria for headache disorders, cranial neuralgias, and facial pain. Cephalalgia 1988;8(Suppl 7):1–96.

Table 7–2 Structural Lesions That Can Cause "Cluster-like" Syndromes and Clues to Their Presence

Lesion	Warning Sign or Symptom
Sinusitis	Fever Prolonged symptoms
Arteriovenous malformations	Decreased vision Prolonged symptoms Papilledema More frequently seen in female patients Lack of full spectrum of autonomic dysfunction
Mycotic aneurysm of intracavemous carotid artery	Continuous headache
Vertebral artery aneurysm	Constant background headache
Nasopharyngeal cancer	Nausea and vomiting Previous treatment for nasopharyngeal carcinoma
Pituitary adenoma	Seizure Progression in frequency Impotence Testicular atrophy Optic atrophy
Chronic subdural hematoma	Progressive frequency History of trauma
Trigeminal neurinoma	Continuous headache
Sphenoidal aspergilloma	Prolonged headache More frequently seen in female patients

various risk factors (hypertension, hyperlipidemia, nicotine addiction),[3, 9, 27, 28] or both. There may also be a higher-than-expected incidence of peptic ulcer disease and alcoholism in the population with cluster headache.[9, 28] These are just a few of the conditions that may complicate, if not contraindicate, certain valuable preparations, which will be described.

Therapy

Although cluster headache is no longer considered a migraine variant, the approach to treatment catalogued in any treatise on the subject displays the vestiges of the former classification. Prophylactic and abortive considerations have clear implications when applied to the migraine sufferer. These terms have little meaning in the context of the modern treatment of cluster headache.

A better characterization of the current approach to cluster headache describes agents used for the ability to either *induce* a remission from the repetitive, short-lived but recurrent attacks of pain or to *maintain* such a remission. Agents in the latter classification, what we label *maintenance therapies,* form the foundation of the rational approach to cluster headache therapy. Agents described in the former category, what we label *induction therapy,* are generally effective in rapidly relieving the suffering of the patient with cluster headache but are not suitable for long-term use. We then describe *palliative* therapies, which are agents that serve to relieve the discomfort associated with an individual attack that has proved to be refractory to the former two approaches.

Maintenance Therapy

The therapy of cluster headache requires an agent that is effective in preventing the volley of attacks that characterize cluster headache and that can be tolerated during the weeks or months occupied by the period of cluster headache. The tolerability of such an agent often is tested indefinitely during the treatment of chronic cluster headache. In 1983, the efficacy of verapamil in cluster headache treatment was reported;[29] based on its usefulness and safety, verapamil has revolutionized the treatment of cluster.

The calcium channel blockers are a heterogeneous group of agents that have been studied and used extensively in the management of cardiovascular disorders.[30] The various agents in this class share the ability to inhibit the movement of calcium ions across the cell membranes of several cell types. Verapamil has well-documented effects on cardiac contractility, as well as vascular reactivity based on this mechanism.[30] The beneficial effects of verapamil in the treatment of cluster (and migraine) headache probably do not result from the rather rapid effects on calcium channels, given the delay in onset of headache relief.[31] It has been suggested that the varying affinity for serotonin receptors explains the differences in activity of the various calcium channel blockers in cluster and migraine headache.[30] Although other calcium channel blockers have been shown to have beneficial effects in the management of cluster headache, efficacy, clinical experience, and cost strongly favor the use of verapamil in this application.[3, 5, 32, 33]

The earliest published report detailing the

efficacy of verapamil in a small number of patients with cluster headache by Meyer and Hardenberg[29] was later confirmed by Gabai and Spierings[34] and others.[35] These studies seem to support the anecdotal experiences of Kudrow and others that verapamil is effective in approximately 70% of cluster headache sufferers.[3, 5, 32, 33]

Bussone and colleagues[35] compared the use of verapamil with the use of lithium carbonate in a double-blind, crossover study in patients with chronic cluster headache. Verapamil not only was better tolerated but had a shorter latency period, with the onset of beneficial effects occurring in more than half the patients at 1 week.[4]

Verapamil is generally well tolerated, with few serious adverse reactions.[3, 5, 30, 33, 36] This is particularly true compared with the alternative agents for the treatment of cluster headache. The most common and troubling side effect noted clinically is constipation. Fiber supplementation and the judicious use of cathartics are warranted in this circumstance.

The more serious of untoward reactions are a direct extension of calcium channel blockade in the heart and peripheral vasculature, leading to cardiac conduction abnormalities, myocardial depression, and hypotension.[30] These effects are unlikely in patients not predisposed by either preexisting illness or drug interaction. Note should be made of a rather complex interaction of verapamil with lithium carbonate, a combination often used in refractory cluster headache.[29] Verapamil may lower lithium serum levels and simultaneously may augment a variety of lithium effects.[31] Lithium may also have calcium channel–blocking properties and therefore enhance the effects of verapamil.[37] Close monitoring of the clinical status of the patient takes priority over serial serum lithium determinations when this combination is used.

Verapamil has been demonstrated to be effective in treating both episodic and chronic cluster. Studies suggest that dosages of verapamil required to control chronic cluster often approach 600 mg/day, as opposed to an average dosage of 360 mg/day to control episodic cluster.[31] A variety of dosage schedules has been proposed. With the advent of several long-acting formulations, compliance may be improved; therefore, a reasonable starting dosage in cluster might be 240 to 360 mg/day in the form of a long-acting preparation given once or twice daily. Although the same dose may be adequate for chronic cluster headache, a dosage of 480 mg/day in divided doses often is necessary.[31] Careful monitoring of blood pressure and heart rate, particularly with the higher doses, is paramount. An indication of maximal dose attainment may be a systolic blood pressure of less than 100 mm Hg, a heart rate of less than 50 beats/min, or both.

In episodic cluster headache, it often is possible to identify cluster periods that designate months during the year that demand treatment. Mathew[3] suggested starting medication early in the cluster period and tapering slowly once the patient is free of headache for a least 2 weeks.

Standard recommendations for the management of chronic cluster are more difficult to support by either controlled study or anecdote. An individualized approach is used, with an attempt to slowly taper off verapamil after the patient has been cluster free for several months. The safety of verapamil, as demonstrated by indefinite use for hypertension and other conditions, permits indefinite use in the chronic cluster headache sufferer who does not tolerate the discontinuation of verapamil.

Lithium Carbonate

Lithium is an alkali metal used primarily in mood disorders.[38] Its mechanism of action in this application, as in cluster headache, is unknown.[31, 38] Proposed beneficial effects in cluster include increased norepinephrine reuptake and increased serotonin receptor sensitivity. The restoration of serotonergic tone is an attractive explanation for lithium effects in cluster headache indirectly supported by effects demonstrated in animal brain.[39, 40]

Ekbom is credited with the earliest report of lithium efficacy in cluster headache management.[41] Larger studies published since the original report in 1978 seem to support the same conclusions: 70% of patients with cluster headache demonstrate a favorable response to lithium, with a greater success generally enjoyed by chronic cluster headache sufferers.[3, 5, 31, 33, 36] The direct comparison of verapamil with lithium by Bussone et al.[35] helps to explain why lithium should be considered an alternative to verapamil in monotherapy for cluster headache; the effects of lithium were realized much later than those of verapamil, with the addition of greater toxicity. A potential benefit of lithium is suggested by anecdotal reports of therapeutic successes manifested by long-term remissions maintained despite the discontinuation of this agent.[41a] This concept probably has a greater impact on an understanding of cluster pathogenesis than on clinical management. Tolerance (tachyphylaxis) to continued therapy with lithium has also been reported, although its frequency is not clear.[5]

The usual dose of lithium carbonate for the treatment of cluster is 600 to 900 mg/day in divided doses.[3, 5, 33] Guidelines for the monitoring of lithium levels, as well as surveillance for potential adverse reactions, have been published by Price and Heninger[38] and are summarized in Table 7–3. Serum lithium levels average 0.5 to 1.0 mEq/L in cluster therapy, somewhat lower than the range encountered in the treatment of mood disorders.[5] Adverse reactions to lithium generally occur with levels of more than 1.5 mEq/L. Some reactions, however, including nausea, fatigue, thirst, edema, weight gain, and polyuria, may occur even with "nontoxic" levels. Tremor is quite common, although it tends to respond to either lowering the dose or adding β-blockers.[31, 38, 41a]

A list of the toxic effects of lithium appears in Table 7–4.[42] A summary of medications and conditions that may complicate lithium therapy appears in Table 7–5.[42]

Table 7–3 Laboratory Evaluation for Patients Receiving Lithium

Before Treatment	During Treatment
Complete blood count	Plasma lithium levels every 5–7 days after initiation of treatment and after any change in the dose; every 1–2 months during maintenance treatment
Serum creatinine and electrolytes	Serum creatinine every 6–12 months
Serum thyroxine, free thyroxine, and thyrotropin	Serum thyroxine, free thyroxine, and thyrotropin every 6–12 months
Urinalysis	Urinalysis every 12 months
Electrocardiogram*	Electrocardiogram
Optional: 24-hour urine volume, creatinine clearance, urine osmolality†	Optional: serum electrolytes, complete blood count, 24-hour urine volume creatinine clearance, urine osmolality‡

*Indicated in patients older than 50 years.

†If clinically indicated.

‡Should be measured more frequently during periods when other factors may alter plasma concentrations; may be measured less frequently (every 6–12 months) in stable patients receiving maintenance treatment.

From Price LH, Heninger GR. Lithium in the treatment of mood disorders. N Engl J Med 1994;331:591–598.

Table 7–4 Clinical Manifestations of Lithium Intoxication

Central Nervous System	*Neuromuscular*
Altered state of consciousness (confusion to coma)	Peripheral neuropathy
Cerebellar symptoms	Myopathy
Dysarthria	***Gastrointestinal***
Ataxia	Nausea, vomiting
Nystagmus	Bloating
Tremors	***Renal***
Basal ganglia symptoms	Polyuria
Choreiform movements	Polydipsia
Parkinsonian movements	Renal insufficiency
Seizures	***Endocrine***
Death	Hypothermia
Cardiac	Hyperthermia
Syncope	

Ergotamine

Ergotamine is a derivative of the rye fungus ergot (*Claviceps purpura*).[46] Its effects on vascular reactivity have received much attention since its application in migraine therapy in 1926.[43] Recently, however, attention has been drawn to its interaction with serotonin receptors.[44] Although the neurochemical model of ergotamine may be the preferred explanation for its beneficial effects, the vascular model

Table 7–5 Factors Predisposing to Lithium Intoxication

- Infection
- Volume depletion
- Gastroenteritis
- Overdose
- Renal insufficiency
- Surgery
- Decreased effective arterial volume
- Congestive heart failure
- Cirrhosis
- Nephrosis
- Drugs
  - Nonsteroidal anti-inflammatory drugs
  - Diuretics
  - Tetracycline
  - Cyclosporine
- Decreased dietary sodium
- Anorexia

continues to explain much of the toxicity of ergotamine.[45] It is this toxicity that tends to limit the use of ergotamine to rather specific circumstances in cluster therapy. Although controlled trials of ergotamine in cluster headache are lacking, the clinical experiences of experts in this field suggest a role in two specific circumstances.

Ergotamine may be useful in the management of the cluster patient who has solely nocturnal attacks. In this situation, a bedtime dose of 2 mg PO may be quite effective. The other accepted indication for ergotamine in cluster treatment is for use in the patient refractory to the therapies mentioned thus far.[3, 36, 38] Kudrow found that the addition of nighttime ergotamine to daily verapamil may increase efficacy by 15%; he also has suggested that the addition of lithium to this combination may boost efficacy by an additional 5% to 10%.[33] Other authors have suggested that any therapy found to be beneficial in migraine (including ergotamine tartrate) may be attempted in the patient resistant to "standard" cluster therapy.[31]

Adverse reactions are fairly common and may not mandate cessation of therapy in an otherwise desirable clinical situation. Nausea and vomiting may occur in up to 10% of patients. Other common side effects include itching, local edema, changes in heart rate, weakness, numbness, paresthesia, or pain in the extremities. Overdosage is generally seen with doses of more than 15 mg/day, although it has been reported with doses of less than 5 mg. In toxic ingestion, central nervous system disturbances such as depression, confusion, and seizures often coexist with vasoconstriction and ischemia in a variety of locations. Drug interaction with β-blockers or macrolide antibiotics may precipitate such a toxic syndrome even in therapeutic doses.[30]

Contraindications to ergotamine include peripheral vascular disease, coronary artery disease, hypertension, hepatic or renal impairment, pregnancy, and sepsis.[30]

Methysergide

Methysergide is a semisynthetic ergot derivative.[30] Like ergotamine, vasoconstrictive properties have been used to explain its therapeutic effects.[45] Methysergide has also been shown to antagonize certain serotonin receptors, perhaps explaining their value in migraine and cluster prophylaxis.[43, 44]

The efficacy of methysergide in cluster management was initially reported by Friedman and Elkind in 1960.[46] Since that time, additional reports, as well as clinical experience, are in agreement that methysergide has efficacy in cluster treatment comparable to that of verapamil[5, 33] or lithium.[47, 48] However, the development of tachyphylaxis to its beneficial effects,[3] in addition to the risk of serious toxicity,[30] precludes the use of methysergide except in the most difficult of clinical circumstances.

The recommended dosage of methysergide is 8 mg/day. Typical adverse reactions occurring early in therapy include leg pain, edema, paresthesia, nausea, and chest pain. The introduction of methysergide at a lower dosage, with a gradual escalation of the dose to 8 mg/day, may limit the severity of the early reactions.[3, 30]

The unusual, often discussed, and controversial question of the toxicity of methysergide is characterized by discussions of the fibrotic reactions about the viscera.[30] It has been debated whether this toxicity, which includes retroperitoneal fibrosis, pulmonary fibrosis, or endomyocardial fibroelastosis, is dose related or idiosyncratic. It is recommended that one or more drug holidays of 2 or more months be taken each year of therapy.[3, 5, 33] Periodic imaging of the chest and abdomen, in addition to the monitoring of renal function, also is recommended for surveillance purposes.[30] Patients with lung disease, as well as connective tissue diseases, are thought to be more susceptible to the fibrotic complications of this agent.[31]

Methysergide may increase gastric acid secretion; therefore, peptic ulcer disease should be considered a relative contraindication to its use. A complete list of contraindications would also include those listed for ergotamine.[30]

Induction Therapy

Although the use of verapamil and lithium has revolutionized the treatment of cluster headache, therapeutic benefits may not be realized for 1 or more weeks. For the patient who is burdened by either an active cluster period or chronic cluster headache, a second agent often is required during this time. As the maintenance drug begins to control the cluster headache, the induction therapy can be discontinued.

Glucocorticoids

The adrenal corticosteroids and their synthetic counterparts have a variety of uses in clinical medicine. Perhaps the most common application of these agents exploits their salutary effects on inflammatory processes. Whether their anti-inflammatory effect is the crucial activity in cluster therapy is not known. The evidence from studies in animals suggesting effects on serotonergic pathways is an attractive explanation that may also apply to the other headache types.[49] The diurnal variation that characterizes physiological steroid production suggests that steroids may be involved in some way with the human biological clock.[31]

In 1952, Horton[50] published a report suggesting the usefulness of steroids in cluster. Since that time, they have had a prominent role in the "prophylactic" treatment of cluster. The rapid relief of symptoms obtained by their administration, their short-term safety, and, alternatively, their toxicities in long-term use all define their role in induction therapy for cluster headache.[3, 5, 31, 33] The ease of outpatient administration and low cost make them the preferred agent in this category.

Kudrow[51] used 40 mg/day of prednisone in 92 patients suffering from cluster headache and obtained meaningful responses in more than 80% of patients. Couch and Ziegler[52] used variable doses of prednisone and found similar efficacy in episodic cluster headache, although only about one half as many patients with chronic cluster headache responded in a similar fashion. As many as 80% of patients in this study suffered relapses of their symptoms as dosages were tapered below 20 mg/day. These studies demonstrate what is known of these agents from clinical experience:

- Steroids are rapidly effective, with effects often within 1 to 2 days.
- Steroids are less effective in chronic cluster headache.
- Attacks of cluster headache tend to resume as the dose of steroids is tapered.

Prednisone may be the preferred agent for cluster headache treatment given the low cost and clinical experience with its use. Some authors report responses with triamcinolone when prednisone was ineffective.[53] The usual dosage of prednisone is 40 or 60 mg/day in either a single or divided dose. Slow reduction in the dose over approximately 3 weeks is generally recommended to allow the selected maintenance regimen time to elicit its effects. There is some evidence that tapering of prednisone to less than 10 mg/day may be less disruptive to the pituitary-adrenal axis.[54]

Contraindications other than serious infections (particularly systemic fungal infections) are relative and are related to the anticipated tolerability of the adverse reactions.[30]

Dihydroergotamine

Dihydroergotamine (DHE) is a synthetic derivative of ergotamine. The subtle structural change provided by hydrogenation makes the substance less vasoconstrictive and less emetogenic.[47] In 1945, Horton et al.[55] demonstrated that DHE was as effective as ergotamine in migraine therapy and had fewer side effects. Raskin[56] introduced the concept of repetitive intravenous dosing of DHE and reported success with the approach in migraine therapy in 1986. Silberstein et al.[57] applied the concept to patients with chronic daily headache. Although the response was impressive in the majority of patients, all 24 patients with cluster headache obtained relief with many fewer side effects than the patients who did not have cluster headache. This success prompted a review of the experiences of 54 patients with cluster headache with repeated intravenous doses of DHE.[58]

All 54 patients with cluster headache, 23 episodic cluster headache patients and 31 chronic cluster headache patients, became headache free during the intravenous DHE therapy. The response rate averaged approximately 30% per day of treatment. Fewer than 20% of patients experienced side effects: eight patients reported nausea without emesis, two patients noted chest tightness without evidence of coronary ischemia, and one patient reported a metallic taste in his mouth. Follow-up was provided at 3, 6, and 12 months because the patients were placed on "prophylactic" (maintenance) therapy with a variety of therapies that have been previously discussed. The long-term response rates do not differ significantly from those reported for the various agents already mentioned.

This study is a useful analysis of repetitive intravenous DHE. Although not a controlled study but a retrospective analysis, it provides documentation for both the short-term efficacy and tolerability of the therapy in a fairly significant number of cluster headache sufferers. The study failed to provide short-term follow-up of the patients soon after discharge. This is of particular interest because we noted frequent relapse of symptoms within a few days of discharge after repeated intravenous DHE. The follow-up provided in this study merely attests to the efficacy of the various maintenance therapies. The low incidence of side effects in cluster patients is intriguing. The authors suggest the higher incidence of side effects in non–cluster headache patients may have been the result of drug withdrawal either alone or in combination with DHE.[57] Perhaps the cluster sufferers themselves are merely more tolerant of adverse reactions.

The role of repetitive intravenous DHE in the induction therapy of cluster headache is not yet well defined. The cost associated with inpatient administration (at least $3000 at our institution) makes it a more expensive alternative to the use of corticosteroids. A potential role might be in the context of patients intolerant of steroids. Patients who have failed to respond to steroid induction may be candidates for admission for intravenous DHE, given the degree of suffering involved in an active cluster headache period. The rapid return of cluster headache soon after discharge that we have noted is a problem that must be dealt with on an individual basis. Early institution of maintenance therapy is paramount. Whether intravenous DHE in some way restores susceptibility to corticosteroids is a subject of further study.

The administration of intravenous DHE with an antiemetic is thought to be crucial. The side effects associated with these agents include consequences of dopamine blockade; intravenous diphenhydramine or benztropine generally provides relief of these extrapyramidal reactions.[58] Contraindications to DHE are those shared with ergotamine and have been listed previously.[30]

Palliative Therapy of Cluster

Attacks of cluster headache tend to occur despite the application of appropriate therapy. As noted, there often is a lag in the onset of efficacy of maintenance therapy. Either induction or maintenance therapy may permit breakthrough attacks of cluster headache. Palliative therapies, also referred to as *symptomatic therapies,* serve to shorten or abort the active cluster headache. Although in general these are the safest of the cluster headache therapies, they are less than ideal. As they are administered on notice of symptoms, several minutes are required for the onset of relief. Although this may shorten an individual cluster headache attack from hours to minutes, these agents generally have no effect on future attacks. Nevertheless, these agents are important tools in allowing the cluster sufferer to cope with a less-than-optimal therapeutic regimen.

Oxygen Inhalation

An association between oxygen desaturation and cluster headache has been described, although the implications of such a finding are unclear.[17] Intracranial and extracranial arterial dilation has been demonstrated during cluster headache attacks.[59] Although oxygen is known to cause cerebral vasoconstriction in normal subjects,[60] Sakai and Meyer[61] demonstrated an exaggerated response to oxygen inhalation in cluster headache patients. A role for serotonin is at least suggested, however, by the finding that its synthesis is stimulated by oxygen.[62, 67] Despite the uncertainties surrounding its behavior in pathogenesis as well as treatment, the value of oxygen in aborting attacks of cluster is well established.[3, 5, 34]

Oxygen inhalation was proposed as a useful treatment for cluster headache by Friedman and Mikropoulos in 1958.[63] In 1981, Kudrow[64] demonstrated the efficacy of oxygen inhalation in treating 51 patients with cluster headache: 75% of patients were successful in relieving at least 7 of 10 attacks within 15 minutes of initiating therapy. In 1985, Fogan[65] studied oxygen in a small number of cluster headache sufferers in a crossover, double-blind fashion using compressed air as placebo: more than half of those using oxygen were successful in relieving their symptoms in at least four of five attacks; only 7% of patients in the control group enjoyed similar success.

The inhalation of oxygen is accepted as the safest and most effective method of aborting attacks of cluster headache. Tolerance to the effects of oxygen does not appear to be a common problem; individual attacks do tend to recur shortly after "successful" treatment, and in many cases the use of oxygen merely postpones the attack.[3, 27]

Guidelines for the use of oxygen therapy in cluster have been proposed by Kudrow[33] and are summarized in Table 7–6. Caution should be used in treating patients with

Table 7–6 Guidelines for Oxygen Use in Cluster Headache

Start oxygen inhalation at the very onset of the attack.
Have the patient assume a sitting position, upright or leaning forward (supine or nearly supine positions may increase cavernous sinus congestion, which may aggravate rather than abate the attack).
Use a facial mask rather than a nasal cannula because associated nasal stuffiness may impede airway flow.
Set the oxygen flow at 7 L/min.
Warn the patient against hyperventilating, which may limit oxyhemoglobin saturation—a high level of oxygen saturation (98–99%) must be sustained for several minutes to achieve relief of the attack.

chronic obstructive pulmonary disease, especially in the context of known carbon dioxide retention. The toxicities of prolonged oxygen administration have been reviewed elsewhere,[66, 71] but these effects are extremely unlikely given the brief periods of administration used in cluster treatment.

Sumatriptan

The development of sumatriptan has revolutionized the treatment of migraine.[67, 72] Its activity at and relative specificity for serotonin receptors often provides the migraineur with rapid relief and few side effects. The same activity and specificity have done much to support the role for serotonin in the modern pathogenetic model of migraine.[68, 73] The application of sumatriptan to cluster headache has met with some success; it seems logical to assume a role for serotonin in the cluster headache process as well.

Since Krabbe published his experience with subcutaneous sumatriptan in a small number of cluster headache patients, two large trials have compared the efficacy of sumatriptan with that of placebo in the symptomatic (palliative) treatment of cluster headache. The Sumatriptan Cluster Headache Study Group published a double-blind, placebo-controlled, crossover trial using the subcutaneous injection of sumatriptan in 39 cluster headache patients.[70, 74] The results did not differ markedly from those published by Ekbom in 1993.[74] Complete relief from cluster headache occurred within 15 minutes of injection in approximately one half of patients in the former study[70, 74] and in approximately three fourths of patients in the latter. The response to placebo was also somewhat higher in the study by Ekbom—35% versus 10%. This study also was able to demonstrate the comparable efficacy of the 6-mg and the 12-mg dose.[74]

The tolerability of sumatriptan has been well established in almost 2000 migraineurs treated with sumatriptan in controlled clinical trials. The most frequently reported adverse reaction in studies with subcutaneous sumatriptan was local discomfort at the injection site. Interestingly, use of the autoinjector device was associated with a much lower incidence of local reactions.[69] The incidence of adverse reactions to subcutaneous sumatriptan appears to be less in patients with cluster headache than in migraineurs.[70] It has been suggested that many of the adverse reactions reported in the migraine population, such as nausea and vomiting, may be related to the underlying condition itself rather than to the treatment. Comparable incidence in placebo and treatment arms offers some support of this concept.[74] Again, the tolerance of the patient with cluster headache to adverse events may be surmised.

In the series by Ekbom,[74] the common adverse reactions reported by patients administered subcutaneous sumatriptan were local injection site reactions (7%), nausea and vomiting (5%), pressure sensation (5%), and a feeling of heaviness (5%). A variety of neurological symptoms such as transient dizziness, tiredness, and paresthesia may occur.[74] In the Sumatriptan Study Group evaluation, there were no changes in either heart rate or blood pressure; there were no electrocardiographic, biochemical, or hematological anomalies identified.

The recommended dose of subcutaneous sumatriptan in the acute treatment of cluster is 6 mg. This dose may be repeated once during a given 24-hour period.[69, 74] It is recommended that the first dose of sumatriptan be administered in a supervised setting so reassurance may follow any transient sensations, such as chest pain, that may develop.

Contraindications to sumatriptan include ischemic heart disease and uncontrolled hypertension. A great deal of caution must be exercised in treating the patient with peripheral vascular disease or known cerebrovascular disease.[69]

The apparent advantages of sumatriptan in the palliative treatment of cluster headache include a high efficacy rate, speed of onset of action, and, compared with oxygen, the relatively small size of the apparatus necessary for its administration. It therefore is useful for the patient who has frequent attacks outside of the home. Cost is considered the major disadvantage of this product. Although tachyphylaxis has not been reported, the use of sumatriptan should be limited to patients who have cluster headache once per day or less often, to avoid exceeding the dosing guidelines.

Local Anesthetics

Reports have been published since 1913 regarding the use of intranasal cocaine in acute pain syndromes thought to be cluster headache. Kittrelle and colleagues[71] suggested the impracticality of using this substance in this way by estimating the requirements of a typical cluster sufferer to be in excess of 3 g of pure cocaine per cluster period. The same authors report on the efficacy of intranasal lidocaine in a small number of cluster patients. Postulating a local anesthetic action on the sphenopalatine ganglion, careful positioning of the patient was undertaken to permit access of the agent to this structure.[71] Further study is warranted based on the favorable response obtained in this study. Although this therapy is uncommonly used, it offers the benefit of a local treatment with little noxious potential.

Alternative Therapy for Refractory Cluster

The patient who continues to have cluster headache despite the approaches and measures recommended merits a trial with any appropriate agent known to have value in treating migraine. Two particular alternative therapies merit consideration before surgical intervention.

Kuritzky and Hering[72] reported encouraging results of an open trial of sodium valproate in 15 patients with cluster headache. Side effects of this agent include drowsiness, tremor, nausea, vomiting, loss of hair, and weight gain. The dosage of sodium valproate generally lies between 600 and 2000 mg/day in divided doses. A periodic assessment of serum levels is necessary to maintain levels in the target range of 50 to 100 μg/ml. Monitoring of liver function and a complete blood count are recommended at periodic intervals; sodium valproate is contraindicated in patients with liver disease.[30]

The application of hot pepper extract to the nasal passages attests to the constitution of the cluster headache patient if not the measures he or she (and the physician) will take in an attempt to lessen his or her suffering. Preliminary reports of the efficacy of intranasal capsaicin are encouraging. Because the application to the naris contralateral to that of symptoms is ineffective in cluster headache, the mechanism of action is presumed to be the depletion of pain-producing polypeptides (substance P) in the peripheral nerves.[75] The optimal dosage schedule has not been elaborated.

Cluster headache remains a medical disorder unless it is chronic, unilateral, and resistant to the therapies discussed in this treatise. In this desperate circumstance, neurosurgical intervention may be successful in providing some relief and improving quality of life. Radiofrequency trigeminal gangliorhizolysis, resulting in the loss of corneal reflexes, is considered the procedure of choice by several authors.[3, 33, 73] Recently, the percutaneous injection of glycerol into the trigeminal cistern was evaluated in a small number of patients at The Cleveland Clinic Foundation. Although the efficacy was respectable (three of eight headache free; five of eight not requiring medication), the safety was notable: none of the patients experienced facial or corneal anesthesia.[76] This procedure may deserve consideration before the institution of the more destructive procedure in the patient desperate for relief.

Intravenous histamine desensitization, which has been used for many years in the treatment of chronic cluster headaches, is discussed in Chapter 23.

References

1. Sacks O. Migrainous neuralgia. *In* Sacks O, ed. Migraine. Berkeley: University of California Press; 1992:99–102.
2. Kunkle EC, Pfeiffer JB, Wilhoit WM, Hamrick LW Jr. Recurrent brief headaches in 'cluster' pattern. Trans Am Neurol Assoc 1952;77:240–243.
3. Mathew NT. Advances in cluster headache. Neurol Clin 1990;8:867–889.
4. Hardebo J. The involvement of trigeminal substance P neurons in cluster headache: An hypothesis. Headache 1984;24:294–304.
5. Mathew NT. Cluster headache. Neurology 1992;42(suppl 2):22–31.
6. Kudrow L, Kudrow DB: The role of chemoreceptor activity and oxyhemoglobin desatu-

ration in cluster headache. Headache 1993;33:484–488.
7. Graham J. Cluster headache: The relation to arousal, relaxation and autonomic tone. Headache 1990;30:145–151.
8. Sutherland JM, Eadie MJ. Cluster headache. Res Clin Studies Headache 1972;3:92–125.
9. Kudrow L. Cluster Headache: Mechanisms and Management. New York: Oxford University Press; 1980.
9a. Sjaastad O, Shen JM, Stovner LT, et al. Cluster headache in identical twins. Headache 1993;33:214–217.
10. Lovshin LL. Clinical caprices of histaminic cephalalgia. Headache 1961;1:3–6.
11. Horton BT. Histamine cephalgia. Md State Med J 1961;10:178–203.
12. Headache Classification Committee of the International Headache Society. Classification and diagnostic criteria for headache disorders, cranial neuralgias, and facial pain. Cephalalgia 1988;8(suppl 7):1–96.
13. Moskowitz MA. Basic mechanisms in vascular headache. Neurol Clin 1990;8:802–816.
14. Moskowitz MA. Cluster headache: Evidence for a pathophysiologic focus in the superior pericarotid cavernous sinus plexus. Headache 1988;28:584–586.
15. Yamamoto M, Meyer JS. Hemicranial disorder of vasomotor adrenoceptors in migraine and cluster headache. Headache 1980;20:321–335.
16. DeBelleroche J, Cook GE, Das I, et al. Erythrocyte choline concentrations and cluster headache. Br Med J 1984;288:268–270.
17. Facchinetti F, Martignoni E, Gallai V, et al. Neuroendocrine evaluation of central opiate activity in primary headache disorders. Pain 1988;34:29–33.
17a. Sicuteri F, Fanciullaci M, Nicolodi M, et al. Substance P theory: A unique focus on the painful and painless phenomena of cluster headache. Headache 1990;30:69–79.
18. Sicuteri F. Antiandrogenic medication of cluster headache. Int J Clin Pharmacol Res 1988;8:21–24.
19. Takeshima T, Nishikawa S, Takahashi K. Cluster headache like symptoms due to sinusitis: Evidence for neuronal pathogenesis of cluster headache syndrome. Headache 1988;28:207–208.
20. Hindfelt LB, Olirecrona H. Cerebral arteriovenous malformation and cluster-like headache. Headache 1991;31:514–517.
21. Todo T, Inoya H. Sudden appearance of a mycotic aneurysm of the intracavernous carotid artery after symptoms resembling cluster headache: Case report. Neurosurgery 1991;29:594–599.
22. West P, Todman D. Chronic cluster headache associated with a vertebral artery aneurysm. Headache 1991;31:210–212.
23. Mani S, Deeter J. Arteriovenous malformation of the brain presenting as a cluster headache: A case report. Headache 1982;22:184–185.
24. Appelbaum J, Noronha A. Pericarotid cluster headache. J Neurol 1989;236:430–431.
25. Tfelt-Hansen P, Paulson OB, Drabbe AE. Invasive adenoma of the pituitary gland and chronic migrainous neuralgia: A rare coincidence or a causal relationship? Cephalalgia 1982;2:25–28.
26. Formisano R, et al. Cluster like headache and head injury: A case report. Ital J Neurol Sci 1990;11:303–305.
27. Olesen J. Cluster headache associated with primary hyperlipidemia. Acta Neurol Scand 1977;56:461–464.
28. Kudrow L. Prevalence of migraine, peptic ulcer, coronary heart disease and hypertension in cluster headache. Headache 1976;16:66–69.
29. Meyer JS, Hardenberg J. Clinical effectiveness of calcium entry blockers in prophylactic treatment of migraine and cluster headache. Headache 1983;23:266–277.
30. Drug Facts and Comparisons. St. Louis: 1994.
31. Solomon SS, Lipton RB, Newman LC. Prophylactic therapy of cluster headaches. Clin Neuropharmacol 1991;14:116–130.
32. Kudrow L. Clinical symptomatology and differential diagnosis of cluster headache. *In* Tollison CD, Kunkel RS, eds. Headache: Diagnosis and Treatment. Baltimore: Williams & Wilkins; 1993:185–189.
33. Kudrow L. Diagnosis and treatment of cluster headache. Med Clin North Am 1991;75:579–593.
34. Gabai IJ, Spierings ELH. Prophylactic treatment of cluster headache with verapamil. Headache 1989;29:167–168.
35. Bussone G, Leone M, Peccarisi C, et al. Double blind comparison of lithium and verapamil in cluster headache prophylaxis. Headache 1990;30:411–417.
36. Freitag FG. Medical management of cluster headache. *In* Tollison CD, Kunkel RS, eds. Headache: Diagnosis and Treatment. Baltimore: Williams & Wilkins; 1993:197–204.
37. Graham JR. Use of a new compound, UML-491, in the prevention of various types of headache. N Engl J Med 1960;263:127.
38. Price LH, Heninger GR. Lithium in the treatment of mood disorders. N Engl J Med 1994;331:591–598.
39. Kafko MS, et al. Effect of lithium on circadian neurotransmitter receptor rhythms. Neuropsychobiology 1982;8:41–50.
40. Treiser SL, et al. Lithium increases serotonin release and decreases serotonin receptors in the hippocampus. Science 1981;213:1529–1539.
41. Ekbom K. Litium vid Kroniska symptom av cluster headache. Opusc Med 1978;19:148.
41a. Ekbom K. Lithium for cluster headache: Review of the literature and preliminary results of long-term treatment. Headache 1981;21:132–139.

42. Okusa MD, Lux Jovita TC. Clinical manifestations and management of acute lithium intoxication. Am J Med 1994;97:383–389.
43. Goldstein J. Ergot pharmacology and alternative delivery systems for ergotamine derivatives. Neurology 1992;42(suppl 2):45–46.
44. Peroutka SJ. Antimigraine drug interactions with serotonin receptor subtypes in human brain. Ann Neurol 1988;23:500–504.
45. Galer BS, Lipton RB, Solomon S, et al. Myocardial ischemia related to ergot alkaloids: A case report and literature review. Headache 1991;31:446–450.
46. Friedman AP, Elkind AH. Appraisal of methysergide in treatment of vascular headaches of migraine type. JAMA 1960;184:125–130.
47. Friedman AP, Losin S. Evaluation of UML-491 in the treatment of vascular headaches. Arch Neurol 1961;4:241.
48. Dubovsky SL, et al. Verapamil: A new antimanic drug with potential interactions with lithium. J Clin Psychiatry 1987;48:371–372.
49. DeKloet ER, Sybesma H, Reul HM. Selective control by corticosterone of serotonin 1 receptor capacity in the raphe-hippocampal system. Neuroendocrinology 1986;42:513–521.
50. Horton B. Histamine cephalgia. Lancet 1952;2:92–98.
51. Kudrow L. Comparative results of prednisone, methysergide, and lithium therapy in cluster headache. *In* Greene R, ed. Current Concepts in Migraine Research. New York: Raven Press; 1978:159–163.
52. Couch JR, Ziegler DK. Prednisone therapy for cluster headache. Headache 1978;18:219–221.
53. Raskin NH. Headache. New York: Churchill Livingstone; 1988:243–244.
54. La Rochelle GE Jr, et al. Recovery of the hypothalamic-pituitary-adrenal axis in patients with rheumatic diseases receiving low-dose prednisone. Am J Med 1993;95:258–264.
55. Horton BT, Peters GA, Blumenthal LS. A new product in the treatment of migraine: A preliminary report. Proc Staff Meetings Mayo Clinic 1945;20:241–248.
56. Raskin NH. Repetitive intravenous dihydroergotamine as therapy for intractable migraine. Neurology 1986;36:995–997.
57. Silberstein SD, Schulman EA, Hopkins MM. Repetitive intravenous DHE in the treatment of refractory headache. Headache 1990;30:334–339.
58. Mather PJ, Silberstein SD, Schulman EA, Hopkins MM. The treatment of cluster headache with repetitive intravenous dihydroergotamine. Headache 1991;31:525–532.
59. Waldenlind E, Ekbom K, Torhall J. MR-angiography during spontaneous attacks of cluster headache: A case report. Headache 1993;33:291–295.
60. Chien S. Cerebral blood flow and metabolism. *In* Kandel ER, Schwartz JH, eds. Principles of Neural Science. New York: Elsevier Science; 1985:845–852.
61. Sakai F, Meyer JS. Abnormal cerebrovascular reactivity in patients with migraine and cluster headache. Headache 1979;19:257–266.
62. Costa E, Meek JL. Regulation of the biosynthesis of catecholamines and serotonin in the CNS. Annu Rev Pharmacol 1974;14:491.
63. Friedman AP, Mikropoulos MD. Cluster headache. Neurology 1958;8:653–663.
64. Kudrow L. Response of cluster headache attacks to oxygen inhalation. Headache 1981;21:1–4.
65. Fogan L. Treatment of cluster headache: A double-blind comparison of oxygen versus air inhalation. Arch Neurol 1985;4:362–363.
66. Nahum A, Sznajder JI. Role of free radicals in critical illness. *In* Hall JB, Schmidt FA, Wood LDH, eds. Principles of Critical Care. New York: McGraw-Hill; 1992:679–692.
67. Solomon GD. Therapeutic advances in migraine. J Clin Pharmacol 1993;33:200–209.
68. Moskowitz MA, Cutrer FM. Sumatriptan: A receptor-targeted treatment for migraine. Annu Rev Med 1993;44:145–154.
69. Plosker GL, McTavish D. Sumatriptan. Drugs 1994;47:622–665.
70. The Sumatriptan Cluster Headache Study Group. Treatment of acute cluster headache with sumatriptan. N Engl J Med 1991;325:322–326.
71. Kittrelle JP, Grouse DS, Seybold ME. Cluster headache local anesthetic abortive agents. Arch Neurol 1985;42:496–498.
72. Kuritzky A, Hering R. The treatment of cluster headaches with sodium valproate: A new approach (abstract). Headache 1987;27:301.
73. Campbell JK, Onofrio BM. Surgical management of cluster headache. *In* Tollison CD, Kunkel RS, eds. Headache: Diagnosis and Treatment. Baltimore: Williams & Wilkins; 1993:205–210.
74. Ekbom K, Monstad I, Prusinski A, et al. Subcutaneous sumatriptan in the acute treatment of cluster headache: A dose comparison study. Acta Neurol Scand 1993;88:63–69.
75. Solomon GD, Kunkel RS, Frame JR. Intranasal capsaicin cream in cluster headache. *In* Rose FC, ed. New Advances in Headache Research 3. London: Smith-Gordon, 1993.
76. Hassenbusch SJ, Kunkel RS, Kosmorsky GS, Covington EC, Pillay PK. Trigeminal cisternal injection of glycerol for treatment of chronic intractable cluster headaches. Neurosurgery 1991;29:504–508.

8

Hormonal Headaches

Seymour Diamond, M.D.

To some extent, hormones probably are involved in most headaches. However, the present discussion is confined to headaches that clearly are related to hormones that govern the menstrual cycle, including headaches that first appear, disappear, or change with pregnancy, oral contraceptive use, and menopause.

Approximately 60% of female migraine sufferers report a menstrual relationship to their migraine attacks,[1, 2] and there is evidence that some tension-type headaches also are linked to the menses. Because men also experience migraines and tension-type headaches, an association with reproductive hormones does not fully explain the etiology of these conditions. Rather, changing levels of these hormones, often in response to other endogenous signals, may be important triggers that set in motion a chain of events culminating in vascular changes and headaches in those who are genetically predisposed.

Menstrual migraine was identified as early as 1666 by Johannis Van der Linden; in *De Hemicrania Menstrua,* Van der Linden described a unilateral headache accompanied by nausea and vomiting that occurred each month during the menstrual flow of the Marchioness of Brandenburg.[3] According to Chaudhuri and Chaudhuri,[4] hormonal treatment of menstrually related headaches has been attempted sporadically for decades. In 1919, for example, there was a report of successful treatment of migraine patients with oral pituitary extract.[5] In 1932, a report stated that injection of an ovarian follicular hormone, oestrin, improved migraine attacks in 23 of 25 patients; another report noted that emmenine, a gonadotropic substance, was effective in the treatment of migraine.[6, 7] Again, 5 years later, the treatment of menstrual migraine with small doses of a gonadotropic extract of pregnancy urine was reported.[8] In 1974, migraine-like headaches in menopausal women were reported to show significant improvement after the administration of pellets of estradiol and testosterone, alone and in combination.[9]

The first careful analyses of the role of reproductive hormones in migraine, however, were carried out by Somerville.[10] Somerville was cognizant that (1) migraines usually occur just before or just after menstruation begins and (2) estrogen and progesterone levels drop from peaks attained approximately 5 days before menstruation to much lower levels immediately before menstrual bleeding. He attempted to determine whether the precipitating event was the decline in estradiol or progesterone level. First, he administered daily injections of progesterone to six women during the premenstrual phase beginning 3 to 6 days before the expected onset of menstruation and continuing until at least the second day of menstruation. The plasma level of progesterone was thus maintained in the usual premenstrual range, although estradiol levels declined normally (Fig. 8–1). Onset of menstruation was delayed in four of six subjects; nevertheless, five of six had migraines at the usual time in their cycles.

In a similar fashion, Somerville administered daily injections of a slow-release form of estradiol to eight women before menstruation. Menstruation occurred on schedule in all subjects, yet the migraine attacks were delayed by 3 to 9 days, until levels of estradiol had attained their preinjection levels (Figs. 8–2, 8–3). Seven women experienced their usual attacks; the eighth subject, who had reported no headache after the progesterone treatment, had a less severe migraine.

In addition, Somerville administered estradiol injections to two women who were no longer menstruating—one because of menopause and the other because of ovarian failure. Both subjects had been migraine free since menstruation had ceased. In both women, migraines developed as the estradiol levels declined. Somerville concluded that

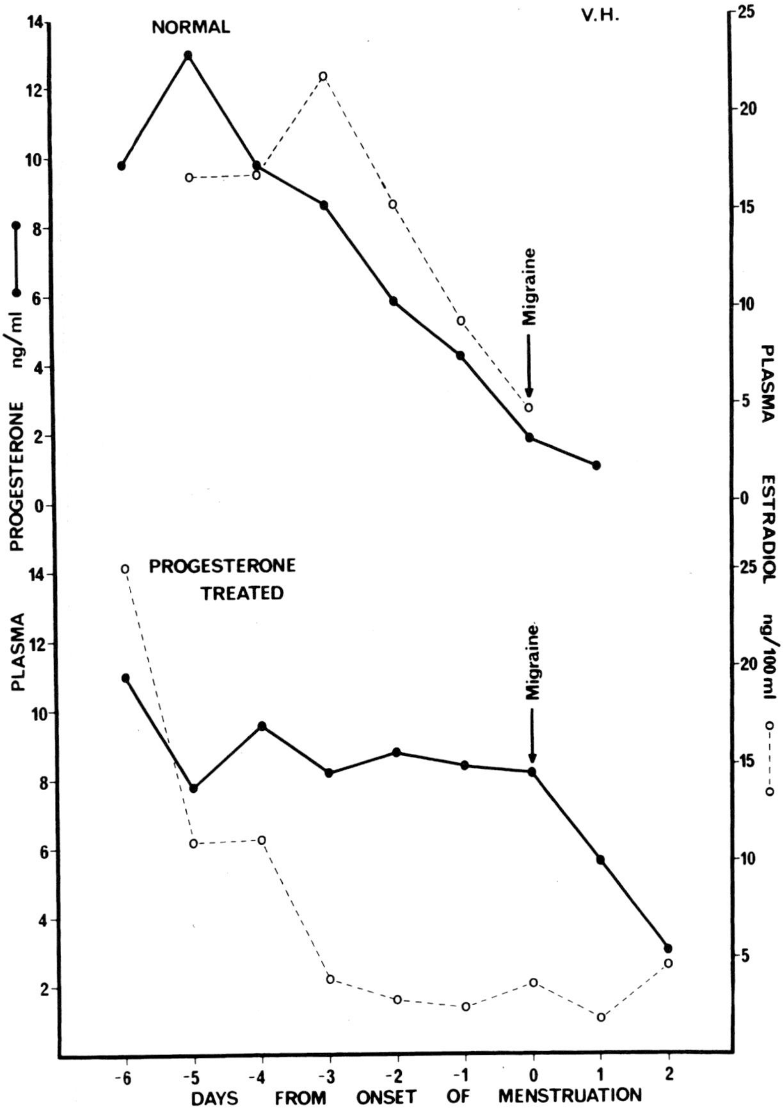

Figure 8–1 Plasma estradiol and progesterone levels during premenstrual phase of normal cycle *(top)* and progesterone-treated cycle *(bottom)*. Note that progesterone treatment has no effect on withdrawal of estradiol and that migraine occurred at the usual time, despite high plasma levels of progesterone. (Reprinted from Somerville BW. The influence of progesterone and estradiol upon migraine. Headache 1972;12:93–102.)

progesterone withdrawal causes menstrual bleeding but not migraine. Somerville notes that estradiol withdrawal, in contrast, "plays a key role in the precipitation of menstrual migraine."

Possible mechanisms for this effect were discussed, including an effect of estradiol on either the cranial vasculature or platelets, causing them to release serotonin. In further studies,[11, 12] Somerville found that several days of exposure to high estrogen levels seemed to be necessary before a declining level of estrogen could result in migraine (Fig. 8–4). His attempts, however, to prevent migraine through premenstrual administration of oral estradiol valerate or conjugated equine estrogens neither affected the normal decline in plasma estradiol levels nor prevented migraine (Fig. 8–5).

In the two decades since the studies of Somerville, additional investigations of headaches associated with the menstrual cycle have been performed, but considering the magnitude of the problem, the literature is surprisingly scant. Nevertheless, valuable contributions have been made.

MacGregor and colleagues[13] studied 55 women between the ages of 17 and 50 years to assess the prevalence of migraine associated with menstruation. The group as a whole had a marked increase in migraine attacks around the first day of menstruation but no increase at the time of ovulation. With a narrow definition of "menstrual migraine" as mi-

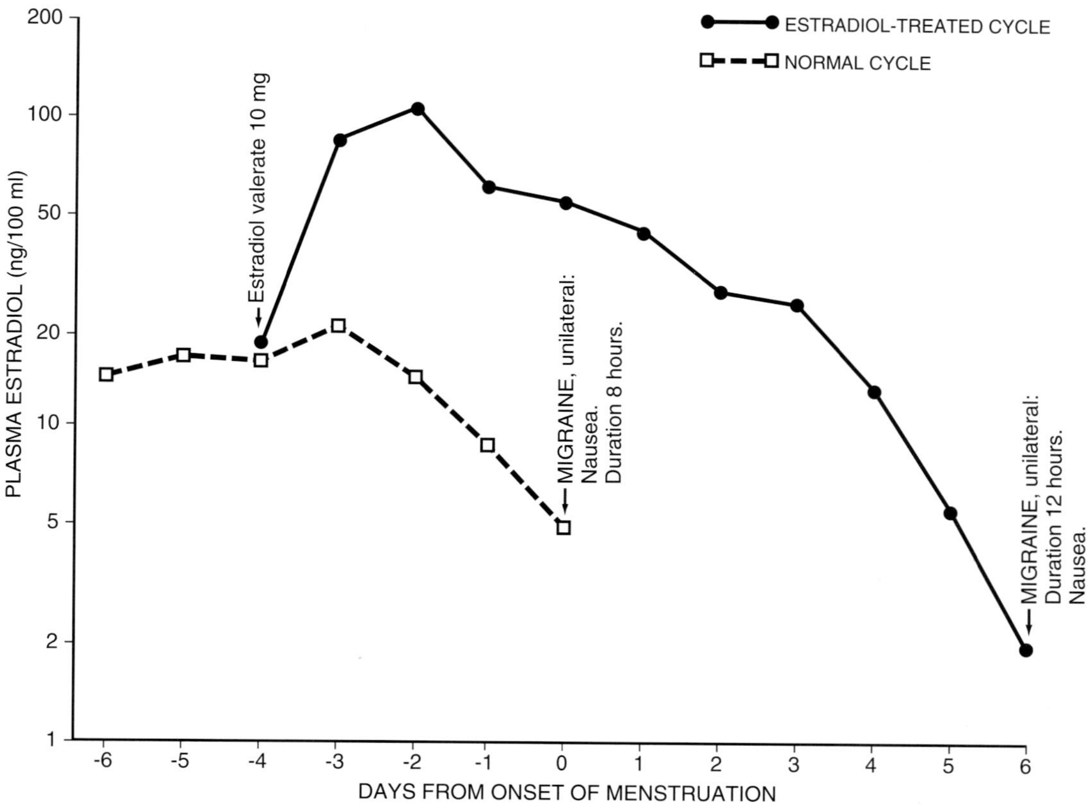

Figure 8–2 Plasma estradiol levels during normal cycle and estradiol-treated cycle. In this patient, treatment with estradiol postponed migraine for 6 days. (Reprinted from Somerville BW. The influence of progesterone and estradiol upon migraine. Headache 1972;12:93–102.)

graine occurring from 2 days before to 3 days after onset of menstruation, MacGregor and coworkers determined that four women (7.2%) fit this category (Fig. 8–6). This compares with the findings by Epstein and colleagues[14] of 14.1% and by Digre and Damasio[15] of 8%, although their definitions of menstrual migraine were broader. Based on my clinical experience, I believe a larger sample may confirm a higher percentage.

Approximately one third of the 55 women in the study were more prone to attacks during menstruation but also experienced attacks at other times during the month; their headaches were considered to be "menstrually related." Another one third had attacks throughout the month with no increase at the time of menstruation, and one fourth of the women had no menstrually associated attacks (Fig. 8–7). The authors hypothesized that hormonal treatment may be effective for the "menstrual migraine" and "menstrually related" groups but not for other headache types.

Types of Hormonally Related Headache

Menstrual Migraine

It is clear that rapid fluctuations in the levels of estrogen and progesterone in particular or changes in the estrogen-to-progesterone ratio play a significant role in triggering menstrual migraine. The ultimate signals may involve, in some way, gonadotropin-releasing hormone (GnRH), which in turn activates the pituitary to secrete luteinizing hormone (LH) and follicle-stimulating hormone (FSH). These two hormones stimulate the production by the ovaries of estrogen and progesterone, which signal the endometrium to produce prostaglandins.

For example, a group from Israel reported in 1990 that when an analogue of GnRH was administered to patients for the purpose of regulating menstrual cycles for in vitro fertilization, some of the subjects experienced se-

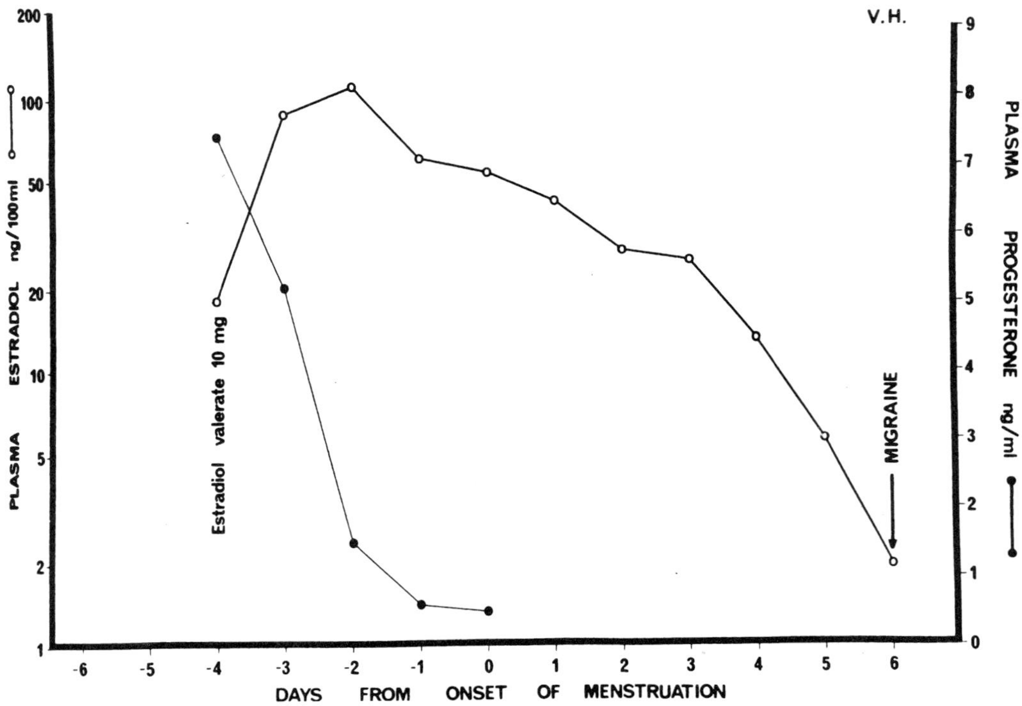

Figure 8–3 Plasma levels of estradiol and progesterone during estradiol-treated cycle showing that estradiol treatment did not affect withdrawal of progesterone during premenstrual phase and that this withdrawal was not accompanied by migraine. (Reprinted from Somerville BW. The influence of progesterone and estradiol upon migraine. Headache 1972;12:93–102.)

vere migraine attacks.[16] The symptoms began between the 8th and 12th days of therapy and subsided over the next 3 to 7 days, despite generally low estradiol levels. The authors hypothesized that estradiol levels fluctuated during the GnRH therapy, resulting in vasospasm of cerebral blood vessels mediated by serotonin, tryptophan, and pyridoxine metabolism. However, they did not rule out a direct effect of the GnRH analogue on the central nervous system vessels.

A similar instance occurred when Lichten administered the GnRH agonist leuprolide acetate to 21 women with intractable severe premenstrual and menstrual migraine attacks in an attempt at treatment (E.M. Lichten, personal communication). Although 11 women reported 50% improvement and 4 reported some improvement, the author was dismayed by the occurrence in 6 patients of severe status migrainosus reactions, lasting in some patients up to 4 weeks.

Secondary Factors

Silberstein and Merriam[17] reviewed the role of prostaglandins, endogenous opioids, and prolactin in menstrual migraine. They noted that dramatic shifts in estrogen levels may boost prostaglandin levels in migraine-susceptible women. Prostaglandins sensitize pain receptors and cause neurogenic inflammation, which also causes pain. In addition, prostaglandin F_2 levels are increased during a migraine attack, and the infusion of prostaglandin E_1 into subjects can generate all the classic symptoms of migraine as well as abdominal cramping pain.

Plasma from menstruating women reinfused at another point in the menstrual cycle will reproduce menstrual symptoms, including headache. Thus, a prostaglandin-generating factor may be present in plasma. Proliferation of arteries in the endometrium is increased in women with migraine, as shown by endometrial biopsies, indicating that the end-organ response of these women to estrogen may be altered. Based on these data, Silberstein and Merriam[17] hypothesized that prostaglandins may mediate the occurrence of migraine that occurs with estrogen withdrawal.

Endogenous pain relief via the endorphins and enkephalins may be more difficult

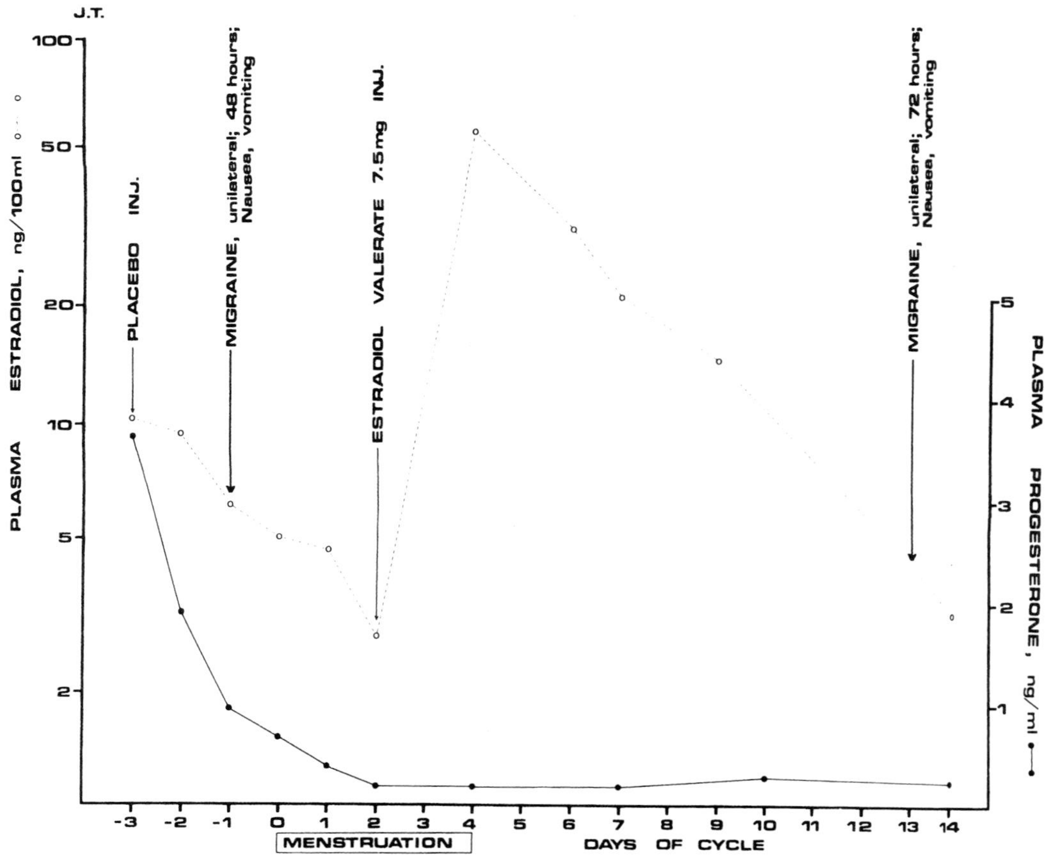

Figure 8–4 Effect of long-acting estradiol administered during follicular phase in one patient. Of four patients who had a preliminary injection of placebo, none received an effect on the usual migraine. In this patient, estradiol valerate injection caused a second rise in plasma estradiol, after which a second migraine attack was observed. (Reprinted from Somerville BW. Estrogen-withdrawal migraine. Neurology 1975;25:239–244.)

for migraine sufferers. Patients with migraine have lower cerebrospinal fluid levels of β-endorphin than normal control subjects. A correlation exists among this, a lack of responsiveness to the narcotic antagonist naloxone, and increasing headache severity. Levels of β-endorphins in the cerebrospinal fluid also are low during menopause or after oophorectomy, but the administration of estrogen restores them to normal.

Regarding the pituitary hormone prolactin, its release may be enhanced by serotonin during migraine attacks. Some of the major migraine triggers (stress, exercise, and oral contraceptives) produce elevated plasma levels of prolactin. In addition, some antimigraine drugs, such as ergot alkaloids and clonidine, suppress prolactin production, lending support to the idea that high prolactin levels are related causally to migraines.

Danazol

Lichten conducted an investigation of the use of danazol in the treatment of patients with severe, menstrually related migraines occurring mostly in the premenstrual period.[18] Danazol, an ethinyltestosterone derivative, suppresses the pituitary-ovarian axis by binding to androgen and progestogen receptors and inhibiting ovarian steroidogenesis. In this four-phase study, 400 mg danazol was administered daily for 25 days to 131 patients who also received the diuretic acetazolamide.

Of the 131 patients, 83 (63.35%) initially reported a 75% decrease in the headache index (a monthly summation of daily headaches graded as to severity). Twenty-seven patients (20.61%) had no improvement, and 21 (16.03%) reported adverse effects (joint pain and acne) that caused discontinuation

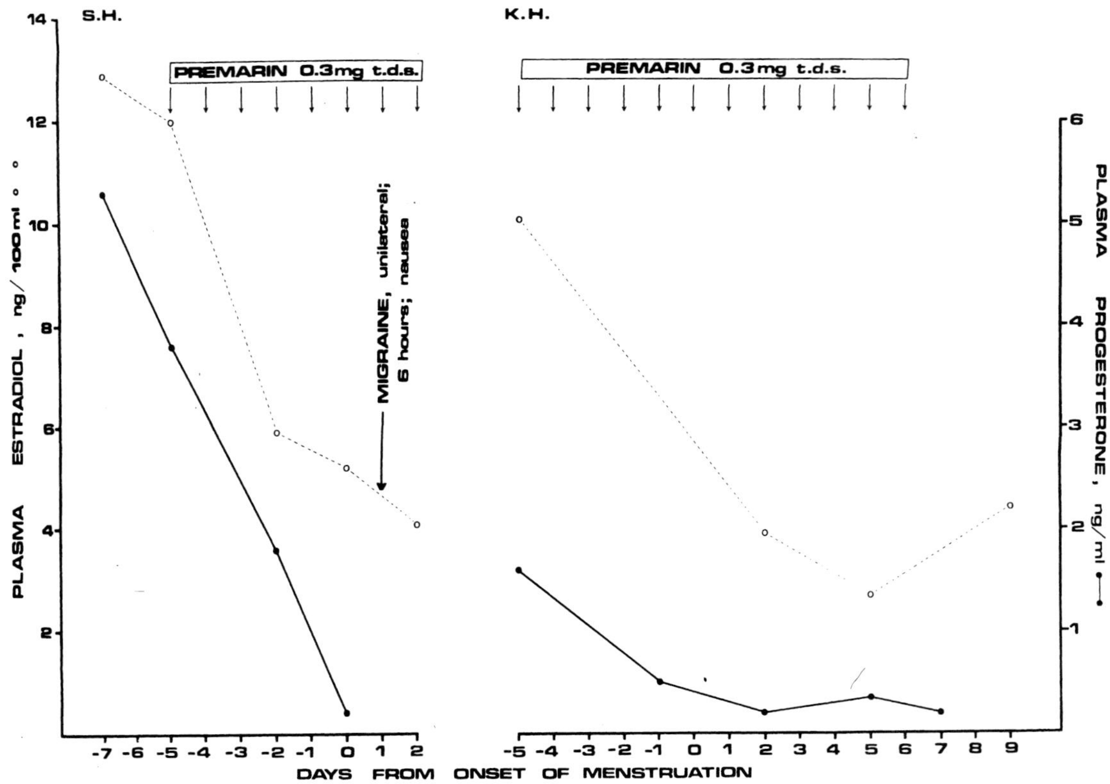

Figure 8–5 Premenstrual treatment with conjugated equine estrogens was ineffective in influencing plasma estradiol levels or preventing migraine. (Reprinted from Somerville BW. Estrogen-withdrawal migraine. Neurology 1975;25:239–244.)

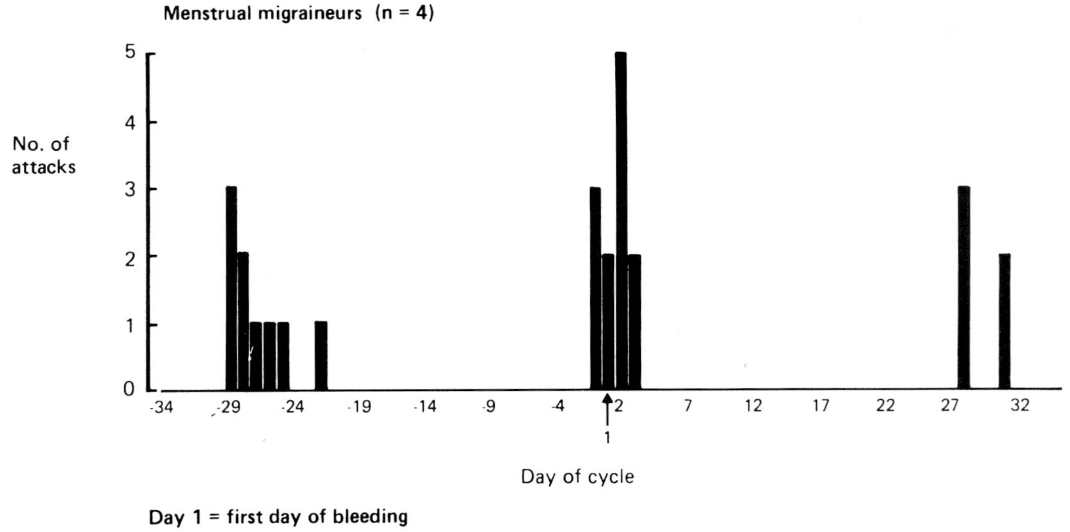

Figure 8–6 Total number of attacks recorded over three complete menstrual cycles by four women with "menstrual migraine." (Reprinted from MacGregor EA, et al. Migraine and menstruation: A pilot study. Cephalalgia 1990;10:305–310.)

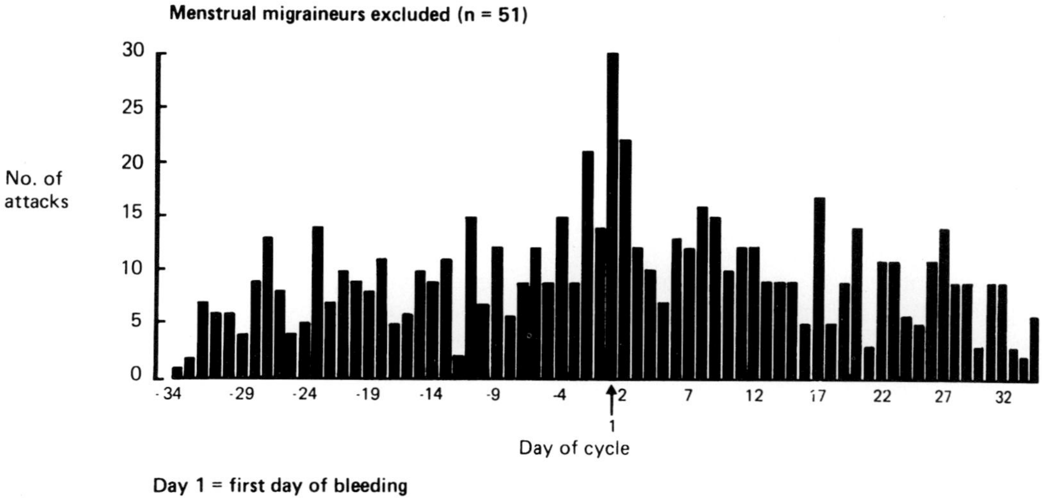

Figure 8–7 Total number of attacks recorded over three complete menstrual cycles by 51 women, excluding the four women with "menstrual migraine." (Reprinted from MacGregor EA, et al. Migraine and menstruation: A pilot study. Cephalalgia 1990;10:305–310.)

of the drug. Later, 81 of 83 women whose headaches had been largely prevented by danazol restarted the agent for another 6 months. In 67 (82.7%) of these women, there was continued control.

The efficacy of danazol was correlated with increasing age of the patient. The agent was most effective for migraines that occurred only premenstrually. Serum estradiol levels dropped markedly with danazol therapy, but the decrease was similar in all subjects.

Menstrual Tension-Type Headaches

In a study of precipitating factors of headache, Rasmussen, found that 39% of women with tension-type headaches that started before age 51 years had experienced attacks related to menstruation.[19] Forty-five percent related more than half of their attacks to menstruation. In these women, headaches were unchanged during pregnancy in 67%, disappeared during pregnancy in 28%, and worsened in 5%.

In another study, 22% of women with tension-type headaches said that menstruation was a provoking factor.[20] Forty-seven percent reported a cyclic influence, with an increase in frequency and seriousness during the premenstrual period.

Premenstrual Syndrome Headaches

Women who experience headaches during the premenstrual portion of their menstrual cycles usually have tension-type headaches or a combination of migraine and tension-type headaches. They may also complain of a wide range of other premenstrual syndrome symptoms, both physical and emotional, including fatigue, joint pain, breast tenderness, and fluid retention. Food cravings are not unusual, and frequently, anxiety and depression, impaired judgment or memory, and paranoia may be present.[21] As with menstrual migraines, fluctuations in estrogen and progesterone levels are linked to both types of headaches.

Migraine and Other Headaches during and after Pregnancy

In about 70% of cases, migraines improve with pregnancy, probably due to sustained high estrogen levels. Even if the migraines persist during the first trimester, they usually disappear during the second and third trimesters. In a study done in Australia involving 200 pregnant women, 31 (15.5%) had a history of migraine.[22] In 7 of the 31 women (22.5%), migraine attacks ceased during pregnancy; in an additional 17 women, there was some improvement. Thus, 77.4% improved during pregnancy. Headaches in another 7 migraine sufferers (22.6%) worsened in either frequency or severity. In the remaining 7 women (3.5%), migraines started for the first time.

Postpartum headaches may be either migraine or tension-type. Although these can occur any time in the first week postpartum, they tend to cluster around days 4 to 6 postpartum. There is a strong association with a previous personal or family history of migraine. Migraines occurring in the postpartum period coincident with the fall in estrogen and progesterone after delivery, however, are commonly milder than usual.

In one study, 39% of 71 women developed postpartum headaches, but 83% of the 71 were known to be susceptible to migraine.[23] In contrast, the women with headaches had significantly more tension and depression than those who did not, suggesting that some of the headaches were tension-type. The headaches often coincided with weight loss, which began 3 or 4 days postpartum. In any case, headaches are known to be part of the postpartum depression complex, which should be treated appropriately.

Menopausal Headaches

Estrogen levels and fluctuations gradually decrease as menopause approaches; therefore, migraines most often lessen in frequency or cease with menopause. However, they can become worse or even occur for the first time in women vulnerable to hormonally mediated vascular changes. Normal versus surgically induced menopause may have varying effects on headaches. According to Neri et al,[24] who studied 47 postmenopausal women with migraines and 29 with tension-type headaches, migraines tended to improve (67%) after physiological menopause but not after surgical menopause (Fig. 8–8). Tension-type headaches, on the other hand, became worse or were unchanged in 70% of cases, regardless of the type of menopause. In addition, hormone replacement therapy (HRT), consisting of a form of estrogen and progesterone, may aggravate migraines that would otherwise stop. Discontinuation of cyclic oral estrogen for 1 week, for example, may precipitate migraine.

The exacerbation of migraine with HRT may occur immediately or gradually as a consequence of prolonged use; however, continuous administration of HRT in low daily doses may relieve persisting or new migraines.

There is an association between the current use of HRT and the risk of venous thromboembolism, but the number of reported cases is only about 1 in 5000.[25]

Lichten and colleagues,[26] who have for some time advocated hormonal treatment of refractory menstrually related migraines, found that continuous oral or transdermal estrogen relieved migraines in 17 of 24 menopausal women. They also found that hormonally influenced migraines in menopausal women with a history of migraines could be prevented by maintaining a serum estradiol level above 50 pg/mL. This could be accomplished by administering 5 mg depo-estradiol cyprionate intramuscularly every 2 weeks.

Oral Contraceptives and Headache

Because oral contraceptives may accentuate hormonal fluctuations, the frequency, duration, severity, and complications of migraine can be increased. These problems are most likely to occur in women with a history of migraine. However, migraine can also occur for the first time in women who have just started oral contraceptives. Frequently, in such cases, there is a family history of migraine.

Migraine headaches are the most common adverse effect of oral contraceptives. In one study, more than one fourth of the women stopped taking oral contraceptives for this reason.[27] Nonvascular headaches also are increased. The incidence of adverse effects, such as headache or other vascular events, has decreased over the years as the newer oral contraceptives have been formulated that contain increasingly lower doses of estrogen. However, women taking these oral contraceptives still have a slightly increased risk of venous thrombosis and venous thromboembolism compared with those not using these agents.[28] In particular, recent reports have suggested that women taking third-generation oral contraceptives—those containing desogestrel or gestodene—are at a slightly higher risk of these events than women taking oral contraceptives containing the progestin levonorgestrel.[29, 30]

According to the US Food and Drug Administration, the risk of nonfatal venous thromboembolism in healthy women not using oral contraceptives is 4 in 100,000. The risk for women using older, low-dose oral contraceptives is 10 to 15 in 100,000; for women using third-generation (containing the progestins desogestrel or gestodene) oral contraceptives, the risk is 20 to 30 in 100,000.

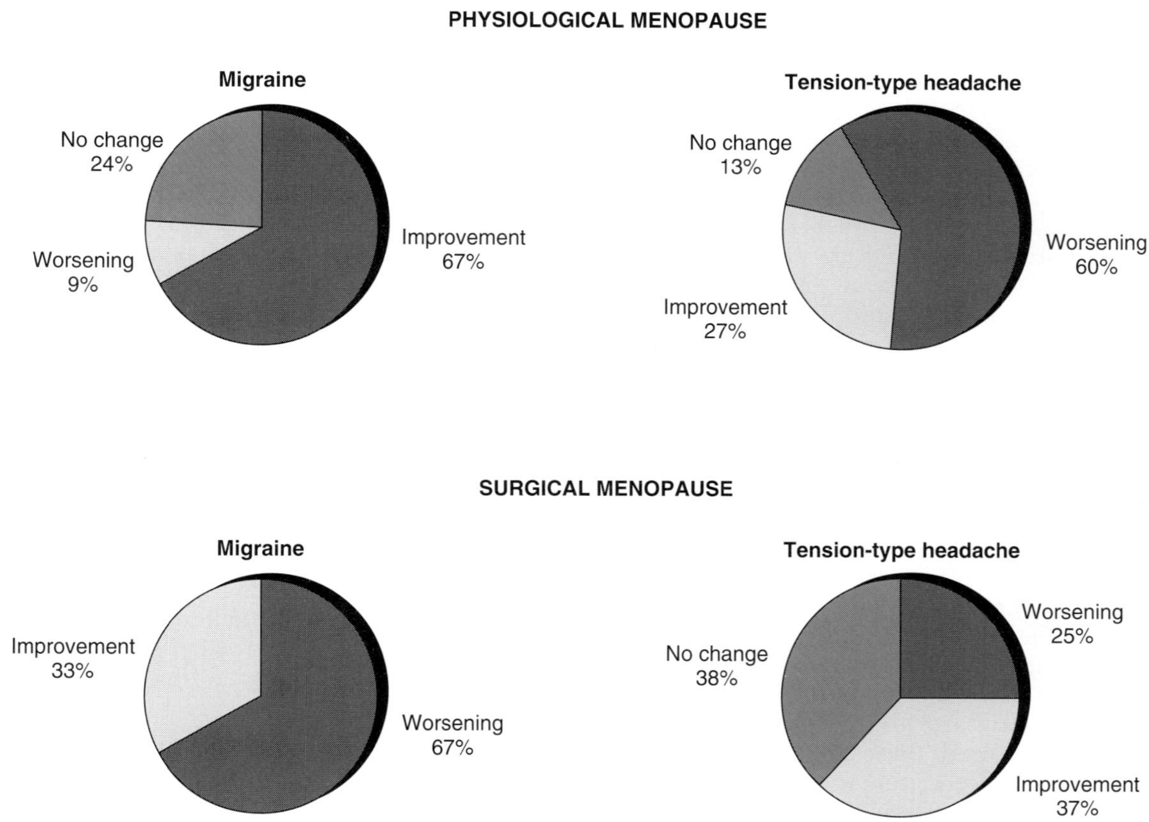

Figure 8–8 Postmenopausal course of premenopause-onset headache, according to type of menopause. Improvement signifies a reduction of more than 50% in the frequency of attacks (course of migraine in physiological versus surgical menopause: $P = 0.003$; course of migraine versus tension-type headache by type of menopause: $P = 0.004$). (Reprinted from Neri I, et al. Characteristics of headache at menopause: A clinico-epidemiologic study. Maturitas 1993;17:31–37.)

In comparison, the risk of such events in pregnant women is 60 in 100,000.

Increased platelet aggregability induced by serotonin has been reported in migraine patients taking oral contraceptives.[31] Can use of the low-dose combined oral contraceptives increase the risk of stroke, transient cerebral ischemia, or venous thromboembolism in women with a history of migraine?[32–35] Despite an array of studies, the answer is not clear. If the question were answered affirmatively, however, the risk would be very small.

Treatment

Menstrual Migraine

The agents of choice in the prevention and treatment of menstrual migraine are the newer nonsteroidal anti-inflammatory drugs (NSAIDs). Therapy should begin 2 to 3 days before the onset of menses and continue through the flow. The NSAIDs prevent platelet aggregation and swelling but also block prostaglandin production. Gastrointestinal adverse effects are limited because the therapy is of short duration. The NSAIDs most often used for menstrual migraine include fenoprofen calcium, naproxen, naproxen sodium, ketoprofen, nabumetone, and ketorolac. If one NSAID is ineffective, another type of NSAID should be tried.

If the patient does not respond to NSAID therapy, small doses of ergotamine agents may be used for prophylaxis without the risk of developing ergot dependence. These agents include ergotamine tartrate taken at bedtime or twice daily. A combination agent, containing 40 mg phenobarbital, 0.6 mg ergotamine tartrate, and 0.2 mg belladonna alkaloids, may be given two or three times a day, starting 3 days before and continuing through the menstrual period. Other agents include methylergonovine maleate and dihydroergotamine maleate, a serotonin receptor agonist that may be quite effective in preventing or terminating severe menstrual migraine. Methysergide also may be considered, and the risks usually associated with this agent (retroperitoneal, pulmonary, or cardiac fibrosis) are minimal due to the short-term therapy—starting 3 days before the menses and continuing through the flow.

Perimenstrual use of other medications also can be effective prophylactically. The β-blockers prevent platelet aggregation and block dilation of cranial arteries and are considered first-line agents for migraine prophylaxis. α-Agonists, antidepressants, calcium channel blockers, neuroleptics (divalproex sodium), and methysergide are other options in migraine prophylaxis. If a patient is already taking one of these agents for other indications, she may increase the dose before the menses. For patients who do not respond to any of these agents, the NSAIDs can be combined with opioids, high-dose corticosteroids, or major tranquilizers.

The standard migraine abortive agents also can be used; these agents include sumatriptan, isometheptene mucate, ergotamine tartrate, and a combination agent of aspirin, acetaminophen, and caffeine.

Hormonal Therapy

Hormonal therapy consists of estrogens, estrogen antagonists, estrogens in combination with testosterone or progesterone, and prolactin-release inhibitors. The goal is to prevent the luteal phase increase in estrogen or its subsequent drop, or both. Agents used in the treatment of endometriosis and cyclic breast pain may be effective, and replacement of estrogen before menstruation has been successful.

The use of percutaneous estradiol gel has achieved good results, as has the use of estradiol transdermal patches, which provide stable plasma estrogen levels.[36] At least one estradiol implant also has stabilized plasma estrogen levels.[37]

Oral contraceptives may help some patients with intractable menstrual migraine, particularly if severe dysmenorrhea is also present. There has been one report of the successful use of a synthetic oral estrogen (0.05 mg ethinyl estradiol) in combination with 2 mg methyltestosterone.[38]

As previously noted, danazol can be effective in prophylaxis of menstrual migraine.[18] Tamoxifen, an antiestrogen used primarily to treat breast cancer, also may be effective in the treatment of intractable menstrual migraine.[39] The agent binds to a cytosol estrogen receptor. When prescribed in a dose of 5 to 15 mg/day for days 7 to 14 of the menstrual cycle (luteal phase), it has yielded significant relief of menstrual headache without side effects.

Premenstrual Syndrome Headaches

Prostaglandin inhibitors, such as aspirin and other NSAIDs, have proved to be remarkably helpful. In severe cases, anovulation therapy, which includes oral contraceptives and depomedroxyprogesterone acetate, is an option. Supplemental doses of progesterone also may be efficacious.[40] An ergotamine combination agent may be useful, particularly in treating aspects of premenstrual syndrome in addition to headache.

Bromocriptine, a dopamine D_2 receptor agonist, inhibits prolactin release. When administered during the luteal phase of the menstrual cycle in a dose of 2.5 to 5 mg/day, this agent may decrease headache and other premenstrual syndrome symptoms.[41]

Migraine during Pregnancy

The gold standard of treatment during pregnancy is no treatment. Because of the oxytocic effects of the ergotamines and other agents with vasoconstrictor actions, most migraine abortive therapy is precluded. However, acetaminophen is helpful for pain relief. Caffeine, most NSAIDs, butorphanol (in the first and second trimesters), and narcotics are relatively safe for acute pain relief. For prophylaxis after the first trimester, a tricyclic antidepressant or fluoxetine may be considered. Another prophylactic agent that can be considered is propranolol.

In this regard, a recent publication is reassuring. Nulman and coworkers[42] showed that in utero exposure to tricyclic antidepressant drugs or fluoxetine had no effect on global IQ, language development, or behavioral development of the children, as measured in preschool years. They also note that when maternal depression is not optimally controlled, there is evidence of adverse effects, including neurodevelopmental, in the offspring.

During the period of lactation, the same drugs listed above are relatively safe for abortive therapy. For prophylaxis, the safest options are β-blockers, calcium channel blockers, divalproex sodium, and prednisone.

Menopausal Headaches

Many women are using HRT on a long-term basis not only to relieve menopausal symptoms but also to help prevent cardiovascular disease and osteoporosis. The lowest dose possible of estrogen on an uninterrupted basis—to maintain a steady state of estrogen—should be used. If problems occur, another form of estrogen can be used. Usually, conjugated estrogens and ethinyl estradiol can pose more problems. The use of an estradiol cutaneous patch seems to be effective in stabilizing plasma estrogen levels.[1] Many gynecologists have voiced concern over the occurrence of uterine cancer in patients who receive estrogen agents without added progesterone or who do not receive cyclic estrogen therapy. Uterine cancer is a rare occurrence; I explain this risk to my patients before the start of therapy, so the patient is involved in the decision-making process about HRT.

For women who do not receive HRT and experience persistent or recent-onset migraine, the administration of a low dose of estrogen, sometimes with testosterone, has been shown in some studies to be helpful.

Headaches Associated with Oral Contraceptive Use

For those women who prefer to continue to receive oral contraceptives, the use of an NSAID from the 20th day of the cycle until the 2nd day of the next cycle is frequently helpful in preventing or lessening the severity of migraines that occur during the week off of oral contraceptives. An alternative for these patients is a newer low-dose oral contraceptive on a noncycling basis (no hiatus or placebo interval) for 3 to 6 months. Estradiol patches also may be used during the 7-day placebo phase. For nonvascular headaches associated with oral contraceptive use, over-the-counter analgesics usually are effective.

References

1. Silberstein SD. The role of sex hormones in headache. Neurology 1992;42(suppl 2):37–42.
2. Fettes I. Menstrual migraine: Methods of prevention and control. Postgrad Med 1997;101:67–77.
3. Van der Linden JA. De Hemicrania Menstrua. London: 1666.
4. Chaudhuri TK, Chaudhuri ST. Estrogen therapy for migraine. Headache 1975;139:139–141.
5. Pardee IH. Pituitary headaches and their cure. Arch Intern Med 1919;23:174–184.
6. Thompson AP. A contribution to the study of intermittent headache. Lancet 1932;2:229–235.
7. Blackie NH, Hossock JC. The treatment of migraine with emmenine. Can Med Assoc J 1932;27:45–47.
8. Mofat WM. Treatment of menstrual migraine with small doses of gonadotropic extract of pregnancy urine. JAMA 1937;108:612–615.
9. Greenblatt RB, Brunteau DW. Menopausal headaches: Psychogenic or metabolic? J Am Geriatr Soc 1974;2:186–190.
10. Somerville BW. The influence of progesterone and estradiol upon migraine. Headache 1972;12:93–102.
11. Somerville BW. Estrogen-withdrawal migraine. I. Duration of exposure required and attempted prophylaxis by premenstrual estrogen administration. Neurology 1975;25:239–244.
12. Somerville BW. Estrogen-withdrawal migraine. II. Attempted prophylaxis by continuous estradiol administration. Neurology 1975;25:245–250.
13. MacGregor EA, Chis H, Vohrah RC, et al. Migraine and menstruation: A pilot study. Cephalalgia 1990;10:305–310.
14. Epstein MT, Hockaday JM, Hockaday TDR. Migraine and reproductive hormones throughout the menstrual cycle. Lancet 1975;1:543–548.
15. Digre K, Damasio H. Menstrual migraine: Differential diagnoses, evaluation and treatment. Clin Obstet Gynecol 1987;30:417–430.
16. Ashkenazi J, Goldman JA, Dicker D, et al. Adverse neurological symptoms after gonadotropin-releasing hormone analog therapy for in vitro fertilization cycles. Fertil Steril 1990;53:738–740.
17. Silberstein SD, Merriam GR. Sex hormones and headache. J Pain Symptom Mgmt 1993;8:98–114.
18. Lichten EM, Bennett RS, Whitty AJ, et al. Efficacy of danazol in the control of hormonal migraine. J Reprod Med 1991;36:419–424.
19. Rasmussen BK. Migraine and tension-type headache in a general population: Precipitating factors, female hormones, sleep pattern and relation to lifestyle. Pain 1993;53:65–72.
20. Bartelink ML, van de Liskonk E, van den Hoogen H, et al. Migraine in family practice: Prevalence and influence of sex hormone status. Fam Med 1993;25:331–336.

21. Barnhart KT, Freeman EW, Sondheimer SJ. A clinician's guide to the premenstrual syndrome. Med Clin North Am 1995;79:1457–1472.
22. Somerville BW. A study of migraine in pregnancy. Neurology 1972;22:824–828.
23. Stein G, Morton J, Marsh A, et al. Headaches after childbirth. Acta Neurol Scand 1984;69:74–79.
24. Neri I, Granella F, Nappi R, Manzoni GC, Facchinetti F, Genazzani AR. Characteristics of headache at menopause: A clinico-epidemiologic study. Maturitas 1993;17:31–37.
25. Daly E, Vessey MP, Hawkins MM, et al. Risk of venous thromboembolism in users of hormone replacement therapy. Lancet 1996;348:977–980.
26. Lichten EM, Lichten JB, Whitty AJ, Piper D. The use of leuprolide acetate in the diagnosis and treatment of menstrual migraine: The role of artificially-induced menopause. Headache Q 1995;6:313–317.
27. Dalton K. Migraine and oral contraceptives. Headache 1976;15:247–251.
28. Jick H, Porter J, Rothman KJ. Oral contraceptives and nonfatal stroke in healthy young women. Ann Intern Med 1978;89:58–60.
29. Pettitti DB, Sidney S, Bernstein A, et al. Stroke in users of low-dose oral contraceptives. N Engl J Med 1996;335:8–15.
30. WHO Collaborative Study of Cardiovascular Disease and Steroid Hormone Contraception. Venous thromboembolic disease and combined oral contraceptives: Results of international multicentre case-control study. Lancet 1995;346:1575–1582.
31. Hanington E, Jones RJ, Amess JAL. Platelet aggregation in response to 5-HT in migraine patients taking oral contraceptives. Lancet 1982;1:968–969.
32. Benson MD, Rebar RW. Relationship of migraine headache and stroke to oral contraceptive use. J Reprod Med 1986;31:1082–1088.
33. Carolei A, Marini C, DeMatteis G, et al. History of migraine and risk of cerebral ischemia in young adults. Lancet 1996;347:1503–1506.
34. Thomas SHL. Mortality from venous thromboembolism and myocardial infarction in young adults in England and Wales. Lancet 1996;348:402.
35. Vandenbroucke JP, Bloemenkamp KWM, Helmerhorst FM, et al. Mortality from venous thromboembolism and myocardial infarction in young women in the Netherlands. Lancet 1996;348:401–402.
36. DeLignières, B, Vincens M, Mauvais-Jarvis P, et al. Prevention of menstrual migraine by percutaneous oestradiol. Br Med J 1986;293:1540.
37. Magos AL, Zilkha KJ, Studd JWW. Treatment of menstrual migraine by oestradiol implants. J Neurol Neurosurg Psychiatry 1983;46:1044–1046.
38. Raskin NH. Headache, 2nd ed. New York: Churchill Livingstone; 1988.
39. O'Dea JPK, Davis EH. Tamoxifen in the treatment of menstrual migraine. Neurology 1990;40:1470–1471.
40. Dalton K. Progesterone suppositories and pessaries in the treatment of menstrual migraine. Headache 1973;12:151–159.
41. Andersen AN, Larsen JF, Steenstrup OR, Svendstrup B, Nielsen J. Effect of bromocriptine on the premenstrual syndrome: A double-blind clinical trial. Br J Obstet Gynecol 1977;84:370–374.
42. Nulman I, Rovet J, Stewart DE, et al. Neurodevelopment of children exposed in utero to antidepressant drugs. N Engl J Med 1997;336:258–262.

9

Complicated and Rare Forms of Migraine

Robert S. Kunkel, M.D.

Introduction

Patients with migraine have migraine with or without aura. Prolonged neurological symptoms can occur with any attack of migraine, and some variants of migraine are always accompanied by neurological symptoms. The term *complicated migraine* is not listed as a diagnosis in the International Headache Society classification of headache;[1] *migrainous infarction* has replaced the term *complicated migraine.* By definition, *migrainous infarction* is a migraine attack with neurological symptoms that are not fully reversible within 7 days and/or there is evidence of an ischemic lesion on neuroimaging in a relevant area of the brain. Criteria for a migrainous infarction also include that other causes of infarction be ruled out. Prolonged neurological or visual symptoms lasting less than 7 days indicate *migraine with prolonged aura.*[1]

Visual or neurological symptoms most often start before the pain as a typical aura, but at times they begin during the painful phase. Very rarely, neurological symptoms begin during the attack and end before the attack is over. This particular situation has been called *migraine accompagnée*, or *interposed migraine.*[2]

The migraine attack is a very complicated phenomenon in which neurogenic, biochemical, and vascular components play a role. Some patients with migraine will have all attacks accompanied by an aura or all attacks without an aura, but most patients will have both kinds of migraine at different times. Any person with migraine can have a complicated migraine attack at any time. The vast majority of patients with migrainous infarction or complicated migraine have had migraine for years; it is very unusual for a migrainous infarction to occur during the initial attack of migraine.

Migraine and Stroke

Migraine and stroke are common conditions and can occur in the same patient. *Migrainous infarction* implies that the neurological symptoms came on during an attack of migraine headache and continued for more than 7 days. Welch and Levine[3] reviewed the various situations in which migraine and stroke can occur and proposed a more detailed classification of migraine-related strokes. The exact incidence of stroke with migraine is not known. There have been several studies, but study patients were those with migraine who sought a physician or headache center because of the severity of their symptoms. In a study from the Mayo Clinic, the records were reviewed of more than 4800 patients diagnosed with migraine who were younger than 50 years.[4] The researchers found that 20 patients of that group had a migraine-associated brain infarction, for an incidence of less than 0.5%. At the last follow-up, 18 of the 20 patients had minimal or no functional impairment. This confirms the clinical impression that the majority of migrainous strokes will clear completely or nearly completely without significant remaining deficit. The same investigators found that 25% of cerebral infarctions occurring in persons less than 50 years of age were associated with a migraine attack.

In a study of cerebral infarctions occurring in 100 persons under age 40, it was found that 27 had no specific etiology.[5] Five of the 27 persons (18.5%) had migraines. This incidence is in the neighborhood of the general incidence of migraine in the community. A somewhat higher incidence was found in a smaller study in which 25% of persons under age 40 with a stroke were found to have migraine.[6] On the basis of International Headache Society criteria for migraine, it was found that overall migraine is not a significant risk factor for ischemic stroke.[7] However, 30% of 20 women under age 45 who had a stroke also had migraine headaches. It should be remembered that 15% to 20% of the population has migraine, and therefore many patients who have strokes will also have migraine. Many older persons who have had strokes have also had migraine when they were younger, but the two conditions have not been found to be related.

Migraine-related stroke appears to be rare among persons with migraine, but migraine is a significant factor in young persons with strokes. Because migraine occurs more frequently in women, migrainous strokes are more common in women. This is contrary to the finding that strokes in nonmigrainous persons under age 50 occur much more commonly in men.

Neurological and visual defects that occur at the time of a migrainous infarction are usually similar to symptoms that have occurred as an aura during previous attacks; therefore, visual defects are much more common and probably occur about twice as often as do neurological abnormalities.[8] Visual defects are usually in the form of quadrantanopsia, hemianopsia, or scintillating scotomata, which is indicative of occipital lobe involvement. Monocular visual symptoms, which indicate problems in the retina *(complicated retinal migraine)*, are very rare but occasionally occur. Vascular abnormalities appear to be much more prevalent in patients with retinal symptoms when they are studied and evaluated.[9] Visual fields were studied in approximately 60 patients with migraine who were asymptomatic for vision problems;[10] 21 of these patients (35%) had some visual field loss on formal testing. The visual field defects were more severe in persons with advanced age who had had migraine for a long time. Another study found small persistent visual field defects in 10 of 23 patients with migraine with aura but intact visual fields in patients with migraine without aura and in control nonmigrainous patients.[11]

The majority of cerebral infarctions are located in the posterior hemisphere in the area supplied by the posterior cerebral artery. This correlates with the fact that visual symptoms are the most common symptoms occurring during the aura of a migraine attack. When a cerebral or retinal infarction occurs in a patient with migraine, a complete investigation must be undertaken to search for any other underlying condition that might be a significant factor.[3] Occlusive cerebrovascular disease, vasculitis, coagulopathy, infection, mass lesions, aneurysm, embolism, and arteriovenous malformation have been reported to cause cerebral infarction in young patients. Because migraine is such a common condition, it is likely that other underlying factors will be found in some patients, and it will be hard to determine which might be the most significant factor in causing the infarction.

In a study by Bogousslavsky et al,[12] 22 patients who had had a stroke at the time of a migraine attack were evaluated for possible underlying cardiac and vascular abnormalities. In matched control subjects who did not have a migraine attack but had had a stroke, only 18% were free of other disease. In migraineurs who had had a stroke that was not associated with a migraine attack, only 9% were free of underlying disease. In patients who had had a stroke at the time of a migraine attack (migrainous infarction), 91% were free of underlying cardiac or vascular abnormalities. The researchers therefore concluded that the cerebral infarction occurring at the time of a migraine attack was usually related to the attack itself rather than to an underlying vascular or cardiac abnormality.

Physiological factors such as decreased blood flow, platelet aggregation, and neuronal depression, all of which occur during many migraine attacks, may play a role in a migrainous infarction. Persons who have visual or neurological symptoms accompanying their migraine attacks should avoid other risk factors for stroke such as smoking, hyperlipidemia, the use of estrogens, and hypertension. When present in a setting of migraine, these known risk factors of cerebrovascular disease can greatly increase the risk of migrainous infarction.

Specific Syndromes of Complicated Migraine

Retinal Migraine

Retinal migraine is thought to be due to ischemia caused by prolonged central retinal artery or branch constriction. Headache may or may not be present. Monocular visual loss, either partial or complete, is often preceded by scintillating scotomata. It is essential to remember that retinal migraine is a very rare condition. The vast majority of monocular visual symptoms are due to vascular lesions along the carotid artery system, emboli from the heart or proximal vessels, or coagulation disorders. If retinal symptoms are accompanied by a unilateral headache, migraine may be suggested, but the diagnosis cannot be made unless all other underlying etiological factors have been ruled out.

Ophthalmoplegic Migraine

Ophthalmoplegic migraine also is very rare; it is a periodic migraine headache that is accompanied by paresis of the ocular nerves. These defects are usually transient, but at times they may be permanent. Ophthalmoplegic migraine usually occurs in children, and it affects males about six times more often than females.[13] Although the third cranial nerve is most often involved in ophthalmoplegic migraine, the fourth and sixth nerves may also be involved. Diplopia is the most common symptom, and it is often accompanied by blurred vision and ptosis. The weakness of the third nerve usually comes on during the attack of pain rather than occurring as an aura. The pupil may remain permanently dilated and fixed, with periodic ptosis and deviation of the eye occurring during the attacks of migraine.

The cause of the ocular nerve paresis in ophthalmoplegic migraine is poorly understood. Research by Bickerstaff[13] has demonstrated narrowing in the internal carotid artery, which was assumed to be due to edema of the wall rather than to vascular spasm. Edema and swelling of the carotid wall might cause some compression of the involved nerve or interfere with blood supply through the vasa nervorum. Although mydriasis of the pupil often occurs, Vijayan[14] reported that the pupil was spared in the majority of patients and therefore suggested that the etiology was most likely due to ischemic neuropathy rather than to compression. Magnetic resonance imaging (MRI) studies on two patients with ophthalmoplegic migraine showed enlargement of the third cranial nerve from the brainstem to the cavernous sinus.[15] Whether this swelling and edema of the third nerve are related to the etiology of the symptoms or are secondary to the headache itself is uncertain.

It is essential to exclude organic causes of ophthalmoplegia. MRI and/or magnetic resonance angiography may be indicated to exclude an aneurysm or a mass lesion. Testing must be done if a patient is seen during the first attack or the symptoms last longer than 2 weeks. If a patient has a history of recurring attacks with interval clearing of symptoms, further diagnostic neurological testing may not be necessary; in all likelihood, patients have had previous studies if they have had recurring attacks.

Because the patient with ophthalmoplegic migraine may have only one or two attacks, it is difficult to recommend any specific treatment. The pain usually subsides within a few days and may not be responsive to the usual abortive drugs used to treat migraine. Large doses of corticosteroids used very early in an attack may be indicated in an attempt to reduce inflammation and edema. If diplopia is distressing, the use of eye patches may be symptomatically helpful. If the attacks occur quite frequently, prevention with one of the usual migraine prophylactic drugs is indicated. Because this condition is so rare, there has been very little written about specific treatment.

Hemiplegic Migraine

Hemiplegic migraine means that the migraine attack is accompanied by unilateral motor deficits. Over the years, unilateral sensory deficits have often been included under this diagnosis. Hemiplegic migraine, however, should be restricted to migraine headaches in which there is weakness. Sensory symptoms often occur along with weakness. Like all of the migrainous conditions, these symptoms are usually transient, but on rare occasions, they can be permanent. Perhaps one third of all migraineurs will at one time experience motor or sensory symptoms during an attack of migraine.[16] It is unusual for motor or sensory symptoms to occur with every attack, but there are a small number of persons who have repeated attacks of migraine with weakness. Frequently, dysphasia, vertigo, and visual abnormalities accompany an attack of unilateral weakness; symptoms of that type implicate involvement of the brainstem during the attack. In a study of aura symptoms in 83 patients with familial hemiplegic migraine, 55 (66%) had symptoms fulfilling the criteria for basilar migraine.[17]

Hemiplegic migraine can be separated into familial and nonfamilial hemiplegic migraine. Episodes of hemiplegic migraine of the nonfamilial type occur sporadically in persons with migraine.[16, 18] It is quite rare for a migraineur to have recurring attacks of unilateral weakness with their headaches.

In persons with familial hemiplegic migraine, the neurological symptoms may begin as an aura to a migraine attack or develop during the attack of migraine and linger for days or weeks. Most patients with familial hemiplegic migraine will consistently have the same pattern with each attack. In the nonfamilial type, neurological symptoms usually precede the pain as an aura and do not last as long after the attack. All of the usual migrainous symptoms, such as nausea, vomiting, visual symptoms, photophobia, phonophobia, and mental aberrations, can occur along with the unilateral weakness. Glista et al[18] reported a family with familial hemiplegic migraine who seemed to have their attacks triggered by minor head trauma.

Researchers have found a locus on chromosome 19 in the majority of the few families with familial hemiplegic migraine who have been investigated.[19] The families with the chromosome 19–linked variety did not differ in clinical symptoms from those who were not linked to chromosome 19.[19] It has been postulated that cerebral edema secondary to ischemia rather than ischemia alone accounts for the prolonged neurological symptoms because the symptoms often resolve completely without residual deficit.[16, 20] Prolonged ischemia with cerebral infarction probably accounts for the few episodes that are followed by permanent neurological deficits. Death has been reported subsequent to attacks of hemiplegic migraine, but it is very rare.[21]

The diagnosis of hemiplegic migraine, particularly of the familial type, is aided by a family history of repeated attacks of weakness. If a typical unilateral sick headache accompanies the neurological symptoms, the diagnosis of migraine is certainly suggested. The diagnosis is made, however, only after exclusion of other causes of vascular and metabolic etiology. Typically, the migrainous neurological symptoms "march," or spread, throughout the area involved rather than hitting suddenly with maximal deficit. The symptoms may begin centrally or peripherally and move in the opposite direction. If several similar attacks have occurred, the possibility of finding an underlying cause is quite unlikely.

Basilar Migraine

Vertebrobasilar migraine or basilar artery migraine was first described by Bickerstaff in 1961.[22] *Basilar migraine* is the term used in the International Headache Society classification.[1] Although Bickerstaff's initial description stated that this condition usually occurs in adolescent females, it does occur in males and in younger children; it may occur as often in males. The symptoms occurring in basilar migraine are symptoms consistent with dysfunction of the posterior part of the brain supplied by the vertebrobasilar artery system. The neurological symptoms usually precede the headache, as occurs with any other aura, but they may also begin during the actual painful phase. As with any migraine attack, the neurological symptoms may linger for hours and sometimes days, but they usually will completely resolve. The headache often is bilateral in the posterior part of the head, but it may radiate into the frontal and temporal areas and perhaps be unilateral. The pain is usually of moderate severity and pulsatile like the usual migraine attack. Nausea is commonly present and may progress to intractable vomiting. As may occur with any migraine syndrome, there are times in which the headache phase is mild or even totally absent, which may delay the proper diagnosis if migraine is not considered.

Common neurological symptoms occurring with a basilar migraine attack include visual disturbances, tinnitus, hearing loss, diplopia, and vertigo. Dysphasia with slurring of speech is not uncommon. Ataxia may be the most common symptom and may not be due to vertigo or visual disturbances. Typically, the paresthesias of basilar migraine are bilateral and begin in the periphery of all four extremities, with gradual spreading up the limbs. Visual and neurological symptoms usually occur at the very onset of the attack before the pain becomes intense. Confusion and disorientation may also occur. This constellation of symptoms, especially if occurring in a teenager, may suggest drug intoxication or encephalitis.

Fluctuating hearing loss and vertigo have been noted to be presenting symptoms of basilar migraine.[23] Sudden hearing loss for which no other etiology can be found may also be due to migraine.[24] Lance and Anthony[25] found that syncope occurred in about 7% of patients with migraine, which was accompanied by symptoms arising from the vertebrobasilar system. Ischemia or decreased function of the reticular activating system may occur in basilar migraine and can cause stupor or even coma that lasts for hours or days. Ischemia involving the brainstem during an attack may cause sympathetic nervous system–induced cardiac arrhythmias.[26, 27]

The differential diagnosis of basilar migraine includes arteriovenous malformation of the pontine angle, posterior fossa tumor, and multiple sclerosis. Freedman and Gray[28] reported that multiple sclerosis may be accompanied by a migrainous type of headache as part of the initial presentation in about 4% in a large group of patients with multiple sclerosis. Multiple sclerosis must therefore be included in the differential diagnosis of complicated migraine because of the neurological symptoms occurring with the headache. The subsequent course will usually make the diagnosis evident, but initially the transient nature of multiple sclerosis symptoms when accompanied by migraine may very closely mimic neurological symptoms accompanying a migraine attack.

Vertigo and Migraine

As mentioned, vertigo very commonly accompanies the attack of basilar migraine. In an evaluation of the neuro-otological manifestations of migraine, isolated vestibular symptoms were found to be much more common than auditory symptoms.[29] Although vertigo usually precedes the attack of basilar migraine, it may not occur until well into the attack. Vertigo may also occur without attacks of pain (migraine aura without headache). It has been estimated that one third of persons with migraine also have vertigo.[30]

In an extensive review of migraine and dizziness, Cutrer and Baloh[31] concluded that some attacks of vertigo are brief and represent an aura with or without headache, whereas other attacks are similar to motion sickness and last longer. They thought that the mechanisms might differ for the two types of symptoms. Some have separated Ménière's disease into cochlear and vestibular types; the former supposedly is without vertigo and the latter is without hearing loss, as opposed to the classic syndrome of vertigo and hearing loss. In a study that separated these two types, migraine was found to be present in 81% of patients with the vestibular type (vertigo only).[32]

The differentiation of vertigo of migrainous origin from other disorders may be difficult. If a typical sick headache along with other migrainous symptoms accompanies the vertigo, the diagnosis very likely is migraine. Episodic vertigo occurring for several years without decreased caloric responses or hearing loss suggests migraine as an etiology as opposed to a peripheral disorder such as Ménière's disease or vestibular neuronitis.[33]

Benign paroxysmal vertigo of childhood, which was first reported by Basser,[34] probably is a precursor of migraine. A review of the literature concerning the vestibular system and migraine in childhood found that 13% of reported cases of patients with benign paroxysmal vertigo of childhood subsequently developed migraine.[35] Also, in about 14% of reported cases of benign paroxysmal vertigo, headache was an accompanying symptom.

It appears quite certain that vertigo is a common symptom accompanying migraine, particularly basilar migraine, and that paroxysmal vertiginous attacks with or without headache often are manifestations of a migraine syndrome.

Dysphrenic Migraine

Decreased mental functioning during an attack of migraine is quite common. Migraineurs find it difficult to concentrate and often are confused. Confusion and mental aberrations may occur in association with a typical attack of migraine or in the absence of a headache. Several forms of dysphrenic migraine have been recognized. Loss of consciousness and syncope occur quite commonly in basilar migraine, as discussed. Loss of memory is prevalent in transient global amnesia, which is probably of migrainous origin. Acute confusional migraine, on the other hand, is accompanied by severe disorientation. These forms of mental aberration may be quite severe, as opposed to the mild, diminished mental function that accompanies the usual migraine attack.

Transient global amnesia is characterized by retrograde amnesia before the attack, inability to form new memories during amnesia, repetitive questioning, and absence of other neurological signs or symptoms.[36] Transient global amnesia may accompany a typical attack of migraine, or more often, it will occur without a headache (migraine aura without headache.) It is likely that transient global amnesia in the pure form without any signs of a neurological deficit represents a migrainous event of the posterior cerebral circulation. Amnesia that occurs due to cerebrovascular disease would more likely be accompanied by neurological findings. Electroencephalographic (EEG) abnormalities consisting of slow waves have been reported during transient global amnesia attacks.[37, 38] These EEG changes are similar to those observed in migraine and ischemia and therefore suggest that transient global amnesia is more likely a migrainous phenomenon than a seizure disorder, as was previously thought.

Acute confusional migraine usually occurs in adolescence and is associated with confusion, disorientation, and agitation.[39, 40] The confusion may last from only a few minutes to several hours and may or may not be accompanied by a significant headache. A family history of migraine is usually present. Minor head trauma, as occurs in contact sports, often is a precipitating event to the attack. Most patients reported in the literature with acute confusional migraine have had only one confusional episode, but they have had subsequent recurring attacks of more typical migraine headaches.

Acute confusional migraine is thought to be caused by cortical or subcortical dysfunction due to transient ischemia with or without subsequent cerebral edema. The EEG taken during an attack of confusion is usually normal but may show the typical slow waves seen in migraine instead of epileptiform discharges.[40] The differential diagnosis includes various metabolic abnormalities due to drug ingestion or toxicity, encephalitis, and postictal states. These conditions must be excluded. The postictal confusion of a seizure tends to be shorter than the confusional state of migraine.

Management of Complicated Migraine Syndromes

Treatment of any type of complicated migraine with neurological symptoms depends on the individual patient and circumstances, as does the treatment of migraine in general. Risk factors that have been implicated in cerebral disorders should be avoided, as should known risk factors of migraine. Estrogens in the form of oral contraceptives or estrogen replacement therapy may aggravate the neurological symptoms of migraine. The low-dose oral contraceptives appear to be less of a problem than the older, higher-dose contraceptives. In general, estrogen should be avoided or used with great caution in patients who have migraine that is accompanied by significant visual or neurological symptoms. Smoking should also be avoided by these patients. Hypertension can aggravate migraine, and vasoconstrictive drugs should be used with extreme caution. Evaluation for coagulation abnormalities, connective tissue diseases, vasculopathies, and cardiac disorders must be done.

If the attacks occur quite frequently, prophylactic therapy is indicated. Calcium channel blockers are the preferred drugs for prevention of complicated migraine. β-Blockers, which are most often used for the prophylactic treatment of routine migraine attacks, are also very effective. There are some, however, who believe that β-blockers should be used with caution when neurological symptoms are present in migraine. Divalproex sodium, which is effective in controlling migraine, may be effective in controlling some of these neurological complications of migraine, but it has not been studied as treatment for these conditions. Tricyclic antidepressants such as amitriptyline or doxepin may be helpful, particularly if there are contraindications to the use of the more vasoactive drugs. Cyproheptadine, an antiserotonin and antihistaminic agent, may be useful, particularly in children who have some of the complicated migraine attacks. It is poorly tolerated in adults because of sedation. Nonsteroidal anti-inflammatory agents, if not contraindicated, are helpful in reducing the number of migraine attacks. Because of platelet aggregation, which may occur in some migraineurs, antiplatelet agents theoretically might be helpful in migraine but have not been proved to be very beneficial in the prevention of migraine attacks. During an attack of migraine that is complicated by neurological or visual symptoms, supportive care with sedation, antiemetics, hydration, and analgesics is indicated. Corticosteroids are usually helpful in shortening the duration of neurological symptoms. They reduce cerebral edema, which is thought to play a role in some of the more prolonged neurological symptoms. Ergotamine tartrate, sumatriptan, and dihydroergotamine, which cause significant constriction of intracranial vessels, are best avoided in patients who have attacks of complicated migraine; however, ergotamines have been frequently used and appear not to have been associated with detrimental effects.

Migraine Aura without Headache (Migraine Equivalents, Acephalgic Migraine)

Migraine aura without headache is the term for what had been called *migraine equivalents* or *acephalgic migraine*.[1] These terms refer to any visual, neurological, or gastrointestinal symptoms that occur episodically without an associated headache. Any symptoms that accompany a migraine attack may occur without pain. The symptoms are usually those occurring as an aura to a typical migraine attack. Any neurological, visual, gastrointestinal, or other symptom may occur at any time in the absence of a headache. Recurring symptoms for which no underlying organic cause has been found should be considered possible manifestations of an underlying migrainous diathesis. Table 9–1 lists symptoms that have been described as representing migraine aura without headache. Disturbances of vascular regulation may occur in any organ system causing these symptoms, but most likely these symptoms are due to neurological, metabolic, and vascular disturbances in various areas of the central nervous system. Migraine aura without headache usually occurs in persons who have previously had migraine attacks or have a strong family history of migraine. Occasionally, they occur in persons who have never had a migraine attack.[41–43] Migraine symptoms occurring without headache are not rare and perhaps are experienced at one time by 20% of all migraineurs and by more than 40% of patients who have migraine with aura.[44, 45]

Table 9–1 Episodic Symptoms That May Represent Migraine Aura without Headache

Visual	Neurological	Other
Photopsia	Amnesia	Abdominal pain
Scotomata	Confusion	Cyclic vomiting
Hemianopsia	Hemiparesis	Coronary artery spasm
Diplopia	Paresthesia	Raynaud's disease
Blindness	Vertigo	
Metamorphopsia	Hearing loss	
	Episodic mood changes	

The diagnosis of migraine aura without headache is always made only after all other causes have been excluded, especially vascular disease and seizure disorders. These migrainous symptoms are paroxysmal and occur sporadically with symptom-free intervals. In general, symptoms will last about 15 to 30 minutes, which is similar to the aura in migraine, but occasionally they may last for a few hours. These symptoms without headache usually do not last for many hours or days, as a migraine headache does. Visual symptoms are the most frequent nonheadache phenomenon of migraine.[41, 43] Alvarez[46] investigated the visual symptoms of migraine and found that 12% of the men in his series had scotomata with no history of a migraine headache.

The most common visual symptom occurring without the headache is *photopsia*, which is the term for bright flashes of light. These flashes may occur episodically, but they usually occur as scintillations with flickering or shimmering bright designs surrounding a defect in the visual field. The classic zig-zag bright lines frequently described are called *fortification spectra*. These bright, shimmering phenomena gradually spread and enlarge as the defect moves across the visual field. A visual field defect, a *scotoma*, will also gradually enlarge or move across the field. The defect in vision may be a round spot, but it often is crescent shaped. Hemianopsia, blindness, and even metamorphopsia (distorted shapes) may occur. Visual defects of migraine are typically bright and "positive" as opposed to the dark, or "negative," defects seen in ischemic retinal disease. Quite typical of migraine are the enlarging defects and movement of these defects across the visual field. Arteriosclerotic ischemic symptoms are usually shorter in duration as well as static. The visual phenomena of migraine are usually homonomous and caused by occipital cortical dysfunction. Monocular defects, which imply retinal dysfunction, are very rare in migraine, as previously discussed. Patients who do have monocular visual defects must be thoroughly evaluated to exclude the presence of other diseases.

The most common visceral manifestation of migraine without aura is abdominal pain, although there is controversy as to whether recurrent abdominal pain can represent a migrainous phenomenon.[47] Abdominal migraine occurs most often in children and seems to be quite rare in adults. There usually is a family history of migraine. Periodic attacks of abdominal pain often accompanied by nausea and vomiting are typical.[48] The attacks of abdominal discomfort may last 1 to 6 hours. Occasionally, a mild headache will occur with these symptoms, but migraine is not thought of because the concern centers around the severe abdominal pain and nausea. Children also may have periodic or cyclic vomiting without the presence of abdominal pain or headache; this also may be a migrainous phenomenon. The child is irritable and photophobic, but the head pain may be minimal or absent. These abdominal attacks usually last several hours and are gone after sleep.

Episodic abdominal symptoms should be considered possible migrainous phenomena only after organic disease has been excluded. It may be impossible to differentiate these attacks from a type of irritable bowel syndrome. If there is a family history of migraine and there are no progressive symptoms, persons with repeated attacks of abdominal discomfort and/or nausea should be considered to have migraine. As with other migrainous symptoms without headache, the diagnosis is that of exclusion by ruling out other diseases.

Neurological symptoms occurring as migraine aura without headache also can take any form and may be quite variable. Any of the neurological symptoms described as accompanying a migraine attack may occur in the absence of a headache. The most common are paresthesias, which Fisher has labeled transient migrainous accompaniments.[41] These sensory symptoms move and spread up or down the limbs as is typical with migraine. They may move up one arm from the fingers to the body and down the opposite arm. These symptoms tend to slowly spread and last the usual 15 to 30 minutes, as does a migraine aura. The march, or spreading nature, of these symptoms is different from the sudden, abrupt onset of symptoms that occurs with a typical transient ischemic attack.

The psychic symptoms of migraine, which have been discussed in the section on dysphrenic migraine, can occur in the absence of a headache. These brief mental aberrations may occur more frequently than is realized. Transient mood disturbances, confusional states, and periodic amnesia can all occur in the absence of head pain. There usually is a prior history of migraine headaches or a strong family history of migraine.

Disorders of altered vasomotor stability, such as Raynaud's disease, flushing, urticaria, and even coronary artery spasm, are often related to migraine. The term *cardiac migraine* was used in 1974 to describe a group of patients with migraine, functional hypoglycemia, and typical anginal-type chest pains.[49] The chest pains were considered to be due to coronary artery spasm related to sympathetic overactivity, which is often seen in the migraine sufferer. Another large study of persons with variant-type angina revealed a 26% incidence of migraine, which is higher than the incidence of migraine in the general population.[50]

As discussed, vertigo, which is so common in basilar migraine, may occur in persons in the absence of a headache. Recurrent vertigo attacks without cochlear or neurological symptoms are probably manifestations of a migrainous disorder.

Treatment of Migraine Aura without Headache

The periodic symptoms occurring without a headache often do not cause significant disruption of an individual's life. Generally, they do not occur too frequently, and because they are quite transient and not accompanied by disabling pain, nausea, or vomiting, treatment often is not necessary. If the attacks do occur frequently, the usual prophylactic agents that are helpful in controlling migraine attacks should be tried.

If the attacks are disturbing to the patient, as loss of vision or vertigo might be, consideration should be given to treatment of the acute attacks. Various vasodilators have been used to abort visual and neurological symptoms occurring as either a prolonged aura or an aura without headache. It was previously thought that these symptoms were due to vasoconstriction, although recent studies on the underlying pathophysiology of migraine have implicated neurogenic factors as well as vasoconstriction. Sublingual nitroglycerin administered promptly at the onset of visual or neurological symptoms preceding a headache or occurring without a headache has been shown to promptly abort these symptoms in about 50% of patients.[51] Isoproterenol, a β-adrenergic agonist, has also been shown to be effective in promptly aborting the visual symptoms of the aura of migraine.[52] The use of sublingual nifedipine, a potent vasodilator, has been shown to be effective in promptly alleviating the neurological symptoms of migraine.[53] I have had good success with the use of both sublingual nifedipine and nitroglycerin in patients who have prolonged auras of headache or aura without headache. It is of interest that the use of these vasodilators is not usually associated with a severe headache, and most of the time the headache does not occur or is lessened. When vasodilators are used at times other than at the onset of an acute attack, they almost always induce a throbbing, pounding, severe headache in a patient with migraine. These vasodilators in all likelihood have properties in addition to their vasodilating effects; other pharmacological actions may account for their beneficial effects.

The use of ergotamine tartrate for symptoms without headache is quite controversial. It has been used for many years to abort acute attacks of migraine. Although there might be concern about prolongation of symptoms due to its vasoconstrictive effect, in practice, ergotamine tartrate usually helps alleviate symptoms and does not aggravate or prolong neurological symptoms. It probably does not reach significant blood levels until the aura is clearing. Injectable sumatriptan should not be used during the acute aura or for the relief of an aura without headache; the oral form of sumatriptan may be used at the onset of an aura to abort the headache pain.

Benign Exertional Headache

Benign exertional headache is a vascular headache brought on by exertion or any activity involving the Valsalva maneuver. There have been specific headache types described that occur with exertion. Common forms of exercise, such as running, playing football, playing tennis, weight-lifting, or sexual intercourse, can cause a vascular type of headache. Other *acute straining* activity, such as coughing, sneezing, straining, and lifting, can at times precipitate a vascular type of headache. These short bilateral headaches are usually called *cough headaches*. The underlying etiology is uncertain, but it is thought that various factors may be involved, including increased venous pressure in the cranium, release of vasoactive substances, transient hypertension, and increased sympathetic tone. The headache that usually occurs with physical exercise is a generalized, throbbing pulsatile pain that does not last more than a few minutes to 1 or 2 hours. It usually occurs at the height of exertion or just after activity.[54, 55]

A more prolonged type of exertional headache has been reported that responds to indomethacin.[56] The majority of patients with exertional headache have or have had migraine headaches. Clinically, an exertional type of headache often occurs after an acute febrile or viral illness. This headache may last for several weeks or even several months. It is aggravated by any Valsalva maneuver but will gradually diminish over the ensuing weeks or months. It is essential that intracranial pathology such as mass lesions, subarachnoid hemorrhage, subdural hematoma, or an Arnold-Chiari malformation be excluded, particularly if the headache is of recent onset. A recent review of exertional headaches revealed intracranial pathology in 42% of 72 patients with cough, exertional, or sexual headaches. Of 30 patients with cough headache, 57% had Chiari type I malformation.[57]

Coital or *orgasmic headache* is a form of exertional headache. Three types of orgasmic headache have been described.[58] (1) The most severe type usually occurs in a person with a background history of vascular headache; it occurs three times as often in males.[59] It is intense but rarely prolonged in duration. It tends to be a transient condition but can occur in cycles or be chronic and recurring. Sudden increases in blood pressure or perhaps sudden rises in vasoactive substances such as prostaglandins have been implicated in the etiology of this type of orgasmic headache. (2) A dull, aching type of headache that is probably due to intense contraction of the neck and scalp muscles during foreplay and intercourse is another type of coital headache. (3) The third type, which is quite rare, is of sudden onset; it is aggravated by standing and may linger for a few weeks.

Management of exertional headache depends on the frequency and severity of symptoms. If the headaches occur quite often, daily prophylactic medication with one of the antimigrainous agents should be considered. The nonsteroidal anti-inflammatory agents are often quite effective in alleviating exertional headache. These agents can be used on a daily prophylactic basis; the faster-acting agents can be used acutely as abortive agents.

Ergotamine tartrate is also effective as an acute measure. Any of these agents may be taken before the physical activity, thereby preventing the subsequent headache, or at the acute onset of the pain.

Cyclic or Cluster Migraine

Cluster migraine is a confusing term and should not be used. Many people use this term when they are actually talking about *cluster headache*, which is a separate entity from migraine. There are patients with migraine, however, who seem to have a "clustering" of their migraine attacks, followed by a relatively long period of remission. These attacks are definitely migraine in type and are not cluster headaches. A better term might be *cyclic migraine*, which has been used to describe this type of phenomenon. The intermittent use of prophylactic agents, such as β-blockers, calcium channel blockers, nonsteroidal anti-inflammatory agents, and methysergide, can be beneficial for this cyclic type of migraine. Lithium carbonate has also been used with good success.[60] The usual acute abortive agents, such as ergotamine tartrate, sumatriptan, isometheptene mucate, and the fast-acting anti-inflammatory agents, can be used for individual migraine attacks.

Carotidynia

Carotidynia is a condition in which the carotid artery in the neck is periodically painful; this can be considered a "migraine in the neck." It is not uncommon, but the diagnosis is often overlooked.[61, 62] The carotid artery periodically swells, distends in the neck, and is quite tender. Typically, the attack lasts for several days and will recur at periodic intervals very similar to a typical migraine pattern. Very often, this dilated, tender carotid artery is mistaken for adenopathy; occasionally, patients are treated for recurring sore throats with antibiotics. If the attacks are frequent, the usual prophylactic migrainous medication should be used. Acutely, nonsteroidal anti-inflammatory drugs and short courses of steroids are usually quite effective if ergotamine tartrate or sumatriptan has been ineffective or is contraindicated.

References

1. Olesen J. Classification and diagnostic criteria for headache disorders, cranial neuralgias, and facial pain. Cephalalgia 1988;8(suppl 7):1–96.
2. Lance JW. Mechanism and Management of Headache, 4th ed. London; Butterworths; 1982:123.
3. Welch KMA, Levine SR. Migraine-related stroke in the context of the International Headache Society classification of head pain. Arch Neurol 1990;47:458–462.
4. Broderick JP, Swanson JW. Migraine-related strokes. Arch Neurol 1987;44:868–871.
5. Hart RG, Miller VT. Cerebral infarction in young adults: A practical approach. Stroke 1983;24:110–114.
6. Spaccavento LJ, Solomon GD. Migraine as an etiology of stroke in young adults. Headache 1984;24:19–22.
7. Tzourio C, Iglesias S, Jean-Baptiste H, et al. Migraine and risk of ischaemic stroke: A case-control study. Br Med J 1993;307:289–293.
8. Bartelson JD. Transient and persistent neurological manifestations of migraine. Stroke 1984;15:383–386.
9. Hedges TR, Lackman RD. Isolated ophthalmic migraine in the differential diagnosis of cerebro-ocular ischemia. Stroke 1976;7:379–381.
10. Lewis LA, Vijayan N, Watson C, et al. Visual field loss in migraine. Ophthalmology 1989;96:321–326.
11. Drummond PD, Anderson M. Visual field loss after attacks of migraine with aura. Cephalalgia 1992;12:349–352.
12. Bogousslavsky J, Regli F, VanMelle G, et al. Migraine stroke. Neurology 1988;38:223–227.
13. Bickerstaff ER. Migraine variants and complications. In Blau JN, ed. Migraine: Clinical and Research Aspects. Baltimore, MD: Johns Hopkins University Press; 1987:61–65.
14. Vijayan N. Ophthalmoplegic migraine: Ischemic or compressive neuropathy? Headache 1980;20:300–304.
15. Ostergaard JR, Moller HU, Christensen T. Recurrent ophthalmoplegia in childhood: Diagnostic and etiologic considerations. Cephalalgia 1996;16:276–277.
16. Bradshaw P, Parsons M. Hemiplegic migraine: a clinical study. Cleveland Q J Med 1965;34:65–85.
17. Haan J, Terwindt GM, Ophoff RA, et al. Is familial hemiplegic migraine a hereditary form of basilar migraine? Cephalalgia 1995;15:477–481.
18. Glista GG, Mellinger JF, Rooke ED. Familial hemiplegic migraine. Mayo Clin Proc 1975;50:307–311.
19. Terwindt G, Haan J, Ophoff RA, et al. Familial hemiplegic migraine: Clinical comparison of families linked and unlinked to chromosome 19. Cephalalgia 1996;16:153–155.

20. Rosenbaum HE. Familial hemiplegic migraine. Neurology 1960;10:164–170.
21. Neligan P, Harriman DGF, Pearce J. Respiratory arrest in familial hemiplegic migraine: A clinical and pathological study. Br Med J 1977;2:732–734.
22. Bickerstaff ER. Basilar artery migraine. Lancet 1961;1:15–17.
23. Love JT. Basilar artery migraine presenting as fluctuating hearing loss and vertigo. ORL J Otorhinolaryngol Relat Spec 1978;86:450–458.
24. Virre ES, Baloh RW. Migraine as a cause of sudden hearing loss. Headache 1996;36:24–28.
25. Lance JW, Anthony M. Some clinical aspects of migraine. Arch Neurol 1966;15:356–361.
26. Gilroy J, Lerman VJ. Cardiac arrhythmia in basilar migraine. Headache 1982;22:140.
27. Petersen J, Scruton D, Downie AW. Basilar artery migraine with transient atrial fibrillation. Br Med J 1977;2:1125–1126.
28. Freedman MS, Gray TA. Vascular headache: A presenting symptom of multiple sclerosis. Can J Neurol Sci 1989;16:63–66.
29. Kayan A, Hood JD. Neuro-otological manifestations of migraine. Brain 1984;107:1123–1142.
30. Selby G, Lance JW. Observations on 500 cases of migraine and allied vascular headache. J Neurol Neurosurg Psychiatry 1960;23:23–32.
31. Cutrer FM, Baloh RW. Migraine-associated dizziness. Headache 1992;32:300–304.
32. Rassekh CH, Harker LA. The presence of migraine in Meniere's disease. Laryngoscope 1992;102:135–138.
33. Harker LA, Rassekh CH. Episodic vertigo in basilar artery migraine. Otolaryngol Head Neck Surg 1987;96:239–250.
34. Basser LS. Benign paroxysmal vertigo of childhood. Brain 1964;87:141–152.
35. Parker W. Migraine and the vestibular system in childhood and adolescence. Am J Otol 1989;10:364–371.
36. Caplan L, Chedra F, Lhermitte F, et al. Transient global amnesia and migraine. Neurology 1981;31:1167–1170.
37. Mathew NT, Meyer JS. Pathogenesis and natural history of transient global amnesia. Stroke 1974;5:303–311.
38. Steinmetz EF, Vroom FQ. Transient global amnesia. Neurology 1972;22:1193–1200.
39. Gascon G, Barlow C. Juvenile migraine presenting as an acute confusional state. Pediatrics 1970;45:628–635.
40. Emery ES. Acute confusional state in children with migraine. Pediatrics 1977;60:110–114.
41. Fisher CM. Late-life migraine accompaniments as a cause of unexplained transient ischemic attacks. Can J Neurol Sci 1980;7:9–17.
42. O'Conner PS, Tredici TJ. Acephalgic migraine. Ophthalmology 1981;88:999–1003.
43. Whitty CWM. Migraine without headache. Lancet 1967;2:283–285.
44. Dalessio DJ. Wolff's Headache and Other Head Pain, 5th ed. New York: Oxford University Press; 1987:5.
45. Ziegler DK, Hassanein RS. Specific headache phenomena: Their frequency and coincidence. Headache 1990;30:152–156.
46. Alvarez WC. The migrainous scotomata as studied in 618 persons. Am J Ophthalmol 1960;49:489–504.
47. Symon DNK, Hockaday J. Is there a place for 'abdominal migraine' as a separate entity in the IHS classification? Cephalalgia 1992;12:345–348.
48. Lundberg PO. Abdominal migraine: Diagnoses and therapy. Headache 1975;15:122–125.
49. Sotomayor LA. Cardiac migraine: Report of twelve cases. Angiology 1974;25:161–171.
50. Miller D, Waters DD, Warnica W, et al. Is variant angina the coronary manifestation of a generalized vasospastic disorder? N Engl J Med 1981;304:763–766.
51. Kunkel RS. Vasodilator therapy for classic migraine headaches. In: Rose FC, ed. Advances in Migraine Research and Therapy. New York: Raven Press; 1982:205–209.
52. Kupersmith MJ, Hass WK, Chase NE. Isoproterenol treatment of visual symptoms in migraine. Stroke 1979;10:299–305.
53. Goldner JA, Leavitt LP. Treatment of complicated migraine with sublingual nefedipine. Headache 1987;27:484–486.
54. Dalessio DJ. Effort migraine. Headache 1974;14:53.
55. Rooke ED. Benign exertional headache. Med Clin North Am 1968;52:801–808.
56. Diamond S. Prolonged benign exertional headache: Its clinical characteristics and response to indomethacin. Headache 1982;22:96–98.
57. Pascual J, Iglesias F, Oterino A, et al. Cough, exertional and sexual headache: An analysis of 72 benign and symptomatic cases. Neurology 1996;46:1520–1524.
58. Paulson GW, Klawans HL. Benign orgasmic cephalgia. Headache 1974;13:181–187.
59. Ostergaard JR, Kraft M. Benign coital headaches. Cephalalgia 1992;12:353–355.
60. Medina JL, Diamond S. Cyclical migraine. Arch Neurol 1981;38:341–344.
61. Lovshin LL. Carotidynia. Headache 1977; 17:192–193.
62. Raskin NH, Prusiner S. Carotidynia. Neurology 1977;27:43–46.

10

Traction and Inflammatory Headache and Cranial Neuralgias

Donald J. Dalessio, M.D.

Mass Lesions

Headache from intracranial sources is most often produced by inflammation, traction, and displacement or distention of the pain-sensitive structures of the head, usually blood vessels. Most of the displacement is the result of traction; hence, the term *traction headache* is used to identify this group. A traction headache can be elicited by hematoma of any type, abscess, nonspecific brain "edema," and lumbar puncture. It is especially a symptom of brain tumor.

Headache, particularly a rapidly expanding lesion producing traction on the pain-sensitive structures of the head, is one of the cardinal signs of brain tumor. This is especially true if the ventricular system is compromised, with obstruction of absorption or flow of cerebrospinal fluid (CSF), and hydrocephalus is produced.

The headache resulting from a brain tumor may be associated with some neurological signs, including seizures (focal or general), progressive loss of neurological function, and mental symptoms. With these headaches, the onset is usually intermittent, and the pain is often dull and aching. The frequency and duration will progressively increase, and the headache will sometimes be altered by changes in posture and tone. Headache is almost always a prominent finding with rapid increase in intracranial pressure. With more slowly growing tumors, headache may be transitory or mild or easily relieved by common analgesics, and the patient's description of head pain in this situation may be desultory. Worse head pains usually are not related to tumor but are related to vascular headaches or the major neuralgias. The following generalizations concerning headache as an aid to localization in patients with brain tumor seem justified:

- Although the headache of brain tumor may be referred from a distant intracranial source, it approximately overlies the tumor in about one third of patients.
- If the tumor is above the tentorium, the pain frequently occurs at the vertex or in the frontal regions.
- If the tumor is below the tentorium, the pain is occipital, and cervical muscle spasm may be present.
- Headache is almost always present with posterior fossa tumor.
- If the tumor is midline, the pain may be increased with cough, straining, or sudden head movement. (This also occurs with migraine.)
- If the tumor is hemispheric, the pain is usually felt on the same side of the head.
- If the tumor is chiasmal, at the sella, the pain may be referred to the vertex.

Quality and Intensity of Brain Tumor Headache

In studies by Kunkle et al,[1, 2] only patients who adequately described their symptoms were reported. The headache was usually a deep, aching, steady, dull pain. It was not rhythmic and was seldom throbbing. It was usually intermittent, but in one tenth of the patients it was continuous. The headache was sometimes severe, but rarely was it as intense as that of migraine or the headache associated with ruptured cerebral aneurysm, meningitis, or certain febrile illnesses or induced by certain drugs. It was usually relieved with acetylsalicylic acid or cold packs applied to the scalp, both indications of its moderate intensity. It rarely interfered with sleep. It was aggravated by coughing or straining at stool, and sometimes it was worse in the erect than in the recumbent position. It also was commonly aggravated by the onset of a minor infection. If there was any variation in intensity during the 24-hour cycle, it was worse in the early morning.

Even when the tumor directly compressed or extensively stretched the cranial nerves containing pain afferents, the pain was not equal in intensity to that of tic douloureux and indeed often was mild or absent.

Unless the pain was severe, nausea with tumor headache was slight. Vomiting occurred with displacement or compression of the medulla and was sometimes "projectile," perhaps because it was unexpected when unaccompanied by nausea. The headache, when occipital or suboccipital, was sometimes associated with "stiffness" or aching of the muscles of the neck and tilting of the head toward the side of the tumor.

Various Types of Tumors in Relation to Headache

Among patients with craniopharyngiomas, headache as an initial symptom was rare, and its location was unpredictable. The hypophysial adenomas also rarely produced headache as an initial symptom, and the site of the headache presented nothing of specific or helpful value.

Among most of the patients with headache due to cerebellopontine angle tumors, the headache was a leading clue in the localization of the lesion, although headache did not occur as an early symptom. Headache solely in the postauricular area was almost specific, especially before gross displacement of the brain occurred. The pain of headaches due to tumors of the posterior fossa is referred to the occipital and neck areas.

Among patients with meningiomas (all except one was supratentorial), headache was a first symptom in one third. In about one half of the 14 patients with headache, the headache was predominantly unilateral and on the same side as the tumor; in all except two of the 14 patients, the headache was due to local traction. Because the meningiomas are situated in contact with pain-sensitive structures at the base and over the convexities, it might be expected that headache as an initial symptom would occur in a higher proportion than indicated by the one third of patients. It is probable, however, that the slow growth and bone invasion offset the effects of proximity to pain-sensitive vascular structures.

Headache was a first symptom of gliomas, despite their lack of direct contact with pain-sensitive structures, in one half of the patients in whom the glioma occurred above the tentorium and even more frequently in those in whom it occurred below the tentorium. Such tumor produced headaches as an early manifestation, probably because of their speed of growth and the likelihood of occluding lateral, third, and fourth ventricles.

Headache from Non-neoplastic Intracranial Mass Lesions

Non-neoplastic intracranial mass lesions, such as hematomas and abscesses, also cause headache and follow the same general rules discussed. Because their clinical presentation is different, however, they are discussed separately.

Headache Resulting from Parenchymal and Epidural Abscess

Because parenchymal abscess is often associated with disease of adjacent nasal and aural structures, it is common to have headache from the latter source long before the actual involvement of brain tissue. Moreover, the brain abscess does not become of adequate size to cause headache by traction and displacement until about 2 months after parenchymatous breakdown has begun. At this time, the abscess is of maximal size and is usually walled off. It is, in essence, then a cystic tumor that has gradually increased in size through the accumulation of fluid. Therefore, headache from the abscess manifests itself with the development of papilledema and other evidence of local traction and generalized displacement of the brain. The mechanisms and clinical features are thus similar to all other parenchymatous tumors. The headache of brain abscess is usually associated with leukocytosis, fever, and pleocytosis. It is noteworthy that brain abscess from infections of the ear may occur either above or below the tentorium. In the latter case, the evidence of brainstem embarrassment—hiccoughing, vomiting, and occipital headache—occurs early in the course of the illness.

Ray and Parsons[3] emphasized that if headache associated with sinus disease and osteomyelitis of the adjacent bony wall persists after drainage of the sinus, it is likely that epidural abscess is also present. Such epidural abscesses occur in the frontal region adjacent to the diseased frontal, ethmoid, and sphenoid sinuses and, after osteomyelitis of the mastoid bone, in the postauricular occipital region.

Headache Resulting from Intracranial Hematoma

The headache resulting from intracranial hematoma cannot be discussed adequately without the division of hematomas into a number of subgroups. These are presented separately, although on some occasions it may not be possible to differentiate them clinically.

Epidural Hematoma

If the patient is conscious, headache may be a prominent early symptom of epidural hematoma because the pain-sensitive vascular structures in the dura are being separated from their natural attachment to the bone. As the mass lesion increases in size, producing brain compression and deteriorating consciousness, the pain input may be manifest as restlessness and combativeness without a specific complaint of headache. The progression of a head-injured patient from headache to restlessness should therefore alert the physician to the possibility of an expanding intracranial mass. Remember that epidural hematoma most frequently appears after injury to the middle meningeal artery on the undersurface of the temporal bone.

Subdural Hematoma

The hematomas that occur between the dura and brain can be classified into five clinical entities.

Acute Subdural Hematomas. Acute subdural hematomas become clinically significant within 48 hours of injury. They occur most commonly in patients who have experienced severe head injury and are unconscious. The complaint of headache is therefore not an important clinical sign.

Subacute Subdural Hematomas. Subacute subdural hematomas become clinically significant 2 to 14 days after injury. They are usually found when a patient fails to recover as expected after a head injury. Headache may or may not be present, but when present it is similar to that described with chronic subdural hematoma. Surgery is almost always indicated. Rarely do the hematomas absorb spontaneously.

Chronic Subdural Hematomas. Chronic subdural hematomas become clinically significant more than 14 days after head injury. The antecedent injury was usually mild to moderate, and in a significant number of cases no history of injury can be elicited.

Headache is the most common complaint in these patients, and it is usually more troublesome than the headache of brain tumor. If the headache is ignored, progressive signs of brain compression may ultimately ensue; these signs may be nonspecific and nonlocalizing, such as apathy, inappropriate behavior, and confusion. The manifestations may result in the patient's admission to a mental hospital.

The intracranial pressure may be normal in a patient with chronic subdural hematoma despite the considerable shift of intracranial structures, and papilledema is uncommon. The headache is presumed to be secondary to the stretching of tributary veins that pass from the cerebral hemispheres to the sagittal sinus. As the subdural collection gradually enlarges from recurrent bleeding or osmotic fluid shifts, the stretching of these veins becomes more marked, and the headache becomes more intense. It is not uncommon for these patients to note that sudden head movement or jolts accentuate the headache, and head tapping can be used as a clinical sign. One can visualize how a stretched vein could easily be stimulated by minor head movement.

Chronic Subdural Hematoma of the Elderly. Chronic subdural hematoma of the elderly should be recognized as a separate entity because it can present as mental deterioration without headache. The existence of brain atrophy may allow this condition to occur because a considerable subdural mass can be accommodated with only minimal shift or stretch of structure. In addition, these lesions are frequently bilateral, and the potential for lateral displacement is counterbalanced.

Infantile Subdural Hematoma. Infantile subdural hematomas are discussed separately because the expansivity of the skull minimizes increases in intracranial pressure and the young child may not be able to complain of headache even if it occurs. Children with subdural hematomas are frequently restless and irritable, however, suggesting that head pain may be present.

Postpuncture Headache

Postpuncture headache is defined as the headache, mild or severe, that may appear a few hours to several days after lumbar puncture, lasting a variable period of days or, rarely, weeks. It is a sequel to lumbar puncture in approximately one of every four patients. The pain is a dull, deep ache and may be throbbing. It is usually bifrontal and often is also suboccipital. In the latter position, it may be associated with moderate stiffness of the neck. Its occurrence when the subject is erect and its virtual elimination when the patient is horizontal are most characteristic. Shaking the head makes the pain more intense. It is usually resistant to all treatment except rest in bed in the horizontal position and the passage of time. Because of the frequency of its occurrence, the occasional severity of the discomfort, and the duration of the disability, headache of this type has been of clinical interest ever since the technique of lumbar puncture was introduced. Although theories concerning postpuncture headache have been clearly contradictory, the weight of the evidence supports the view that it is usually related to a loss of CSF secondary to leakage through the dural hole.

Lasater[4] described a syndrome of primary intracranial hypotension, with symptomatology that is identical to that of postpuncture headache. Headache is present in the upright position and is relieved by recumbency. Nausea, vomiting, vertigo, pallor, and sweating may accompany the headache. CSF pressure is always very low. The symptoms last from 2 to 16 weeks and subside spontaneously. There is no specific therapy, and to date, the cause is unknown. Lasater suggests that the syndrome may be the result of leakage of CSF from a tear in the arachnoid or the dural sheath of a spinal nerve root.

Other Causes of Low Cerebrospinal Fluid Pressure Headache

Headache can occur with any condition resulting in decreased intracranial pressure, such as CSF rhinorrhea or an inappropriately functioning ventricular shunt. In the former, there usually is a history of head injury, and in the latter, of course, there is a history of shunt insertion. In both instances, as one would expect, the headache is aggravated by the subject being erect or by rapid head movements and is relieved by the subject lying down. The appropriate therapy is correction of the offending lesion.

Headache with Chronic or Marked Elevations of Intracranial Pressure

Although it has been stated that headache does not always occur with mild to moderate elevations of intracranial traction or distortions of pain-sensitive structures, at least two conditions in which this is not the case—acute hydrocephalus and essential intracranial hypertension—must be recognized. The mechanisms underlying the cause of head pain are not understood, but because of the severity or chronicity of the pressure change, one must assume that shift of structures does occur and is sufficient to put traction on pain-sensitive areas.

Acute Hydrocephalus

The acute increase in intracranial pressure that occurs with ventricular obstruction or shunt malfunction in a treated hydrocephalic patient usually causes severe headache followed by visual disturbances. Because vascular perfusion of the brain is reduced as intracranial pressure approaches mean systemic arterial pressure, permanent neurological deficit or death can result if emergency ventricular drainage is not instituted. Lumbar puncture is contraindicated if this situation is suspected, and papilledema may not occur.

Benign Intracranial Hypertension

The term *benign intracranial hypertension* refers to a syndrome of increased intracranial pressure for which no specific cause can be determined. Definitive diagnosis cannot be made without excluding brain tumors and other intracranial mass lesions, infection, hypertensive encephalopathy, pulmonary encephalopathy (related to chronic CO_2 toxicity), and obstruction of the cerebral ventricles from any cause. The adjective *benign* is used because spontaneous recovery usually occurs, although this is not invariable; indeed, permanent visual loss may occur. Etiological factors that may be associated with benign intracranial hypertension include (in addition to intracranial venous occlusion) menstrual dysfunction, deficiency of the adrenals, corticosteroid therapy, hypoparathyroidism, vitamin A intoxication, administration of tetracycline in infants, poison, and insecticide.

Papilledema (sometimes with retinal hemorrhages) that reflects the increased intracranial pressure is often present. Generalized headache, giddiness, and vomiting occur in the majority of cases, but these symptoms are usually mild. The headache is generalized, nonthrobbing, or of low intensity and is usually increased by sudden jolting or rotating of the head. Some degree of blurring of vision develops with persistence of papilledema; occasionally, visual acuity is significantly diminished, but blindness is rare. Perimetry discloses only enlargement of blind spots and minimal restriction of peripheral vision. Diplopia as a result of abducens nerve palsy secondary to increased intracranial pressure sometimes occurs. Convulsions are rare. The patient's feeling and appearance of well-being are striking. They are out of keeping with the papilledema and increased intracranial pressure and are in contrast to what is so commonly observed in patients with papilledema due to brain neoplasm or subdural hematoma.

The term *otitic hydrocephalus* arose because of the once-frequent association of the syndrome with an infectious process of the ear. Accumulated evidence has indicated that increased intracranial pressure in conjunction with ear infection results from thrombosis of the dural venous sinuses (transverse or superior sagittal sinus). Thrombosis or phlebitis of these sinuses has also been implicated in the presence of systemic infections and in conjunction with phlebothrombosis or thrombophlebitis elsewhere in the body.

In the syndrome of pseudotumor, the resting spinal pressures vary from 220 to 600 mm of water. The fluid is always clear, colorless, and without any abnormality of cellular or chemical constituents. Indeed, the protein content of the CSF may be unusually low.

The electroencephalogram is usually normal. Occasionally, diffuse slowing with high-amplitude waves has been reported. The computed tomography scan of the head shows small or narrowed ventricles, with little or no displacement.

Srensen et al[5] reviewed the clinical course and progress of pseudotumor cerebri. Twenty-four consecutive patients were studied over a period of 49 months. Most patients responded well to acetazolamide, but approximately one fourth had a protracted course with persistent headache, asthenia, and memory impairment. A shunt operation was required in five patients. Almost half of the patients had chronic changes of the optic discs, and one patient developed optic atrophy and severe visual impairment.

For a full discussion of the etiology and treatment of the subject, see Corbett and Thompson.[6]

Arteritis and Infections

Headaches can be caused by arteritis and infections. These headaches are related to inflammatory processes within or without the skull, in particular to meningitis, intracranial arteritis, and phlebitis. The pain is evoked by inflammatory responses that include those of the pain-sensitive structures of the head. The head pain is, in most instances, coincident with the course of the disease, usually abating as the disease is brought under control, and is not recurrent or paroxysmal.

Much of headache pain relates to changes in blood vessels. In particular, arterial inflammation is considered to be painful, and angiitis occurs as a frequent complication of immunological disorders (Table 10–1). Headache is especially associated with periarteritis nodosa and giant cell arteritis. It is not com-

Table 10–1 Immunological Diseases and Angiitis

Periarteritis nodosa (polyarteritis nodosa)
Giant cell arteritis (temporal arteritis)
Connective tissue disease ("collagen disease") associated with
Rheumatoid arthritis
Scleroderma
Polymyositis and dermatomyositis
Rheumatic fever
Erythema nodosum
Sjögren's syndrome
Hypersensitivity angiitis
Drug reaction
Henoch-Schönlein purpura
Systemic lupus erythematosus
Mixed cryoglobulinemia
Goodpasture's syndrome
Hypergammaglobulinemic purpura
C2 deficiency with vasculitis
Australia antigenemia with vasculitis

monly associated with systemic lupus erythematosus unless there are other signs of involvement of the central nervous system.

In temporal arteritis, a similar pathological picture occurs, except that the inflammatory reaction may be limited to the cranial arteries. The elastic tissues appear frayed or fragmented, and giant cells within the vessel walls are almost a constant feature of the pathological findings. The giant cells are most numerous in the region of the deranged internal elastic lamina.

Not all patients with temporal arteritis have headache, but when present, the headache is of high intensity, of a deep aching quality, throbbing, and persistent. In addition to the aching and throbbing, there often is a burning component, unlike most other vascular headaches. The headache is slightly worse when the patient lies flat in bed and is diminished in intensity with the upright or half-upright position. It is somewhat reduced in intensity by digital pressure on the common carotid artery on the affected side and is made worse by stooping over. There is hyperalgesia of the scalp, and the distended arteries are extremely tender, so any pressure greatly increases the pain.

Some patients may have pain on mastication, and in some it may be the initial symptom. Facial swelling and redness of the skin overlying the temporal arteries, with the addition of the burning component of pain, are usually noted after the onset of headache. Immediate relief from burning pain and headache may follow biopsy of the inflamed temporal artery, and it is assumed that this is due to the interruption of the afferents for pain about the vessel.

Before the onset of the full-blown picture of temporal arteritis, there often is pain in the teeth, ear, jaw, zygoma, nuchal region, and occiput. The distribution of these symptoms suggests primary involvement of other branches of the external carotid artery, notably the external and internal maxillary arteries.

Other arteries may also be involved, including the major vessels of the aorta, coronaries, and arteries of the limbs. Large- and medium-sized arteries are the principal sites of the inflammatory process. Aneurysm formation may occur in association with the arteritis.

The presenting complaint may be of ocular symptoms. It has become evident that more than one third of patients with temporal arteritis are threatened with partial or even complete loss of vision. Diplopia and photophobia have been noted, and ophthalmoscopic evidence of occlusion of the ophthalmic artery has been apparent in some cases.

Some patients have presented with signs suggestive of cerebral damage and encephalitis during the acute stage of the illness. I have observed several patients with thrombotic strokes related to cranial arteritis. Other atypical presentations of temporal arteritis have been reported by Paulley and Hughes.[7]

If loss of vision is the presenting complaint, a medical emergency is in progress, and the patient requires urgent treatment. Treatment should not wait on the specific method used to make the diagnosis—temporal artery biopsy. Prednisone or another corticosteroid is the treatment of choice. As soon as the diagnosis is made, 40 to 60 mg should be administered. The sedimentation rate should be followed as a guide to management with prednisone. It is generally necessary to continue therapy with prednisone at a low maintenance dose of approximately 10 to 20 mg for a prolonged period.

Granulomatous Angiitis

Younger et al[8] described four patients with headache and granulomatous angiitis. In three patients, the angiitis was due to Hodgkin's lymphoma, herpes zoster, and neurosarcoidosis, respectively; a fourth patient had no obvious associated illness. Vasculitis was limited to the brain in all of the patients and involved large and small arteries and veins. The chief features were headache, fever, or mental dysfunction followed by weakness, coma, and death. None of the computed tomograms, spinal fluids, or cerebral angiograms were diagnostic. Histological evaluation of a biopsy specimen is the only way to establish the diagnosis during life.

Cranial Neuritis and Neuralgias and Temporomandibular Joint Disease

Some forms of facial pain are considered to be related to the cranial nerves, excluding the trigeminal and glossopharyngeal neuralgias. They commonly include the atypical facial neuralgias, lower-half headache, vidian neuralgias, carotidynia, and buccal neuralgia. Some of these syndromes are poorly developed and may not deserve a separate status. Some of them probably represent vascular pain or a form of migraine perceived in an unusual location. This is particularly true of lower-half headaches, which may respond to prophylaxis such as lysergic acid derivatives like methysergide.

Which symptoms are related to temporomandibular joint (TMJ) disease? The question is still being debated. I believe that facial pain can occur with TMJ disease that is usually best appreciated locally, with radiation to the jaw, the neck, and behind the ear; it is not neuritic. The syndrome consists of localized facial pain, limitation of jaw motion, muscle tenderness, and joint crepitus. Usually, the joint itself has a normal radiological appearance.

The TMJ is the only moveable joint in the head if junction of the head with the atlas is excluded. The most common complaint in TMJ disease is headache, of moderate intensity and located at the vertex, occiput, or in the face overlying the joints. Diagnosis can be difficult. The clinician should certainly palpate and auscultate the joints with significant pressure, with the patient opening and closing his or her mouth. If crepitus can be heard, osteoarthritis in the joint can be assumed. The clinician can then inject a local anesthetic (e.g., 1 mL of 2% lidocaine solution) into the joint to determine whether there is alteration in facial pain. Again, consultation with a dentist who is knowledgeable in this field is essential. Patients with TMJ disease have pain primarily from muscular tension related to dental occlusive disease. Because of localized pain, the patient begins to use the opposite side of the mouth to chew, attempting to splint the painful side, yet this has exactly the opposite effect and makes the painful joint do all the work. For example, with right TMJ disease, chewing on the left side moves the right TMJ excessively. There is no evidence that hearing loss, damage to cranial nerves, disturbances of equilibrium, development of Ménière's syndrome, or difficulty with the eustachian tubes is in any way related to this syndrome. Current concepts of etiology are that occlusal disharmony and psychophysiological factors play primary roles, with most of the dysfunction resident in the masticatory muscles rather than in the TMJ itself. Pathological changes that affect the joint, such as rheumatoid arthritis, may cause similar complaints but are by definition different problems.

Attempts to relieve pain should be directed toward relief of the muscle spasm. Mouth reconstructions are not usually indicated in this situation, and extensive surgery of the oral area should be undertaken with the greater caution because such procedures tend to reinforce the pain syndrome rather than relieve it. I suggest the use of simple sedatives and muscle relaxants if these prove to be helpful after a therapeutic trial. Placebo effects are very evident in this condition. Physical methods of pain relief, including heat, hot packs, and massage, should also be used. The physician should work closely with a dentist in therapy of this condition. The application of dental splints and similar maneuvers may prove helpful.

Reik and Hale[9] surveyed 100 consecutive headache clinic patients prospectively for features of the TMJ pain-dysfunction syndrome. They identified this syndrome in 14 of the 100 patients, mainly young women. The authors noted that the clinical characteristics of patients with TMJ disease resemble those of patients with ordinary muscle contraction headache, with a high incidence of associated depression that responded to tricyclic antidepressants as well as to physical therapy. They note that joint abnormalities were rarely seen on radiographs of the TMJ. They conclude that the TMJ pain-dysfunction syndrome appears to be a frequent, easily diagnosed, and easily treated headache.

Headache Related to Pain in the Teeth and Jaws

In addition to the TMJ syndrome, pain in the face may be related to dental disease, particularly to retrograde pulpal disease, pulpal inflammation, and periodontal disease. The practicing dentist should be able to evaluate these diseases adequately and to eliminate their source, particularly if there is radiological demonstration of a specific lesion. If there is any question regarding dental disease, the patient should be referred to a specialist who has had experience dealing with patients with chronic head and face pain.

Odontalgia may be due to pulpal disease or to inflammatory or degenerative diseases that have clear-cut clinical courses. In the early phases of such diseases, a neuralgic type of pain may occur and the patient may complain of headache, but generally there is no confusion as the process continues. As pulpal degeneration proceeds, putrefactive products result in pressures within the closed tooth, and incision and drainage of the tooth relieve the symptoms.

Another syndrome that may cause localized facial pain is the *cracked tooth syndrome*, or *incomplete tooth fracture*.[10] Often, the affected teeth are mandibular molars, with the second molar by far the most commonly involved. These teeth are seldom carious and are sensitive primarily to cold. Periodic compression may lead to an erratic clinical description of headache and face pain that may be persistent, and the etiology may not be recognized by physicians and dentists. Nevertheless, the management of such a problem is dental, and if there is a question regarding this matter, a second dental opinion should be obtained.

Chronic facial pain, particularly when unilateral, may be of dental origin or related to a disorder of the TMJ. Management of such facial pain often requires close cooperation between physician and dentist.

The syndromes delineated as trigeminal neuralgia (tic douloureux) and glossopharyngeal neuralgia are better characterized than headache due to dental and TMJ disturbance.

The Major Neuralgias

Trigeminal Neuralgia (Tic Douloureux)

The major neuralgias include trigeminal neuralgia and glossopharyngeal neuralgia. *Trigeminal neuralgia (tic douloureux)* is an episode-recurrent unilateral pain syndrome that occurs in the elderly. It almost never begins before the age of 30 years unless the patient has concomitant multiple sclerosis. The pain is of high intensity and particularly occurs in association with trigger zones. These are areas of increased sensitivity on the face, particularly about the nares and mouth, that set off the attack when they are stimulated, often by trivial sensations. Thus, the behavioral characteristic of patients with trigeminal neuralgia is to avoid touching the face or washing, shaving, biting, or chewing—any of the other maneuvers that stimulate the trigger zones and produce the pain. This avoidance technique is an invaluable clue to the diagnosis. In almost every other facial pain syndrome, patients are found massaging the painful area, abrading it, or applying heat or cold, but in trigeminal neuralgia, exactly the opposite occurs, and the patient goes to great lengths to avoid any stimulation of the face or mouth. The pain is usually a high-intensity jab that lasts less than 20 to 30 seconds, followed at times by a period of relief lasting a few seconds to a minute and then by another jab of pain. Repeated episodes of pain may occur, but the pain is not long lived, as is usually the case with other chronic facial pains.

Fromm et al[11–14] proposed a theory of the etiology and pathogenesis of trigeminal neuralgia that includes both peripheral and central mechanisms. They suggest that trigeminal neuralgia has a peripheral cause and a central pathogenesis; that is, some damage to the peripheral trigeminal ganglion leads to both a failure of segmental inhibition in the trigeminal nucleus and ectopic action potentials of the trigeminal nerve. Thus, a combination of increased firing and impaired efficiency of inhibitory mechanisms leads to paroxysmal discharges in the trigeminal nucleus, which may be provoked by trivial sensory stimuli. These are then perceived as attacks of trigeminal neuralgia when they proceed antidromically down the trigeminal nerve, where they are appreciated by the patient as pain in the face.

Glossopharyngeal Neuralgia

Glossopharyngeal tic is a similar phenomenon, with the symptoms related to the anatomic base of the glossopharyngeal nerve. In this situation, a pain similar to that described for trigeminal neuralgia is usually appreciated in the pharynx, tonsils, and ear and is often initiated by swallowing, yawning, or eating. Syncope may occur during glossopharyngeal neuralgia, presumably related to asystole as a result of stimulation of the vagus system as well.[15]

Treatment of Trigeminal and Glossopharyngeal Neuralgia

It should now be possible, in almost all cases, to relieve the pain of patients with trigeminal neuralgia (tic douloureux). Given a series of observations of a medical and surgical nature made over the past decade, a patient with this disease can be encouraged by the specific forms of treatment that should produce permanent or at least semipermanent pain remission. Therapy should require medical or surgical expertise, or more likely, both. Thus, cooperation is mandatory between physician and surgeon in the management of patients with trigeminal neuralgia.

Most authorities agree that medical treatment is indicated first, if for no other reason than that its use constitutes a therapeutic challenge to the diagnosis. If a patient presumed to have trigeminal neuralgia does not rapidly respond to carbamazepine (Tegretol) (e.g., within 24 to 48 hours), the diagnosis is in serious doubt.[16] After all, the diagnosis is made on the basis of history alone, and the patient may not be a good observer of pains or sensations unless he or she has the sensitivity of Proust.

If the patient does respond to carbamazepine, that is the treatment of choice. Clinicians who have followed patients with trigeminal neuralgia for more than a decade realize that this disease is often remitting, and it may be possible, with the use of drugs, to nudge the patient into remission, after which medication can sometimes be stopped. If this is not the case and response to carbamazepine is only partial, other drugs may be useful in the treatment of this condition, such as phenytoin and baclofen.[16] Some neurosurgeons suggest that frequent unpleasant side effects occur with carbamazepine, implying that 20% to 30% of patients taking this drug should discontinue its use. This suggestion is surprising because the drug seems to be better tolerated when used in epilepsy. Nevertheless, carbamazepine may produce undesirable sedation or idiosyncratic reactions (including, rarely, blood dyscrasias), and caution must be used. Carbamazepine should be used like a rapier, not like a bludgeon (Tables 10–2 and 10–3).

To inhibit or reduce synaptic transmission and relieve pain, one naturally turns to the anticonvulsants.[11] These drugs reduce the sensitivity of the trigger zones and relieve the pain within 4 to 24 hours, often dramatically. Generally, treatment is begun with carbamazepine (100 to 200 mg BID or TID). If this dose is well tolerated and the pain is rapidly relieved, it may be continued for several weeks or months, depending on the course of the disease. One should attempt to titrate the medication to the severity of the patient's pain. It may be necessary to continue the carbamazepine at a maintenance level, such as 200 mg/day, to keep the patient pain free.[13, 14]

If symptoms persist with an adequate dose of carbamazepine with therapeutic blood levels, I add another drug to the regimen. Usually, baclofen is the choice, beginning with 10 mg/day and increasing to 60 to 80 mg/day, in divided doses, and taken with carbamazepine. Rarely, if pain persists, a third drug such as phenytoin is added in a therapeutic dose. (Other drugs, including sodium valproate and chlorazepam, are mentioned in passing, but formal studies of therapeutic efficacy have not been done with these agents.) By the time the three-drug treatment level is reached, one should be considering referring the patient for appropriate surgery. In general, parenteral doses of drugs are not used.

Serum levels of anticonvulsants are a useful way of monitoring treatment. For carbamazepine, at least initially, levels of 6 to 12 μg/mL (25 to 50 μmol/L) are usually required to relieve the pain. For phenytoin, therapeutic levels are 10 to 20 μg/mL (40 to 80 μmol/L).

In addition to the therapies described above, other drugs for trigeminal neuralgia have been reported to be efficacious, but their effects have not been repeatedly confirmed. Lechin et al[17] described the use of pimozide for trigeminal neuralgia. In a double-blind, crossover trial in 48 patients described as "refractory to medical therapy," pimozide was

Table 10–2 Medical Therapy of Trigeminal Neuralgia

Drug Name		Dosage		
Generic	*Brand*	(mg/day)	Precautions	Preparation
Carbamazepine	Tegretol	200–600	Monitor for blood disorders	Oral
Phenytoin	Dilantin	200–400	Central nervous system, hemopoietic	Oral
Baclofen	Lioresal	30–80	Drowsiness, weakness, nausea, vomiting	Oral

superior to carbamazepine for relief of pain. Pimozide is administered in a dose of 4 to 12 mg/day. The drug is described as an antipsychotic of the piperidine series, which blocks dopaminergic receptors in the brain. Multiple side effects occur with this medication, which the physician must review carefully before considering its use in trigeminal neuralgia. I have not had experience with this drug.

A keto derivation of carbamazepine, oxcarbazepine, has also been tested in patients with trigeminal neuralgia who are refractory to medical treatment.[18] Six patients were treated over 6 months and had an "excellent therapeutic response." The authors suggest that oxcarbazepine has potent antineuralgic properties in the absence of significant side effects and therefore may be useful in intractable trigeminal neuralgia. This drug is not available in the United States. A more recent review confirms these observations.[19]

Fusco and Alessandri[20] described an alternative pharmacological approach to trigeminal neuralgia. Twelve informed and consenting patients were studied to determine the influence of capsaicin, the pungent component of the red pepper, on trigeminal neuralgia. All of the patients had idiopathic trigeminal neuralgia. These patients were followed for 1 year after the topical application of 1.0 g of capsaicin TID over the painful area for several days. Six patients had complete relief and four patients had partial relief of pain; the remaining two patients had no relief of pain. Of the 10 patients who were responsive to therapy, four had relapses of pain within 95 to 149 days. There were no relapses after the second treatment for the remainder of the year. A more recent study casts doubt on the efficacy of capsaicin therapy.[21]

Table 10–3 Pharmacological Activity of Baclofen, Phenytoin, and Carbamazepine

	Baclofen	Phenytoin	Carbamazepine
Anticonvulsant	+	+ + +	+ +
Muscle relaxant	+ + +	+	+ +
Sedative	+ +	+	+ +
Anesthetic	0	0	0
Analgesic	0	0	±

A number of patients with trigeminal neuralgia (25% to 50%) will eventually become unresponsive to medical therapy and will need some form of neurosurgical treatment. The type of operation performed varies widely. Patients must be completely and clearly apprised of the nature of the operations proposed, procedures to be undertaken, possible side effects, costs, morbidity, and mortality. Informed consent regarding these neurosurgical procedures, given their many differences, is mandatory (Table 10–4).

Two operations—local ablation of peripheral nerves and wide section of the sensory roots of the trigeminal nerve—are rarely done because better methods are usually available for surgical pain relief.

Selective lesioning of the trigeminal root through the use of a radiofrequency electrode placed in the root under radiographic control *(radiofrequency rhizotomy)* is a surgical procedure that has gained wide acceptance.[22, 23] It has the advantages of safety and simplicity. The anesthesia used is light. The patient is awake during some of the procedure, recovers rapidly, and often is found eating supper a few hours after the operation. Almost always, the patient can be discharged the next day. However, there is a recurrence rate of about 25%, occasional corneal anesthesia occurs, and, rarely, uncomfortable dysesthesias or jaw weakness is produced. Altered sensation in the face is reported by many patients, but only a few are bothered by it. At present, there has been no mortality associated with this operation.

A variation on this procedure was proposed by Hakanson.[24] He injects 0.3 to 0.4 mL of glycerol via the anterior percutaneous route in the trigeminal cistern (Meckel's cave), which is visualized through the use

Table 10–4 Operative Comparisons

Procedures	Advantages	Disadvantages
Radiofrequency rhizotomy	90% Effective; "minor" procedure; brief hospital stay	Facial sensory loss; facial weakness; corneal hypesthesia (10–15%)
Glycerol injection	No craniotomy; 85% effective; minor procedure	Masseter weakness; facial sensory loss
Microvascular decompression	90% Effective; *no* sensory loss	±4% Serious postoperative complications; 1% mortality; long hospital stay; major craniotomy

of contrast medium (metrizamide). Hakanson reports an excellent response to this procedure, with only minimal disturbance of facial sensitivity. Sweet et al[25] have also reported their experience with this procedure. They describe greater pain on injection and more sensory loss than Hakanson. The presumption is made that glycerol is neurotoxic, acts on partially demyelinated nerve fibers, and eliminates the compound action potentials in the trigeminal rootlets that are associated with pain.

An alternative procedure is microvascular decompression of the trigeminal root.[26, 27] The neurosurgeon assumes that he or she will find a lesion (usually an arterial loop) compressing the trigeminal root close by the brainstem. With current neuroradiological techniques, it may be possible to demonstrate these lesions before surgery.[28]

Trigeminal neuralgia may also be produced by vertebrobasilar compression. Linskey et al[29] described this anatomic arrangement in detail. Thirty-one of 1404 consecutive patients (2%) with typical trigeminal neuralgia who underwent microvascular decompression between 1972 and 1993 were found to have vascular compression by the vertebral artery (VA) or basilar artery (BA). Compared with the remaining 1373 patients, this subgroup was older (mean age, 62 versus 55 years, $P<.001$), was predominantly male (68% versus 39%, $P<.002$), demonstrated left-sided predominance (65% versus 39%, $P<.002$), was more likely to be hypertensive (65% versus 18%, $P<.001$), and was more likely to have ipsilateral hemifacial spasm (16% versus 0.6%, $P<.001$). The trigeminal nerve was compressed by the VA in 18 cases (the VA alone in three and the VA plus other vessels in 15), by the BA in 12 cases (the BA alone in four and the BA plus other vessels in eight), and by the vertebrobasilar junction in one case. Twenty-nine of the 31 patients underwent vascular decompression of the trigeminal nerve, one had complete trigeminal root section, and one underwent partial root section with vascular decompression of the remaining nerve. All 31 patients were pain free and off medication immediately after surgery, and this pain-free, medication-free status was maintained at 1 year after surgery in 96% of cases, at 3 years in 92%, and at 10 years in 86%, based on life-table analysis. Minor trigeminal hypesthesia/hypalgesia was present before surgery in 52% of cases. New or worsened minor hypesthesia/hypalgesia developed in 41% of patients, whereas transient diplopia as well as hearing loss developed in 23% and 13% in the overall series, respectively. No patient developed major trigeminal sensory loss or masseter weakness after vascular decompression alone. There was no operative mortality.

The authors concluded that vascular decompression is an effective treatment for patients with trigeminal neuralgia who have vertebrobasilar compression of the trigeminal nerve. Patients should be warned that decompression of a tortuous vertebrobasilar system carries a higher risk of mild trigeminal dysfunction, diplopia, and hearing loss than standard microvascular decompression. If and when it is found, the offending compressing lesion is lifted from the trigeminal root, often by interposition of a sponge; by deduction, it then is suggested that in most cases, trigeminal neuralgia is a compressive cranial mononeuropathy, although other abnormalities in the trigeminal ganglion itself may contribute to its pathogenesis.

There are, of course, significant differences in costs among these operations. Radiofrequency lesions and glycerol injections are done rapidly, and almost always the patient is quickly discharged. With microsurgical decompression of the trigeminal root, a formal craniotomy is required, and the patient frequently spends 4 to 10 days in the hospital and a similar period of time in convalescence.

Meglio and Cioni[30] described percutaneous microcompression of the trigeminal ganglion as a variation on the usual surgical techniques. They used a small balloon filled to about 1 mL and introduced percutaneously through the foramen ovale; it is inflated against the ganglion for time periods of 1 to 10 minutes. The results reported were in the range of 90% improvement in pain and compare favorably with other standard neurosurgical procedures. In effect, this is a variation on older concepts of compressing the trigeminal ganglion to achieve pain relief.

Although some neurosurgeons continue to favor percutaneous radiofrequency rhizotomy, the trend is to use glycerol rhizolysis of the trigeminal ganglion. I routinely suggest the glycerol procedure for patients who want to avoid craniotomy.

Other Cranial Neuralgias and Atypical Facial Pain

Historical Note

Osler[31] made brief mention of a form of cervico-occipital neuralgia, a subject that is still controversial. He does not mention other categories of facial pain. Clark and Taylor[32] described a woman with geniculate neuralgia, with pain just in front of the left ear, that was relieved by surgical section of the seventh and eighth cranial nerves, leaving her with a complete peripheral facial palsy. Cushing[33] reported five cases of painful tic convulsif characterized by periodic contractions of one side of the face and accompanied by great pain that had been treated surgically. In modern times, the concept of atypical facial neuralgia (atypical facial pain) has been formulated to cover a series of facial pain syndromes that are generally chronic and not well defined and lack a specific definable etiology. Trigeminal neuralgia and glossopharyngeal neuralgia are not included under this classification.

Clinical Manifestations

The head and face pains included for consideration in this section differ from the typical or major facial neuralgias chiefly as follows:

1. In the atypical neuralgias, the pain is seldom limited to the distribution of the fifth or ninth cranial nerve but usually spreads over the area supplied by the cervical roots.
2. The pain is not significantly reduced or eliminated by division of the fifth or ninth cranial nerve.
3. The pain is of a steady, diffuse, aching quality lasting hours or days. It does not occur in paroxysms of short duration (1 to 30 seconds) followed by freedom from pain, as occurs with trigeminal neuralgia.
4. Patients with atypical facial neuralgia syndromes do not have trigger zones.
5. These disorders occur in a younger age group than the major neuralgias and far more commonly in women than in men.
6. Attacks are not precipitated by cold, drafts, cold water in the mouth, swallowing, talking, chewing, shaving, or washing the face, as occurs with typical neuralgias.

Many factors may be responsible for these complaints. A careful search should be made for local pathology of the eyes, nose, teeth, sinuses, and pharynx. In particular, nasopharyngeal cancer should be excluded by magnetic resonance imaging (MRI).[34]

The relatively uncommon painful states of tic-like neuritides of the fifth cranial nerve associated with brain tumors and other pathological processes resemble trigeminal neuralgia but usually can be differentiated because each painful paroxysm is commonly a sustained high-intensity ache of several minutes' duration, whereas the true tic is characterized by recurrent, brief, painful jabs lasting about 30 seconds. In describing neuralgias resulting from tumor involvement of the sensory root, trigeminal ganglion, or fifth nerve, Cushing[33] classified them into four groups on the basis of the site of the tumor, as follows.

1. Tumors of the cerebellopontine angle involving the trigeminal root may rarely be accompanied by paroxysms of pain that resemble tic douloureux. The pain is not eliminated by trigeminal ganglion operation. Sometimes, there is a low-intensity, steady, dull ache, but usually little or no pain is produced by such tumors, and there is a gradual hypesthesia in the distribution of the fifth cranial nerve.
2. Tumors of the middle fossa that involve the trigeminal ganglion by direct pressure from above, mainly on the dura overlying the ganglion, are growths with a meningeal attachment, such as endothelial tumors, granulomas, and occasional gliomas. Again, the pain rarely resembles tic douloureux in its temporal features. Furthermore, it is an inconspicuous symptom of the underlying disor-

der. When pain occurs, it usually is of a sustained aching and burning character and is associated with hypesthesia of an appropriate area of the skin. Paroxysms of high-intensity pain of 10 to 15 minutes' duration may occur.

3. Tumors that grow in the cranium or extracranial tissues beneath the ganglion, often metastatic, are almost certain to eventually involve the ganglion. Occasionally, the nerve may be completely destroyed, resulting in total anesthesia in its territory, without production of pain. More often, however, the process is accompanied by aching and burning pain of high intensity, occurring in paroxysms lasting 10 to 15 minutes.

4. Endothelial tumors originating from the envelopes of the trigeminal ganglion give rise to pain in the region supplied by one or more branches of the fifth nerve. The character of the pain—a more-or-less sustained, steady ache—readily distinguishes it from true trigeminal neuralgia. It also is inevitably accompanied by a hypesthesia, if not anesthesia, and motor paralysis. Also, the third, sixth, and eighth nerves may be involved by the tumor.

Geniculate Neuralgia of Herpetic Origin

Geniculate neuralgia is generally related to herpes zoster infection of the geniculate ganglion and is characterized by severe pain in the tympanic membrane, walls of the auditory canal, external auditory meatus, and external structure of the ear. The pain is typically deep and may be associated with a herpetic rash in the auricle, or the rash may be present in the external auditory canal. The disease may be associated with facial palsy (Ramsay-Hunt syndrome), difficulty with hearing, vertigo, and tinnitus.

Hemifacial Spasm

Maroon[35] reviewed the literature on hemifacial spasm and described his therapy of this syndrome. Recent surgical observations indicate that hemifacial spasm is most likely caused by normal or pathological vascular structures that cross-compress the facial nerve. The critical area of compression is found at the brainstem exit zone of the seventh nerve. In this area, the central glial investment of the facial nerve changes to peripheral or schwannian myelin. It is suspected that this anatomic junction zone may be of pathophysiological significance when directly compressed or irritated. Maroon recommends a retromastoid craniectomy and vascular decompression operation to relieve hemifacial spasm, while at the same time preserving facial nerve function. This is in contrast to commonly used destructive operations for hemifacial spasm. He emphasizes, however, that microsurgical techniques must be used, or high morbidity and mortality may occur with use of the retromastoid approach. Interestingly, in Maroon's series of cases, facial pain or headache associated with chronic facial spasm was rare. He emphasizes that the problem is primarily a muscular one related to predominant contraction of the orbicularis and zygomatic muscles.

Hemifacial spasm should be differentiated from blepharospasm and the synkinesis that may occur after a Bell's palsy. In my experience, blepharospasm is always bilateral, affects primarily the periorbital muscles, but may spread to the upper facial muscles as well. In a small number of patients with Bell's palsy, hemifacial synkinetic movements may develop as the patient recovers from the episode but is left with persisting weakness. This history is clearly different from that of hemifacial spasm. Also, facial myokymia may appear as a form of fascicular twitching of the facial muscles, especially the orbicularis oculi.

Facial pain of a chronic nature may occur with each of these conditions but, conversely, may also be absent.

Headache and Diabetic Neuropathy

Isolated cranial nerve palsies, especially of the third and sixth nerves, are known to occur in diabetes. Neuralgia of the fifth nerve may occur with diabetic ocular paresis. No suitable explanation for the pain is available. It appears likely that the third, fourth, and sixth cranial nerve defects stem from vascular occlusive disease of the vasa nervorum and that the fifth cranial nerve may rarely become similarly involved.

Herpetic and Postherpetic Neuritis of the Trigeminal Nerve

The pain of herpes zoster is steady and sustained, which is in contrast to paroxysmal pain of trigeminal neuralgia. Although the pain often regresses spontaneously within 2 or 3 weeks, it may persist for several months; when it occurs in persons more than 70 years old, as it frequently does, its duration may be 1 year or longer. Rarely, it may persist indefinitely. The pain is unilateral, and the quality of the pain is both burning and aching. It may be experienced in any part of the distribution of the fifth cranial nerve, although involvement of the forehead is most common. The pain is nonthrobbing and relatively uniform, and it usually diminishes gradually in intensity. Examination soon after onset reveals erythema and the typical herpetiform lesion of the skin associated with hyperalgesia and paresthesia. Examination later reveals hypesthesia and paresthesia of the involved areas and sometimes scarring and pigmentation of the skin. There may be weakness of the masseter and pterygoid muscles ipsilaterally. The judicious use of codeine and salicylates with reassurance of better days to come makes the period of spontaneous regression tolerable. Sensory root section does not usually give complete relief and often may have no effect.

In atypical facial pain due to herpes zoster and related disorders, steady pain in the face and ear, back of the head, and neck, associated with vertigo and ipsilateral palsy of the face, results from widespread inflammation involving the gasserian and glossopharyngeal and the first two or three dorsal root ganglia and the dorsal horns of the cervical spinal cord. The pain has the quality and duration described above. There may be a slight or moderate palsy with or without herpetiform lesions.

Occipital Neuritis Due to Herpes and Other Infections and Cervical Cord Tumors

Occipital headache due to inflammation, injury, or pressure on the occipital nerves, upper cervical spinal roots, dorsal horn, or dorsal root ganglia is a long-lasting, sustained, nonthrobbing ache of moderate intensity. It is difficult to distinguish it from tension-type headache because it is always associated with muscle contraction and tenderness. The characteristic feature is paresthesia or analgesia of the tissues of the scalp and skin of the neck. Discoloration or scarring of the skin, such as occurs after herpes, may also occur. When the headache is postherpetic, section of nerves or roots probably will not eliminate the pain but may reduce it. Procaine injections involving the sensory roots may have a slight effect in reducing the intensity of pain. Anthony[36] reviewed in detail the subject of occipital pain and its treatment.

Occipital headache caused by tumors of the upper cervical cord, especially by those masses attached or adjacent to the first two or three roots, closely resembles that described above. In most instances, there is disturbance in sensory perception within the dermatomes involved in addition to the pain. MRI is the diagnostic procedure of choice after plain cervical spine radiography is done. Removal of the tumor, or rhizotomy when removal is impossible, eliminates or reduces the intensity of headache.

Sustained contraction of the neck on a radiograph of a straight cervical spine may also be associated with a variety of cervical defects, including herniated cervical intervertebral discs. Unilateral neckache extending to the occiput and sometimes including the temple and forehead may appear in patients with mid- and upper-cervical joint disorders.

Painful Tic Convulsif

Painful tic convulsif is characterized by periodic contractions of one side of the face, accompanied by great pain. It may be confused with the facial contortions and masticatory movements on the involved side that rarely accompany the paroxysms of true trigeminal neuralgia.

Painful tic convulsif is reported to be more severe in women than in men. It may begin in or about the orbicularis oculi as fine intermittent myokymia with some spread thereafter into the muscles of the lower part of the face. Occasionally, strong spasms involve all of the facial muscles on one side almost continuously; rarely, the face may become weak, and some of the facial muscles may atrophy.

A more recent report of tic convulsif by Harsh et al[37] is of interest. A 54-year-old patient is described with a 5-year history of left hemifacial spasm and a 2-month history of left trigeminal neuralgia. MRI with enhancement showed massively ectatic vertebral and basilar arteries, distorting the brainstem and trigeminal and facial nerves. Surgical therapy included selective trigeminal rhizotomy (the patient had not responded to carbamazepine), decompression of the seventh nerve, and "cushioning" of the residual trigeminal nerve at the point of maximum distortion by the underlying basilar artery. Postoperatively, the patient did well, with neither facial pain nor movement.

Carotidynia

Fay[38] introduced the term *carotidynia* to describe a variety of pain that arises in the neck.

He suggested that the pain originated in the common carotid and external carotid arteries and its maxillary branches and that the course of afferent impulses to the central nervous system was indirect, involving in part the vagus nerve. Carotidynia is a syndrome that is characterized by tenderness, swelling, and sometimes conspicuous pulsation of the common carotid artery on the affected side. If the thumbs are placed on the common carotid arteries just below the bifurcation and the structures pressed back against the transverse cervical processes with a rolling movement, a severe pain is produced. Patients who already have a dull aching pain that is referred to the eye, deep in the malar region, spreading back to the ear, behind the ear, and down the neck, have the pain accentuated. The attacks are usually periodic, more likely to occur on the same side, and not associated with visual disturbances.

Roseman[39] reviewed the literature on carotidynia and reported his observations in young and middle-aged adults. He describes a unilateral or bilateral neck pain of high intensity but of relatively short duration, lasting 11 days on the average. In 90% of cases, the disease was self-limited. Systemic signs of illness were absent. Treatment of carotidynia is usually supportive. Simple analgesics such as aspirin may be helpful; corticosteroids are rarely necessary.

Lovshin[40] reported on a series of 100 patients with carotidynia from the Cleveland Clinic. All of the patients were examined, treated, and followed by the author. There were 82 women and 18 men, and 67 patients had a history of vascular headache. Forty-five patients volunteered the information that the glands in the neck had been swollen. Lovshin found that the most common form of carotidynia is related to overdistention, relaxation, and increased pulsation in the carotid artery. This syndrome of vascular neck pain is closely associated with various forms of extracranial vascular headache. It is more common in women than in men, with a ratio of about 4:1. The syndrome occurs at almost any age but is more prevalent during the fourth and fifth decades, and there often is a history of vascular headache. The only significant abnormality on physical examination is the presence of a tender, throbbing, often dilated carotid artery. The condition is frequently misdiagnosed and therefore not properly treated. Lovshin stated that preferred treatment is similar to that of migraine and other painful vasodilating conditions of the head. In particular, he suggested the use of various oral preparations of ergotamine tartrate or methysergide (2 mg TID or QID) in a short course. Apparently, carotidynia is not characterized by an inflammatory arteritis. The condition is not related to cranial arteritis.

Raeder's Syndrome and the Pericarotid Syndrome

Raeder's paratrigeminal syndrome[41] is a rare illness characterized by oculosympathetic paralysis, the sudden onset of severe frontotemporal burning, and aching pain of rapid onset, with associated ptosis and meiosis, often in a periorbital distribution; no previous history of headache; and normal sweating in the supraorbital area of the ipsilateral forehead. Raeder based his conclusions on five cases in whom there were cranial nerve dysfunctions, usually involving the optic, oculomotor, trochlear, trigeminal, and abducens nerves. Raeder's first patient had a tumor arising from the region of the trigeminal ganglion that infiltrated all of these cranial nerves. Two of his patients had multiple cranial nerve lesions and sympathetic paralysis related to head injury. In two cases, no particular cause could be identified. In essence, then, Raeder's patients had multiple cranial nerve involvements, primarily parasellar, associated with oculosympathetic paralysis and intact facial sweating. Others have since described almost any lesion in which there is oculosympathetic paralysis associated with head pain as Raeder's syndrome. Given this confusion, it is probably best to abandon the eponym and more precisely classify patients with oculosympathetic paralysis and headache, who may or may not have disturbances of sweating as well.

Many patients with cluster headaches have an associated oculosympathetic paralysis, but in this situation the tempo of the cluster headache rather than the autonomic dysfunction establishes the diagnosis.

Vijayan and Watson[42] described a pericarotid syndrome characterized by oculosympathetic paralysis, ipsilateral head pain, and anhidrosis over the forehead with otherwise intact facial sweating. They suggest that the site of the lesion involving the oculosympathetic fibers in their patients is pericarotid. Their patients had no previous history of headache. They were able to establish a pathogenesis in only one of their six patients in whom a left internal carotid artery occlusion had occurred; in the other five patients, the etiology was unknown.

Other reports stress the diversity of illness that may produce facial pain. Golding-Wood and Brookes[43] describe a form of posttraumatic nasal pain. Garen et al[44] report on intracranial fibro-osseous lesions that produce chronic facial pain. Lepore[45] described a series of patients with pain related to optic neuritis. Moffat et al[46] reported mastoid ache with unilateral acoustic neuroma.

Sjaastad et al[47, 48] described a headache syndrome characterized by short-lasting (usually 15 to 120 seconds), untreated head pain paroxysms localized about the eye, accompanied by unilateral conjunctival injection, lacrimation, nasal obstruction and lacrimation, and forehead sweating, all on the symptomatic side. This is termed the *SUNCT syndrome.* It may be best understood as a cluster headache variant. Treatment is symptomatic and often not particularly effective.

Etiology

As noted, multiple etiologies are involved in the production of facial pain, including inflammation, neoplasia, neuropathy, and structural changes of the skull itself. Some patients with atypical pains may have a form of vascular or common migraine that involves the face. This is particularly true if the pain is throbbing in nature, and a trial with an ergot-type vasoconstrictor agent may be helpful. If autonomic symptoms, including cutaneous pallor, sweating, flushing, rhinitis, and so forth, occur, responses to autonomic stimuli with β-adrenergic blockers such as propranolol can be used. Many patients with chronic, long-standing, atypical facial pains require intensive inpatient evaluation. A pain center approach to the problem is indicated to identify, if possible, the origins of the pain.

Biological Basis

With multiple etiologies responsible for the chronic facial pain, several disparate factors underlie the biological mechanisms. Often, with atypical facial pain in particular, no discrete biological basis for the pain can be discerned.

Epidemiology

No epidemiological information is available.

Precautions, Risk Factors, and Associated Conditions

Often, patients with atypical facial pain will have had extensive dental procedures, raising the question of possible alveolar neuritis. This diagnosis is, however, difficult to prove. No prevention or risk factors are identified.

Differential Diagnosis

The history and physical examination should direct the subsequent investigation of the patient. The major neuralgias are characterized by episodic pains in a stereotypical manner, often evoked by the patient. Generally, these can be eliminated quickly. It is incumbent on the examiner to rule out underlying disease; almost always, this involves a diagnostic workup.

Diagnostic Workup

For investigation of the face and sinuses, a coronal computed tomography is suggested. For investigation of the brain, MRI and magnetic resonance angiography should be done. Consultation with other specialties, including head and neck, ophthalmology, and dentistry, may be indicated.

Prognosis and Complications

For chronic facial pain regardless of the cause, the prognosis is guarded.

Management

Treatment depends on the diagnosis. When there is chronic infection, the use of appropriate antibiotics, surgical debridement, or both may be indicated. Neoplasia is usually investigated through biopsy, and therapy is determined by cell type. If no disease is found, a pain clinic approach is indicated to identify, if possible, the origins of the pain as medical or otherwise, to isolate factors contributing to the pain problem, and to quantify or measure the severity of the pain. In this situation, psychological testing and pain measurements should be included in the evaluation. Treatment can include pain-relieving or analgesic medications, attitude-influencing or psychotropic medications, nerve blocks, electrical neurostimulation, biofeedback techniques for reduction of muscle spasm, activity management, and family counseling.

Pregnancy

No information is available; the use of teratogenic drugs during pregnancy should be avoided.

Anesthesia

Anesthesia may be used as indicated or necessary. Medications should be stopped 1 day before anesthesia and resumed as soon as recovery from anesthetic has occurred.

References

1. Kunkle EC, Ray BS, Wolff HG: Studies on headache: The mechanisms and significance of headache associated with brain tumor. Bull NY Acad Med 1942;18:400.
2. Kunkle EC, Ray BS, Wolff HG: Experimental studies on headache: Analysis of the headache associated with changes in intracranial pressure. Arch Neurol Psychiatry 1943;49:323.
3. Ray BS, Parsons H: Subdural abscess complicating frontal sinusitis. Arch Otolaryngol 1943;37:536.
4. Lasater G: Primary intracranial hypotension. Headache 1970;10:63–66.
5. Srensen PS, Krogsaa B, Gerris F: Clinical course and prognosis of pseudotumor cerebri. A prospective study of 24 patients. Acta Med Scand 1988;77:164.
6. Corbett JJ, Thompson HS: The rational management of idiopathic intracranial hypertension. Arch Neurol 1989;46:1049.
7. Paulley JU, Hughes JP: Giant-cell arteritis of the aged. Br Med J 1960;2:1562.
8. Younger DS, Hays AP, Brust JC, et al: Granulomatous angiitis of the brain: An inflammatory reaction of diverse etiology. Arch Neurol 1988;45:514.
9. Reik L, Hale M: The temporomandibular joint pain-dysfunction syndrome: A frequent cause of headache. Headache 1996;21:151–156.
10. Cameron CE: Cracked tooth syndrome. J Am Dent Assoc 1964;68:405.
11. Fromm GH: Pharmacological consideration of anticonvulsants. Headache 1969;9:35–41.
12. Fromm GH, Terrence CF, Maroon JC: Trigeminal neuralgia: Concepts regarding etiology and pathogenesis. Arch Neurol 1984;41:1204–1207.
13. Fromm GH: The pharmacology of trigeminal neuralgia. Clin Neuropharmacol 1989;12:185.
14. Fromm GH: Trigeminal neuralgia and related disorders. Neurol Clin 1989;7:305.
15. Chawla JC, Falconer MA: Glossopharyngeal and vagal neuralgia. Br Med J 1967;2:527.
16. Dalessio DJ: Wolff's Headache and Other Head Pain, 6th ed. New York: Oxford University Press; 1990:345.
17. Lechin F, Vander Dijs B, Lechin ME, et al: Pimozide therapy for trigeminal neuralgia. Arch Neurol 1989;46:960.
18. Zakrzewska JM, Patsalos PN: Oxcarbazepine: A new drug in the management of intractable trigeminal neuralgia. J Neurol Neurosurg Psychiatry 1988;52:472.
19. Grant SM, Faulds D: Oxcarbazepine: A review of its pharmacology and therapeutic potential in epilepsy, trigeminal neuralgia, and affective disorders. Drugs 1992;43:873.
20. Fusco BM, Alessandri M: Analgesic effect of capsaicin in idiopathic trigeminal neuralgia. Anesth Analg 1992;50:621.
21. Epstein JB, Marcoe JH: Topical application of capsaicin for treatment of oral neuropathic pain and trigeminal neuralgia. Oral Surg Oral Med Oral Pathol 1994;77:135.
22. Sweet WH, Wepsic JG: Controlled thermocoagulation of trigeminal ganglion and rootlets for differential destruction of pain fibers: I. Trigeminal neuralgia. J Neurosurg 1974;40:143–156.
23. Tew JM, Keller JT: The treatment of trigeminal neuralgia by percutaneous radiofrequency technique. Clin Neurosurg 1977;24:557–575.
24. Hakanson S: Trigeminal neuralgia treated by injection of glycerol into the trigeminal cistern. Neurosurgery 1981;9:638.
25. Sweet WH, Poletti CE, Macon JB: Treatment of trigeminal neuralgia and other facial pains by retrogasserian injection of glycerol. Neurosurgery 1981;9:647–653.
26. Jannetta PJ: Treatment of trigeminal neuralgia by suboccipital and transtentorial cranial operations. Clin Neurosurg 1977;24:538–549.
27. Voorhies R, Patterson RH: Management of trigeminal neuralgia (tic douloureux). JAMA 1981;245:2521–2523.
28. Meaney JF, Miles JB, Nixon TE, et al: Vascular contact with the fifth cranial nerve at the pons in patients with trigeminal neuralgia: Detection with 3DFISP imaging. AJR 1994;163:1447.
29. Linskey ME, Jho HD, Jannetta PJ: Microvascular decompression for trigeminal neuralgia caused by vertebrobasilar compression. J Neurosurg 1994;81:1.

30. Meglio M, Cioni B: Percutaneous procedures for trigeminal neuralgia: Microcompression versus radiofrequency thermocoagulation. Pain 1989;38:9–16.
31. Osler W: The Principles and Practice of Medicine, 8th ed. New York: D. Appleton and Co; 1912:1090.
32. Clark LP, Taylor AS: True tic douloureux of the sensory filaments of the facial nerve. JAMA 1909;53:2144.
33. Cushing H: The major trigeminal neuralgias and their surgical treatment, based on experiences with 332 gasserian operations: The varieties of facial neuralgia. Am J Med Sci 1920; 160:157.
34. Dunteman ED, Swarm RA: Atypical facial neuralgia. Anesth Analg 1995;80:188.
35. Maroon JC: Hemifacial spasm. Arch Neurol 1978;35:481–483.
36. Anthony M: Headache and the greater occipital nerve. Clin Neurol Neurosurg 1992;94:297.
37. Harsh GR, Wilson CB, Hieshima GB, et al: Magnetic resonance imaging of vertebrobasilar ectasia in tic convulsif. J Neurosurg 1991; 74:999–1003.
38. Fay T: Atypical facial neuralgia: A syndrome of vascular pain. Ann Otol 1932;41:1030.
39. Roseman DM: Carotidynia: A distinct syndrome. Arch Otolaryngol 1967;85:81.
40. Lovshin LL: Carotidynia. Headache 1977; 17:192–195.
41. Raeder JG: Paratrigeminal paralysis of oculopupillary sympathetic. Brain 1924;47:149–158.
42. Vijayan N, Watson D: The pericarotid syndrome. Headache 1978;18:244.
43. Golding-Wood DG, Brookes GB: Posttraumatic external nasal neuralgia: An often missed cause of facial pain. Postgrad Med J 1991;67:55.
44. Garen PD, Powers JM, King JS, et al: Intracranial fibro-osseous lesion. J Neurosurg 1989; 70:475.
45. Lepore FE: The origin of pain in optic neuritis. Arch Neurol 1991;48:748.
46. Moffat DA, Baguley DM, Evans RA, et al: Mastoid ache in acoustic neuroma. J Laryngol Otol 1989;103:1043.
47. Sjaastad O, Saunte C, Salvesen R, et al.: Short-lasting, unilateral, neuralgiform headache attacks with conjunctival injection, tearing, sweating, and rhinorrhea. Cephalalgia 1989; 9:147–156.
48. Kruszewski P, Sand T, Shen TM, Sjaastad O.: Short-lasting, unilateral, neuralgiform headaches with conjunctival injection and tearing. Headache 1992;32:377–383.

11

Tension-Type Headache

Merle L. Diamond, M.D.

Glen D. Solomon, M.D.

Introduction

The tension-type headache is the most common form of headache in Western populations. Tension-type headache is typically described as a bandlike pressure headache without associated symptoms. The International Headache Society (IHS)[1] defines tension-type headache as a bilateral headache with a pressing or tightening quality of mild-to-moderate severity. Unlike migraine, it is not aggravated by physical activity, nor is it associated with vomiting. Phonophobia or photophobia may be present but not both. In chronic tension-type headache, but not episodic tension-type headache, patients may experience nausea. By definition, chronic tension-type headache occurs at least 15 days per month for at least 6 months,[1] although in clinical practice, it is usually a daily or almost-daily headache.

Previously used names for tension-type headache included muscle contraction headache, psychogenic headache, and chronic daily headache. The term *muscle contraction headache* was abandoned because electromyographic evidence failed to show consistent changes in muscle tone in patients with tension-type headache. Furthermore, it suggested a pathophysiological mechanism for the headache that has yet to be proved.

The concept that tension-type headache is a "psychogenic" headache also has been questioned. Patients with chronic tension-type headache, like patients with other chronic pain disorders, have about a 25% likelihood of developing secondary depression. Half of these patients develop depression simultaneously with the pain, whereas in the other half, the development of depression is more insidious.[2] Tension-type headache may be present in almost all psychiatric disturbances.[3] This should not suggest, however, that most tension-type headache is associated with psychiatric or psychological disorders.

The term *chronic daily headache* usually refers to headaches that meet IHS criteria for tension-type headache and for migraine (usually without aura). This group of patients often includes those with analgesic abuse or ergotamine rebound headaches. Other well-defined headaches can occur on a daily basis, such as cluster headache, chronic paroxysmal hemicrania (CPH), and idiopathic stabbing headache, but they are not considered chronic daily headaches.

Epidemiology

In surveys of the general population, the prevalence of tension-type headache has ranged from 30% to about 80%. This wide disparity may reflect the fact that tension-type headache may vary in frequency and severity from rare episodes of head discomfort to frequent, severe, and debilitating headaches.

In the most detailed epidemiological study of headache, the Danish Glostrup Population Studies,[4] the 1-year prevalence of episodic tension-type headache was 63%: 56% in men and 71% in women. The prevalence of chronic tension-type headache was 3%: 2% in men and 5% in women. Differences according to sex were significant, with a male-to-female ratio of 4:5. The prevalence of tension-type headache decreased with increasing age.

Most people with tension-type headache had it once monthly or less, but about 40% had it several times per month. Headache occurring at least half the days of the year was reported by 4% of people. The severity of tension-type headache increased significantly with frequency. In 59% of people with tension-type headache, their daily activities were impaired because of the headache.

Tension-type headache sufferers rarely sought medical attention. Only 16% consulted a general practitioner, and 4% consulted a specialist. Consultation rates were higher in women than in men and correlated with the frequency of attacks.[4]

Because of the large number of persons in the general population with tension-type headache, the economic impact is enormous. On average, 5% of the total employed population between the ages of 25 and 64 were absent for 4 days per year, 2% were absent for 11 days, and 2% were absent for about 20 days. The number of days lost from work that were attributable to tension-type headache was 820 work days lost per 1000 employed persons per year.[4]

Pathophysiology

The pathophysiology of tension-type headache is poorly understood. It is probable that episodic tension-type headache is predominantly a disorder of peripheral mechanisms, whereas chronic tension-type headache reflects a central pain disturbance.

Episodic tension-type headache is thought to be caused by increased nociception from strained muscles, as occurs with inadequate rest or poor posture, or by increased muscle tension, as occurs with stress. Increased pain impulses may cause an increased sensitivity of neurons of the trigeminal tract, and pain then may propagate itself to some extent.[5] Recurrent bouts of tension-type headache may lower the threshold for new episodes by altering the myofascial tissues, potentiating nociceptive neurons, or decreasing the activity of the antinociceptive system.

Chronic tension-type headache appears to be one of a group of disorders marked by low levels of brain serotonin. Like other chronic pain disorders, chronic tension-type headache also is associated with hypofunction of the central opioid system.[6] Patients with chronic tension-type headache commonly report symptoms of constant headache, generalized myalgias and arthralgias, difficulty initiating and maintaining sleep, chronic fatigue, carbohydrate craving, decreased libido, irritability, and disturbed memory and concentration.[7] This disorder is similar to the disease depression; however, in chronic tension-type headache, anhedonia is not present, the mood disturbance is less marked or may even be absent, and the primary symptom is headache pain. It also resembles the disease fibromyalgia, with generalized myofascial pain and sleep disturbance.

Treatment

Despite its frequency in the population and its societal impact, there are very few well controlled studies of treatment of tension-type headache. Many earlier trials included patients with combined tension-type and migraine without aura and patients with medication-overuse headache.

Given the chronic nature of the disorder and the risk of medication-overuse headache in patients with frequent headaches, prophylactic therapy is warranted for most patients with chronic tension-type headache.

Antidepressant Drugs

Antidepressants are the drugs of choice for chronic tension-type headache, and several of these agents are also effective in migraine prophylaxis. The antidepressants that have been tested in double-blind, placebo-controlled studies of patients with chronic tension-type headache include amitriptyline, doxepin, and maprotiline. Although other antidepressants have not been studied in chronic tension-type headache, clinical experience suggests that there are only minimal differences in efficacy between agents; however, differences in side effects can be significant.

Of the antidepressants, the tricyclic drugs and the newer selective serotonin reuptake inhibitors (SSRIs) are usually the agents of first choice because of the lower incidence of side effects and the decreased likelihood of serious drug interactions compared with the monoamine oxidase inhibitors (MAOIs).

The selection of a specific antidepressant drug should be based primarily on whether the patient has a sleep disturbance. Patients who initiate and maintain sleep easily generally tolerate nonsedating drugs better than sedating agents. The patients who have difficulty initiating or maintaining sleep respond better to sedating drugs. Patients often will note an improvement in headaches within 1 or 2 weeks after their sleep disturbance is corrected.

The nonsedating antidepressant drugs include fluoxetine, sertraline, bupropion, venlafaxine, nefazodone, protriptyline, and desipramine. The MAOIs are nonsedating and may induce insomnia.

The sedating antidepressant drugs include amitriptyline, doxepin, nortriptyline, imipramine, trimipramine, and trazodone. Of these drugs, nortriptyline appears to cause the least amount of morning sedation.

The second consideration after the effect on sleep is whether the patient is likely to be intolerant of anticholinergic side effects. The common anticholinergic side effects that occur with tricyclic antidepressants are dry mouth, blurred vision, urinary retention, and constipation.

All tricyclic antidepressants have anticholinergic side effects; doxepin appears to cause the least anticholinergic side effects. SSRIs and atypical antidepressant drugs, such as fluoxetine, sertraline, paroxetine, bupropion, venlafaxine, nefazodone, and trazodone, are generally free of anticholinergic effects.

Tricyclic antidepressants have several potential cardiac effects.[8] These drugs may cause orthostatic hypotension, although they do not have negative inotropic effects on the heart. The orthostatic hypotension is mediated through α_1-adrenergic receptor blockade and is most commonly reported with tertiary amines such as amitriptyline and imipramine. Cardiac conduction problems can occur with all tricyclic antidepressants but do not occur with the nontricyclic drugs such as trazodone, fluoxetine, sertraline, paroxetine, venlafaxine, nefazodone, and bupropion. Tricyclic drugs slow the process of depolarization and prolong repolarization, a quinidine-like effect. On electrocardiogram, there may be prolongation of PR, QRS, and QT intervals. This effect is of clinical significance only in patients with second-degree heart block, right or left bundle-branch block, or intraventricular conduction delays (QRS width of more than 0.11 second). In patients with first-degree heart block, treatment with tricyclic drugs does not cause the development of higher degrees of heart block. Patients with advanced heart block or intraventricular conduction delays who require therapy with antidepressant agents should be treated with fluoxetine, sertraline, paroxetine, bupropion, venlafaxine, nefazodone, trazodone, or MAOIs.

The SSRIs have become the most commonly prescribed antidepressant drugs due to their adverse effect profile. These drugs are generally well tolerated and lack the sedation, increased appetite, and anticholinergic side effects of the tricyclic drugs. These agents have unique adverse effects and are significantly more expensive than the generic versions of the tricyclic antidepressants.

Fluoxetine is the most activating of the currently available SSRIs. As such, it is most useful in patients who sleep well but complain of chronic fatigue. Nervousness and insomnia are common side effects, in addition to the gastrointestinal upset and diarrhea that are common to all SSRIs. Fluoxetine may also exacerbate migraine. A recent study[9] of fluoxetine in patients with headache suggests that it has moderate benefit in chronic tension-type headache but does not reduce the frequency or severity of migraine. There are no controlled studies of fluoxetine in children with headache, and pediatric dosing has not been established. In adolescents, a 10-mg dose given in the morning is a reasonable starting dose. In adults, the usual starting dosage is 20 mg/day.

Due to their inhibition of the cytochrome P450 enzyme system, fluoxetine and other SSRIs can increase the effects of tricyclic antidepressants, some β-blockers (propranolol and metoprolol), trazodone, diazepam, codeine-containing drugs, cough medications containing dextromethorphan, and highly protein bound drugs. Fluoxetine is contraindicated in patients receiving MAOIs currently or within the past 2 weeks. It has a half-life of 2 to 3 days.

Sertraline is not as stimulating as fluoxetine, nor as sedating as paroxetine. It can be given in the morning or at bedtime. Published experience with sertraline in headache or chronic pain is quite limited. We[10] have found sertraline to be moderately effective in patients with chronic tension-type headache and coexisting migraine and tension-type headache (mixed headache). The common adverse effects with sertraline are nausea and diarrhea, which often resolve within 1 or 2 weeks. Of the SSRIs, sertraline has the lowest inhibitory effect on the cytochrome P450 system and is less likely to increase the effects of other drugs. There is no established pediatric dosing for sertraline. Adolescents may be treated with 25 to 50 mg/day.

Paroxetine is mildly sedating and often is taken at bedtime. There is no published experience of paroxetine in headache disorders, nor is there an established pediatric dose. The usual adult and adolescent dose is 20 mg at bedtime.

Some antidepressant drugs have unique adverse effects. Trazodone has been reported to cause priapism in some men. Fluoxetine and sertraline may cause anorexia and weight loss in a small percentage of patients. Although the medical literature does not support the contention, reports of suicide and violent behavior with fluoxetine have been widely heralded by the lay media.

In children and elderly patients, the usual starting dose of amitriptyline (or a similar drug) is 10 mg at bedtime. In adults, the usual starting dose is 25 mg at bedtime. The dosage can be increased until a therapeutic result is obtained or side effects become intolerable. Antidepressants usually take from 4 to 6 weeks to show beneficial effects.

Muscle Relaxants

Cyclobenzaprine is a muscle relaxant that is related structurally to amitriptyline. In a 1972 double-blind study,[11] 10 of 20 patients receiving cyclobenzaprine showed a 50% or greater improvement in tension-type headache, whereas only 5 of 20 patients receiving placebo improved.

NSAIDs

Nonsteroidal anti-inflammatory drugs (NSAIDs) are widely prescribed in the treatment of arthritis and as analgesics and antipyretics. They are valuable in both the adjunctive therapy for tension-type headache and for the prophylaxis of migraine headache.[7]

Adverse effects from NSAIDs are relatively common and can include gastrointestinal symptoms such as dyspepsia, heartburn, nausea, vomiting, diarrhea, constipation, and generalized abdominal pain. Most NSAIDs can cause bleeding of the upper gastrointestinal tract. The renal effects of NSAIDs can include decreased glomerular filtration rate with sodium, chloride, and water retention. These renal problems are most likely to occur in patients who are elderly, are hypertensive, have renovascular or advanced atherosclerotic disease, or take diuretics. Indomethacin and fenoprofen appear to be more nephrotoxic than other NSAIDs. Analgesic nephropathy, the most common cause of drug-induced renal failure, has been associated with the excessive use of NSAIDs along with phenacetin or acetaminophen.

Valproate

For the adult or older adolescent patient for whom conventional therapy has failed, alternatives include MAOIs or valproate. Because of the potential for serious toxicity, prescription of these agents for headache should be limited to physicians experienced in their use.

Valproate, a γ-aminobutyric acid (GABA) agonist anticonvulsant, has been evaluated for efficacy in migraine[12, 13] and "chronic daily headache."[14]

GABA is an inhibitory neurotransmitter present in the small neurons of the suprachiasmatic nucleus. GABA dilates the cerebral arteries, influences human circadian rhythm, and may play a role in the regulation of the secretion of hormones from the anterior pituitary gland. Valproate (sodium valproate) is a GABA agonist that may affect migraine through an influence on cerebral arteries and circadian rhythms.[13]

Mathew and Ali[14] evaluated the efficacy of valproate (1000 to 2000 mg/day) in 30 patients with intractable chronic daily headache (migraine without aura and chronic tension-type headaches) in an open-label trial. Blood levels were maintained between 75 and 100 μg/mL. By the third month of therapy, two thirds of the patients improved significantly. They reported common side effects of weight gain, tremor, hair loss, and nausea.

Abortive Therapy

Treatment of the daily, tension-type headache with abortive medications is difficult. Muscle relaxants such as chlorzoxazone, orphenadrine citrate, carisoprodol, and metaxalone, either alone or in combinations with aspirin, acetaminophen, caffeine, or a combination, are generally helpful. NSAIDs also are useful as analgesics for daily headache. Benzodiazepines, butalbital combinations, and narcotics should be avoided or their use should be carefully controlled because of the risk of habituation and analgesic-rebound headache.

Medication Overuse

An extremely important condition contributing to the development of headaches in a chronic daily pattern is overuse of medication. This is most likely to occur in patients with frequent headaches, especially tension-type headache. The most common medications associated with analgesic-rebound headache are ergotamine preparations, butalbital combination analgesics, opiates, and caffeine-containing combination analgesics. Simple analgesics such as aspirin, acetaminophen, and NSAIDs probably do not induce analgesic-rebound headache. The diagnosis of medication overuse is dependent on a careful history of medication ingestion, including over-the-counter medications. Effective treatment of headache associated with drug overuse requires withdrawal from the offending agents.

Nonpharmacological Therapy

Many clinical studies have supported the use of relaxation and electromyographic biofeedback therapies in the management of chronic tension-type headaches.[15] In averaging of the results of 37 trials that used daily headache recordings to evaluate relaxation or electromyographic biofeedback therapies, each therapy or the combination yielded a 50% reduction in tension-type headache activity. Studies have not found that relaxation, biofeedback, or the combination is preferable.

Stress management therapy using cognitive-behavior therapy is as effective as relaxation or biofeedback therapy in reducing tension-type headache. Cognitive therapy may be most likely to enhance the effectiveness of relaxation or biofeedback therapies when chronic stress, depression, or adjustment problems aggravate the patient's headaches.[15]

Nonpharmacological therapy may be used in conjunction with pharmacotherapy. Nonpharmacological therapy is particularly useful for patients who are reluctant to take medications due to desire for pregnancy, previous adverse reactions to medications, or concomitant medical problems.

References

1. Headache Classification Committee of the International Headache Society. Classification and diagnostic criteria for headache disorders, cranial neuralgias, and facial pain. Cephalalgia 1988;8(suppl 7):1–96.
2. Bech P, Langemark M, Loidrup D, et al. Tension-type headache: Psychiatric aspects. *In* Olesen J, Schoenen J, eds. Tension-Type Headache: Classification, Mechanisms, and Treatment. New York, Raven Press, 1993:143–146.
3. Goncalves JA, Monteiro P. Psychiatric analysis of patients with tension-type headache. *In* Olesen J, Schoenen J, eds. Tension-Type Headache: Classification, Mechanisms, and Treatment. New York: Raven Press; 1993:167–172.
4. Rasmussen BK, Jensen R, Olesen J. Epidemiology of tension-type headache in a general population. *In* Olesen J, Schoenen J, eds. Tension-Type Headache: Classification, Mechanisms, and Treatment. New York: Raven Press; 1993:9–13.
5. Olesen J, Schoenen J. Synthesis. *In* Olesen J, Tfelt-Hansen P, Welch KMA, eds. The Headaches. New York: Raven Press; 1993:495.
6. Schoenen J. Session IV discussion summary: Central mechanisms of tension-type headache. *In* Olesen J, Schoenen J, eds. Tension-Type Headache: Classification, Mechanisms, and Treatment. New York: Raven Press; 1993:207–208.
7. Solomon GD. Pharmacology and use of headache medications. Cleve Clin J Med 1990; 57:627–635.
8. Solomon GD. Concomitant medical disease and headache. Med Clin North Am 1991; 75:631–639.
9. Saper JR, Silberstein SD, Lake AE, Winters ME. Double-blind trial of fluoxetine: Chronic daily headache and migraine. Headache 1994; 34:497–502.
10. Solomon GD, Pearson E. Sertraline in the management of headache. Clin Pharmacol Ther 1994;55:130.
11. Lance JW, Anthony M. Cyclobenzaprine in the treatment of chronic tension headache. Med J Aust 1972;2:1409–1411.
12. Sorensen K. Valproate: A new drug in migraine prophylaxis. Acta Neurol Scand 1988; 78:346–348.
13. Herring R, Kuritzky A. Sodium valproate in the prophylactic treatment of migraine: A double-blind study versus placebo. Cephalalgia 1992;12:81–84.
14. Mathew NT, Ali S. Valproate in the treatment of persistant chronic daily headache: An open label study. Headache 1991;31:71–74.
15. Holroyd KA. Behavioral treatment strategies. *In* Olesen J, Schoenen J, eds. Tension-Type Headache: Classification, Mechanisms, and Treatment. New York: Raven Press; 1993:245–254.

12

Coexisting Migraine and Tension-Type Headaches (Mixed Headache Syndrome)

Merle L. Diamond, M.D.

Glen D. Solomon, M.D.

Introduction

Coexisting migraine and tension-type headaches were previously termed the mixed headache syndrome and also are known as tension-vascular headache or combination headache. Patients with this condition are those most frequently seen by the neurologist or headache specialist. This patient has both migraine and tension-type headache. The International Headache Society, (IHS) Committee on Classification noted that these patients should be considered to have both forms.[1]

We believe these patients have the combination of migraine and depression (Fig. 12–1). The depression becomes "masked" by a chronic, daily tension-type headache complicated by periodic migrainous headaches. Although very common, this syndrome has been poorly defined, causing many patients to be misdiagnosed, improperly treated, and ultimately referred from the arena of primary care to more specialized centers. This scenario need not be the rule.

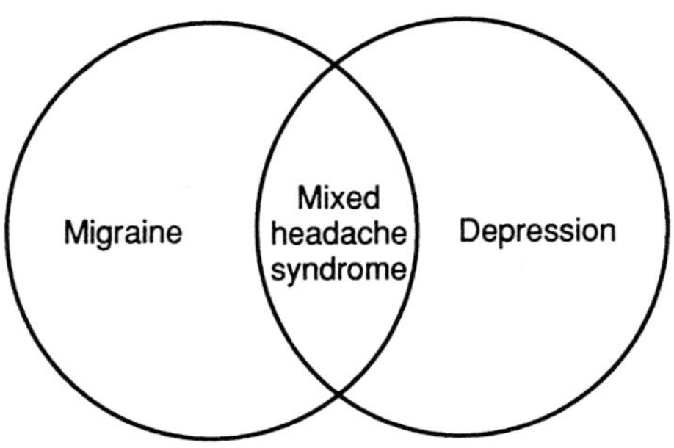

Figure 12–1 Combination of migraine and depression in mixed headache syndrome.

Definition

Typically, coexisting migraine and tension-type headache consists of the following symptomatology: (1) daily chronic tension headache, (2) hard, or "sick," migrainous headache, and (3) an increased susceptibility of habituation to over-the-counter or prescribed analgesics, ergotamine tartrate, or both.[2]

The most common history obtained is one of periodic migraine headaches, occurring from one to more than eight times per month, superimposed on an essentially daily, lower-grade, tension-type headache. Other patients report a history of daily headaches that demonstrate characteristics of both migraine and tension type, but are void of a clear distinction between the two components. The third reported form consists of a long-established history of definite migrainous headaches, lasting over a period of years, that become less clearly migrainous and begin to increase in frequency. The patient develops essentially a daily tension headache pattern devoid of migrainous component. Other variations are likely to occur.

Many patients with coexisting migraine and tension-type headaches seek medical attention for their periodic "sick" headaches while at the same time accept their daily lower-grade headaches as part of their normal existence. Therefore, in taking a headache history, it is essential to determine the number of types of headaches that the patient experiences. Specific questioning about a daily or almost daily headache in addition to a migraine-like headache will enhance diagnosis of the problem and guide treatment planning for many patients.

Most frequently, the patient with coexisting migraine and tension-type headaches present with a history of migraine without aura. However, migraine with aura and other less common migraine variants may occur. For some patients with coexisting migraine and tension-type headaches, visual or neurological auras may present as antecedents to only some headache attacks. Throbbing pain, usually unilateral, and associated symptoms such as anorexia, nausea, vomiting, polyuria, photophobia, phonophobia, and blurred vision are usual components of the migraine headache.

Common Ground

Many investigators have examined the association between headaches and depression.[3–6] In an epidemiological study of a general population of adults, using the diagnostic criteria of the IHS,[1] migraine was found in 10% of the subjects, and tension-type headache was reported by 74%.[7, 8] In the population-based study,[7] 83% of persons with migraine also experienced tension-type headaches. Thirteen percent of persons with migraine have never had a tension-type headache. For those with severe tension-type headaches, 77% did not have concomitant migraine. The male-to-female ratio in migraine is 1:3, whereas as in tension-type headache, it is 4:5.[9]

In 1873, Liveing commented on the psychic manifestations of migraine, including depression, decreased memory, and drowsiness. In the late 1930s, Wolff associated the occurrence of migraine with personality traits such as meticulousness, being well dressed and hard-working, and perfectionism.[10] According to Wolff, the personality functions of these migraineurs precipitate attacks. Although most controlled studies have failed to support the conclusions of Wolff,[11] it is possible that self-selection due to personality traits has caused some migraineurs to seek help, whereas migraineurs without rigid personalities self-medicate.

Other investigators[5] have examined the relationship of migraine and depression from a different perspective; they examined the rate of occurrence of migraine headaches in patients with a depressive disorder. Their results indicated a greater prevalence of migraine in depressed men than in men in the general population.

The association and familial transmission of migraine and depression were reviewed in a 1988 study of a group of 133 patients with major depression, a group of 82 normal community control subjects, and 400 first-degree relatives of the depressed patients and control subjects.[7] The association between migraine and depression was significant in the depressed subjects and their relatives, as well as in the relatives of the normal control subjects. Both disorders were shown to be strongly familial. Through their model, they were unable to conclusively determine whether the association between the two disorders was transmissible, but their findings did suggest a shared liability to depression and migraine, as well as evidence to support an environmental association between the two disorders.

In a 1987 study, 788 depressive patients were evaluated from three different psychiatric services: inpatient, outpatient, and a mobile unit population.[12] With the exception of typical migrainous attacks or the rarely occurring space-occupying lesion, tension-type headache was found to be the most cited symptom in both the outpatient and mobile unit populations, with both groups reporting the complaint more than 60% of the time. The inpatient unit had a lower percentage (56%) of patients reporting headache as a complaint. The authors inferred that these inpatients were more concerned about their depressed moods and psychomotor retardation than about any somatic complaint.

Clinical Picture

Patients with the coexisting migraine and tension-type headache usually present with an extensive past medical history. They have been unsuccessfully treated by many professionals, including primary care specialists, neurologists, and chiropractors and often nontraditional healers. Most of their care has been focused on the migraine headaches, and they have had adequate trials of most antimigrainous agents without achieving success. They have tried self-medication with excessive amounts of over-the-counter drugs and commonly are experiencing the effects of withdrawal from the caffeine in many of these products. When asked which medications seemed most helpful, these patients recall predominantly the narcotic agents as providing the greatest relief. In an analysis of 61 patients with the mixed headache syndrome, neuroticism, stress, excessive use of narcotic and caffeine-containing analgesic agents, ergot dependency, and hypertension were identified as provocateurs, in addition to depression, in the development of this condition in patients with a previous history of migraine.[13] Many patients also are dependent on the habit-forming benzodiazepines.

Their outlook can vary greatly. Many are hopeful that they will finally be helped or "cured" of their dreadful condition, whereas others are skeptical and believe that the current caregiver will only repeat the mistakes of the previous physician. They are hesitant to discontinue their narcotic agents because of the real fear of the pain that withdrawal will precipitate.

These patients, however, do not appear depressed. They do not possess the *sine quo non* of depression—a sad and dysphoric mood. Their depression is masked by their major somatic complaint, a headache, rather than a depressed mood. A sensitive historian will also be able to disclose complaints of insomnia, decreased ability to concentrate, low energy or fatigue, and loss of interest in pleasurable activities. The term "masked depression" must be constantly considered when a practitioner agrees to provide service to individuals with the coexisting migraine and tension-type headache.

Treatment

The cornerstone of treatment is twofold. First, continuity of care is essential. Most patients have seen numerous practitioners and have either self-referred or been referred to another provider. The patient must be confident that he or she will remain under the care of one professional and that seeking additional help will only sabotage the treatment. The second essential element of treatment is education. The patient will experience great relief when advised that the condition is a recognized entity and that treatment is available. Patients should be instructed that some agent that they tried previously will be tried again, only this time in combination therapy. Patients also must be advised that withdrawal from narcotic agents is mandatory and that these agents will not be used in their future care.

Antidepressants

In the area of headaches and depression, the tricyclic antidepressants (TCAs) have been studied extensively. As early as 1964, the successful use of amitriptyline in the treatment of chronic tension headache had been described.[14] The use of antidepressants in the treatment of migraine was suggested by Friedman in 1968[15] and Mahloudji in 1969.[16] In 1969, Diamond[17] studied 167 patients presenting with a chief complaint of headache and treated them with TCAs. The patients were diagnosed as having migraine (91), depression (52), and migraine and depressive overlay (24). Excellent results were demonstrated in 80% of these patients.

The role of the antidepressant compounds in both the prophylaxis and relief of pain has become increasingly recognized. It has been suggested that if the antidepressant drugs had been studied for pain relief before they were experimentally administered to depressed patients, these agents would have been classified as analgesics. The relevance of antidepressant drugs to pain control has been attributed to their effects on the synthesis and metabolism of serotonin (5-hydroxytryptamine) and norepinephrine. Neurons containing serotonin and norepinephrine have been identified as part of the analgesia system of the brain.[18, 19] Virtually all the antidepressants alter the synthesis or reuptake of the neurotransmitters serotonin and norepinephrine. Because of this mechanism, these agents would be expected to play a role in the modulation of pain.

The antidepressants are becoming recognized for their analgesic properties due to the results of many previous studies[20–22] that documented a decrease in the severity, frequency, and duration of migraine headaches during tricyclic therapy. However, these studies did not include control for subjects who were depressed, rendering the efficacy of TCAs in the therapy of "pure migraine" as moot.

The TCAs also have been investigated in comparison studies of TCAs and β-blockers in the prophylactic treatment of migraine.[23, 24] Pizotifen and cyproheptadine, which are structurally similar to the TCAs, decreased the severity and frequency of attacks in many patients.[25]

In a double-blind crossover trial, doxepin was compared with amitriptyline in the treatment of coexisting migraine and tension-type headache.[26] Significant reductions were demonstrated in all headache indexes, as well as in the consumption of analgesics and ergotamine preparations. Another study compared the use of amitriptyline and dihydroergotamine (DHE) in 41 outpatients diagnosed with coexisting migraine and tension-type headache.[19] The prophylactic effect of a timed-release DHE formulation was tested versus that of amitriptyline. During the month before the initiation of therapy and after 2 months of treatment, the patients maintained a daily diary that itemized the hours of headache and degree of pain. Although amitriptyline was found to be more effective than DHE in reducing headache intensity, time-release DHE was found to be significantly more effective than amitriptyline in reducing "migraine"-type attacks. To prevent the rebound phenomena associated with this therapy, ergotamine or its derivatives should not be used clinically on a daily basis.

Many of the reports on the response of migraine patients to the TCAs have been sporadic, anecdotal, or contradictory. However, it is generally thought that these agents are effective in migraine prophylaxis; this is further supported by the results of open trials.[15, 16, 19, 27] Of the 2000 new patients seen annually at the Diamond Headache Clinic, 425 will be diagnosed with either coexisting migraine and tension-type headaches, which are responsive to antidepressant therapy. The drugs of choice are amitriptyline, doxepin, and fluoxetine.

Monoamine Oxidase Inhibitors

Patients with migraine who are refractory to the TCAs and other forms of interval therapy may be helped with the monoamine oxidase inhibitors (MAOIs). The MAOIs block the oxidative deamination of numerous monoamines, including epinephrine, norepinephrine, serotonin, and dopamine. The prevailing theory in depression is that these monoamines are decreased in the brain and other tissues. The MAOIs function to replenish these neurotransmitters, and thus the depression created by their deficiency is ameliorated. It is commonly recognized that the MAOIs produce adverse effects that may be severe. Their clinical use declined markedly with the introduction of the TCAs. The MAOIs are often used in the event of TCA failure and, in some cases, in combination therapy with a TCA, although the latter regimen generally is not recommended. MAOI therapy may be indicated in the elderly because these agents are safer than the TCAs in terms of cardiovascular and anticholinergic effects.[28, 29]

In severe and intractable migraine, MAOIs are a vital therapeutic resource, and MAOIs are sometimes used in migraine prophylaxis.[30] As early as 1969, the MAOIs were found to be effective in the treatment of migraine, with a striking reduction in the frequency of headaches.[31] Anthony and Lance reported on 25 patients who were subject to frequent and severe attacks of migraine and who had not responded to conventional therapy. The patients were treated with the MAOI phenelzine sulfate (Nardil) at 45 mg/day for periods up to 2 years. The frequency of headache was reduced to less than one half that of the preceding 12 months in 20 of 25 patients.

A review study at the Diamond Headache Clinic was conducted on the use of MAOIs alone or in combination with TCAs in the treatment of the patient with recidivist headache.[32] Nineteen patients diagnosed with pure migraine were treated with MAOI therapy alone, and 11 of those patients reported improvement of 50% or greater. With coexisting migraine and tension-type headaches, improvement of more than 50% was reported by 12 of 16 patients. The results were dramatically improved compared with the patients with pure migraine.

Thus, MAOIs are a useful group of drugs in the management of migraine, depression, and coexisting migraine and tension-type headaches. Because of their potentially severe side effects, they should be reserved for those patients resistant to other forms of prophylactic therapy.

The use of MAOIs and TCAs as combination pharmacotherapy for the treatment of resistant depression has been gaining acceptance,[33] based on evidence suggesting synergism between the agents.[34] The increasing use of combined treatment has continued despite warnings from pharmaceutical firms and the U.S. Food and Drug Administration. The safety and effectiveness of combined therapy have been demonstrated in an extensive report[35] that included a review of all reported cases of complications or death associated with their use. These researchers found that the combination of any of several MAOIs with the TCA imipramine was responsible for the complications. Another report suggested that amitriptyline may prevent the reaction between the MAOIs and tyramine-containing foods.[36]

As previously mentioned,[32] MAOIs used in combination therapy with the TCAs in the patient with recidivist headache showed more than 50% improvement in 75% of patients with coexisting migraine and tension-type headaches. In addition, none of these patients experienced any significant reactions, thus confirming the findings of previous reports dealing with the safety of combination MAOI and TCA therapy.

Careful patient selection is essential in determining the appropriate form of therapy, especially in singular MAOI treatment or in combination with a TCA. The potential for serious drug and food interactions does exist, and the patient should have adequate trials on standard therapies before MAOI therapy or combination therapy is considered. Patients selected for MAOI therapy should be clearly motivated to strictly adhere to the necessary dietary and medication restrictions essential for use of the MAOIs. It is essential that patients receive thorough instruction on these restrictions and periodic reinforcement of these precautions. The physician must be cognizant of the need to carefully select patients who will have a high degree of compliance. Admission to an inpatient headache treatment unit should be considered for the initiation of combination therapy with an MAOI and a TCA.

Polytherapy

The issue of combination therapy is rarely discussed in most major textbooks and handbooks on headaches. Polypharmacy[37] is a pejorative term indicating unjustified and chaotic administration of several, often similar, drugs in an attempt to demonstrate intensive treatment. However, polytherapy is defined as a purposeful procedure being used to intensify the effect of a single drug and to affect the different elements of the complex pathophysiology of any given disease. Polytherapy is used commonly for the acute treatment of migraine, whereas very few researchers have studied polytherapy for migraine or mixed headache prophylaxis.[2, 32, 38] Because the pathophysiology of migraine, chronic tension headache, and especially the two in combination is not only complex but also not completely understood, polytherapy is justified.

The addition of the more traditional prophylactic agents for pure migraine, such as β-blockers or calcium channel blockers, can aid in the overall treatment of patients with coexisting migraine and tension-type headaches. Abortive agents, such as the triptans, ergotamine, and NSAIDs, including ibuprofen, fenoprofen (Nalfon), naproxen sodium (Anaprox), diflunisal (Dolobid), and ketoprofen (Orudis), may have several uses in patients with coexisting migraine and tension-type headaches. Naproxen sodium at an initial dose of 875 mg may be useful in aborting an acute migrainous episode.[39] However, strict control of vasoconstrictors and over-the-counter or prescribed analgesics must be emphasized.

Withdrawal Therapy

In a study of 139 patients with migraine or tension headache, or both, who had developed chronic headaches occurring at least 20 days per month for at least 6 months along with consumption of analgesic or antimigraine drugs on more than 20 days per month,[40] the mean number of tablets or suppositories taken weekly by patients before withdrawal therapy was 34.6, with the majority being ergots, caffeine, and barbiturates. Patients were hospitalized for 10 to 14 days, and all drugs were abruptly stopped. Withdrawal headache was not treated. On discharge from the hospital, 45% of patients had no headache, and 33% had improvement of 50% or greater compared with before treatment; however, fewer than 8% were headache free on a long-term basis. At a 3-month follow-up, 39% of patients were not taking any drugs, and the overall drug intake had decreased dramatically. The authors concluded that the regular intake of analgesics or antimigraine drugs can precipitate a chronic daily headache in addition to causing a deterioration of the underlying headache, whether migraine or tension.

Conclusion

A common ground exists between migraine headaches and depression. Masked depression often manifests as chronic daily headache. The TCAs or MAOIs are the agents of choice in the prophylactic treatment of coexisting migraine and tension-type headaches. For refractory cases, combination therapy consisting of a TCA and an MAOI may be indicated and should be undertaken cautiously. The recognition of this complicated headache condition offers an explanation of the overlap between depression and migraine, enhances understanding of effective therapy, and helps many patients.

References

1. International Headache Society. Classification and diagnostic criteria for headache disorders, cranial neuralgias and facial pain. Cephalalgia 1988;8(suppl 7):1–96.
2. Mathew NT. Prophylaxis of migraine and mixed headache: A randomized controlled study. Headache 1981;21:105–109.
3. Cassidy WL, Flanagan NB, Spellman ME. Clinical observations in manic depressive disease. JAMA 1957;164:1535–1546.
4. Diamond S. Depressive headaches. Headaches 1964;4:255–259.
5. Garvey MJ, Tollefson GD, Schaffer CB. Migraine headaches and depression. Am J Psychiatry 1984;141:986–988.
6. Merikangas KR, Risch NJ, Merikangas JR, et al. Migraine and depression: Association and familial transmission. J Psychiatr Res 1988; 22:119–129.
7. Rasmussen BK, Jensen R, Schroll M, Olesen J. Interrelations between migraine and tension-type headache in the general population. Arch Neurol 1992;49:914–918.
8. Rasmussen BK, Jensen R, Schroll M, Olesen J. Epidemiology of headache in a general population: A prevalence study. J Clin Epidemiol 1991;44:1147–1157.
9. Rasmussen BK. Migraine and tension-type headache are separate disorders. Cephalalgia 1996;16:217–223.
10. Wolff HG. Personality features and reactions of subjects with migraine. Arch Neurol Psychiatry 1937;37:895–921.
11. Linet MS, Stewart WF. Migraine headache: Epidemiologic perspectives. Epidemiol Res 1984; 6:107–139.
12. Ierodiakonou CS, Iavocides A. Somatic manifestations of depressive patients in different patients in different psychiatric settings. Psychopathology 1987;20:136–143.
13. Mathew NT, Stubits E, Nigam MP. Transformation of episodic migraine into daily headache: Analysis of factors. Headache 1982;22:382–383.
14. Lance JW, Curran DA. Treatment of chronic tension headache. Lancet 1964;1:1235–1239.
15. Friedman AP. The migraine syndrome. Bull NY Acad Med 1968;44:45–62.
16. Mahloudji M. Prevention of migraine. Br Med J 1969;1:182–183.
17. Diamond S. The psychiatric aspects of headache. *In* Cochrane AL, ed. Background to Migraine. New York: Springer-Verlag; 1970:60–64.
18. Diamond S. Depression and headache. Headache 1983;23:122–126.
19. Pfaffenrath V, Kellhammer U, Pollman W. Combination headache: Practical experience with a combination of a beta blocker and an antidepressive. Cephalalgia 1986;6(suppl 5): 25–32.
20. Couch JR, Ziegler DK, Hassanein R. Amitriptyline in the prophylaxis of migraine. Neurology 1976;26:121–127.
21. Noone JR. Psychotropic drugs and migraine. J Int Med Res 1977;5:66–67.
22. Couch JR, Hassanein RS. Amitriptyline in migraine prophylaxis. Arch Neurol 1979;36:695–699.
23. Langohr HD, Gerber WD, Kdetzki E, et al. Clomipramine and metoprolol in migraine prophylaxis: A double-blind cross-over study. Headache 1985;25:107–113.
24. Ziegler DK, Hurwitz A, Hassanein RS, et al. Migraine prophylaxis: A comparison of propranolol and amitriptyline. Arch Neurol 1987;44:486–489.
25. Speight TM, Avery GS. Pizotifen (BC105): A review of its pharmacological properties and its therapeutic efficacy in vascular headache. Drugs 1972;3:153.
26. Morland TJ, Starli OV, Mogstad TE. Doxepin in the prophylactic treatment of mixed 'vascular' and tension headache. Headache 1979;19:382–383.
27. Anderson PG. Treatment of migraine patients with amitriptyline. Nord Psykiat 1974;28:227–229.
28. Ashford JW, Ford CV. Use of MAO inhibitors in elderly patients. Am J Psychiatry 1979; 36:1466–1477.
29. Robinson DS. MAOIs and the elderly. *In* Friedman E, Mann J, Gershon S, eds. Depression and Antidepressants: Implications for Cause and Treatment. New York: Plenum Press; 1981.
30. Diamond S. Headaches: Method of Seymour Diamond. *In* Rakel R, ed. Conn's Current Therapy 1998. Philadelphia: WB Saunders; 1998: 895–909.

31. Anthony M, Lance JW. Monoamine oxidase inhibition in the treatment of migraine. Arch Neurol 1969;21:263–268.
32. Freitag FG, Diamond S, Solomon GD. Antidepressants in the treatment of mixed headache: MAO inhibitors and combined use of MAO inhibitors and tricyclic antidepressants in the recidivist headache patient. *In* Rose FC, ed. Advances in Headache Research. London: John Libbey; 1987:271–275.
33. White D, Simpson G. Combined MAOI-tricyclic antidepressants treatment: A reevaluation. J Clin Psychopharmacol 1981;1:264–282.
34. Schildkraut JJ, Kety SS. Biogenic amines and emotions. Science 1967;156:21–30.
35. Schuckit M, Robins E, Feighner J. Tricyclic antidepressants and monoamine oxidase inhibitors, combination therapy in treatment of depression. Arch Gen Psychiatry 1971;24:509–514.
36. Pare CMB, Hallstrom C, Kline N, Cooper TB. Will amitriptyline prevent the 'cheese' reaction of monoamine oxidase inhibitors? Lancet 1982;2:183–186.
37. Prusinski A. Monotherapy or polytherapy in migraine. Neuroepidemiology 1987;6:186–189.
38. Dexter JD, et al. The concomitant use of amitriptyline and propranolol in intractable headache. Headache 1980;20:157 (Abstract).
39. Johnson ES, et al. Naproxen sodium in the treatment of migraine. Cephalalgia 1985;5:5–10.
40. Diener HC, Dichgans J, Scholz E, et al. Analgesic-induced chronic headache: Long-term results of withdrawal therapy. J Neurol 1989;236:9–14.

13

Post-traumatic Headache

Mitchell S. Elkind, M.D.

Arthur H. Elkind, M.D.

Introduction

Headache is a common symptom after injury of the head, face, and neck. It frequently coexists with other symptoms as a symptom complex referred to variously as the *postconcussion* or *post–head trauma syndrome*. The cause of the syndrome remains somewhat controversial because many persons may have chronic pain and other symptoms despite the absence of a readily identifiable structural brain injury and obvious abnormalities on medical or neurological examination. The pathophysiology of the disorder also remains cryptic, though many investigators continue to study this issue. Despite these limitations in our understanding of the entity, there are treatments available to help the many patients who have this disorder.

Historical Perspective

Trimble[1] and Evans[2] provide good reviews of the early history of the postconcussive syndrome. Early descriptions of the persistence of headache and other symptoms after head injury can be attributed to Maty in 1766 and Boyer, Astley Cooper, and Dupuytren in the early nineteenth century. John Erichsen, Professor of Surgery at University College Hospital in London, published the first extensive reviews of the subject in 1866 and 1875, when the term *railway spine* came into use. Erichsen believed that symptoms after railway collisions and other accidents, such as falls, resulted from organic damage to the nervous system. Several other physicians of the time, however, including another London surgeon, Herbert Page, refuted Erichsen's arguments. Page helped establish the notion of a functional disorder as the cause of persistent symptoms.

The controversy spread throughout continental Europe.[1, 2] When it was recognized that passage of a law allowing compensation of passengers injured on the railroad in Prussia greatly increased the number of claims, many physicians expressed their opinion that such symptoms were due to a desire for compensation. Others, however, argued that the symptoms were directly attributable to the trauma. Various mechanisms, including hysteria, neurasthenia, and disordered cerebral circulation, were proposed.

The disagreement persisted in late nineteenth-century America, much as it does today.[1, 2] Writing in the *Boston Medical and Surgical Journal*, Hodges and Putnam questioned the organic basis of the syndrome, whereas others, including Walton, suggested that the syndrome might be due to injury to the brain rather than the spine because the brain is more susceptible to damage. In 1893, Landon Carter Gray, a New York neurologist, suggested that although the nervous system may be injured as a result of an accident, the possibility of litigation and compensation exacerbates and prolongs the symptoms. This controversy persists today.

Epidemiology

Accurate determination of the incidence of head injuries is complicated by the variability among study designs and case definitions. Mild head injury in particular is difficult to assess because individuals frequently do not come into contact with the health care system. Although the Glasgow Coma Scale[3] (GCS) (Table 13–1) is frequently used to define cate-

Table 13–1 Glasgow Coma Scale Score

Eye opening (E)	
Spontaneous	4
To speech	3
To pain	2
Nil	1
Motor response (M)	
Obeys	6
Localizes	5
Withdraws	4
Flexion	3
Extension	2
Nil	1
Verbal response (V)	
Oriented	5
Confused	4
Inappropriate	3
Unintelligible	2
Nil	1

Glasgow Coma Scale score = E + M + V (range, 3–15).

gories of severity after brain injury, there are limitations to its use, particularly with regard to mild head injury. In some studies,[4] scores as low as 8 (of 15) on the GCS are used to indicate mild injury, whereas in others,[5, 6] only scores above 12 are so used. In addition, several studies define mild head injury in a negative fashion only, suggesting that patients without any neurological examination or neuroradiological abnormalities have mild injury; these patients, however, may in fact have no injury at all. Imaging criteria are themselves subject to limitation; both computed tomography (CT) and magnetic resonance imaging (MRI) may reveal abnormalities not detected by the other.[7, 8] These methodological problems, as reviewed by Kraus et al,[9] pose significant obstacles to assessment of the true incidence of head injury, mild and otherwise.

With data from the National Health Interview Survey for 1985 through 1987, Collins[10] estimated the incidence of nonfatal head injuries in the United States to be 1,975,000 for 1990. The proportion of mild brain injury cases, variously defined, among all cases of head injury ranges from 49% to 88% of all cases of patients hospitalized for head injury in different populations.[5, 6] Most studies since 1980 indicate that about 80% of head injuries are mild.[9] One detailed study from San Diego County in 1981[11] showed that the group at highest risk of head trauma is males between the ages of 15 and 24 years and that in general at ages younger than 75 years, men are at higher risk than women. Motor vehicle accidents accounted for the highest proportion of brain injuries (42%), with falls (23%) and assaults (14%) next in order. Bicycle collisions (6%) and other sports or recreational-related activities (6%) were responsible for many of the other injuries. One third of patients older than age 15 were tested for alcohol; of these, 64% were at or above the legal limit for intoxication.

Estimates of the incidence of post-traumatic headache among patients with head injuries vary depending on the population sampled, criteria used for diagnosis, and time of assessment. Denker[12] found that as many as 90% of patients had headache at 1 month after injury, whereas Rutherford[13] found a prevalence as low as 8% at 1 year. In the classic study by Brenner et al,[14] 69% of patients had post-traumatic headache, with one third lasting longer than 2 months. Most investigators suggest that about 80% of patients will develop headache of some duration. Approximately 10% to 20% of patients with head injury will develop chronic symptoms. The incidence of persistent headache after minor head injury in children appears to be lower than that in adults, from 7% to 29% in various studies.[15–17]

Of note, the severity of the head injury appears to be inversely correlated with the presence of headache. Uomoto and Esselman,[18] for instance, found that 89% of patients with mild head injury developed headache compared with only 18% of moderate or severely injured patients ($P<.0001$). They also found that other pain syndromes, including back, neck, and shoulder pain, were significantly more common among mildly head–injured patients. Yamaguchi,[19] using a different set of criteria for severity of head injury in a group of patients in Japan, also found a statistically significant inverse correlation between severity of injury and headache. He showed that findings on CT scan correlated inversely with headache. Some have suggested that this inverse relationship between severity of injury and presence of post-traumatic symptoms indicates a functional cause of the symptoms, but others have disputed this claim.

Pathogenesis

The pathogenesis of post-traumatic headache and its related symptomatology, termed the *post-traumatic syndrome,* is a controversial topic. Although experimental, pathological, radiological, and clinical studies have shed light on the mechanisms of brain injury, their relationship to common post-traumatic symptoms is less clear.

The mechanisms of head injury are of several types. They may involve only the extracranial structures of the scalp and face or the neuraxis itself. Injuries that involve the brain may lead to direct mechanical disruption of neural tissues, such as occurs in penetrating brain injuries, or they may result in indirect damage to the brain because of movement and distortion of brain tissue within the rigid skull, as occurs in closed head injury. This movement of the brain within the skull may in turn result in several types of pathological injury, including contusion, hemorrhage, vascular injury, and diffuse axonal injury (DAI).

Extracranial injuries may result in post-traumatic pain. The scalp is extremely well vascularized, and lacerations of scalp vessels may cause profound bleeding, resulting in shock or death in cases in which it is not recognized in time. Children in particular are at risk of this complication, and they may exsanguinate while frantic attempts are made by emergency personnel to find a more common cause of acute post-traumatic hypotension. Scar tissue and disruption of local nerves with subsequent neuroma formation may contribute to post-traumatic pain in the setting of scalp or facial injury or laceration. Temporomandibular joint injury may also occur if the jaw is flung open as the mandible rotates away from the maxillary structures, resulting in persistent pain.

Open or penetrating brain injuries generally result in moderate-to-severe brain injury. They may result in one of several types of hemorrhage due to injury to blood vessels or in necrosis of brain tissue itself. When a skull fracture results in laceration of the middle meningeal artery, for example, it may cause rapid bleeding into the epidural space, resulting in rapid decline of neurological function, often after an initial lucid interval of several minutes to hours (Fig. 13–1). Surgical intervention is life-saving. Subdural hematomas may occur, as well, due to the shearing of meningothelial cells within the dural space itself. Tearing of bridging veins connecting the cortical surface to the venous sinuses can result in more slowly progressive, but still very dangerous, hematomas. These chronic subdural hematomas may occur as sequelae of even minor, unrecognized head trauma, particularly in elderly patients (Fig. 13–2). Hematomas result in symptoms and signs primarily by acting as focal masses, inducing elevations in intracranial pressure and tissue shifts within the cranial vault. Brain lacerations due to bullets or other penetrating foreign bodies result in tissue necrosis and hemorrhage. Of note, the extent of these injuries is more significantly affected by the velocity of the penetrating missile than by its mass because the energy imparted to the brain tissue is a function of the square of the missile velocity (i.e., $E = \frac{1}{2} mv^2$).[20]

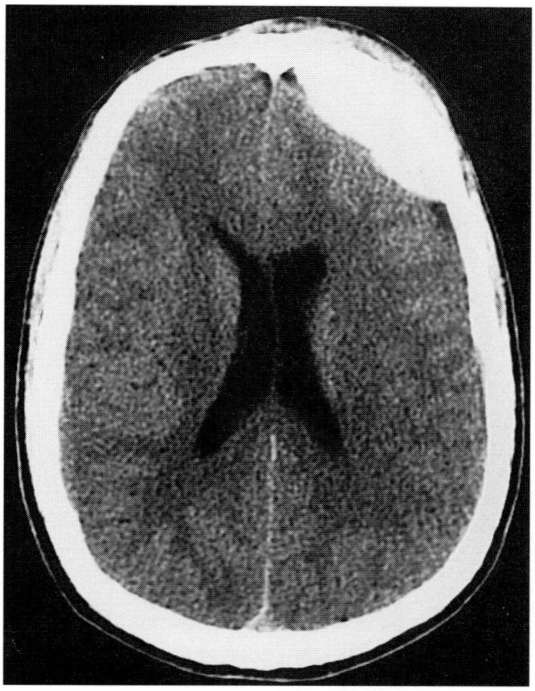

Figure 13–1 Axial CT scan shows left frontal epidural hematoma in a 23-year-old construction worker struck in the head by a cinder block. At surgery, a left frontal sinus fracture was found. The sinus was packed, and the epidural was drained. He continued to experience headache at the site of the injury for several months before spontaneous resolution.

Closed-head injury may be conceptualized best by considering the brain as a nearly noncompressible gel-like substance enclosed in a rigid shell.[21] In addition, there is liquid cerebrospinal fluid and an outlet at the base of the skull, the foramen magnum, both of which serve to buffer impact forces. Biomechanical studies involving experiments on nonhuman primates and human cadavers and computer modeling have afforded insight into the mechanisms of such injuries.

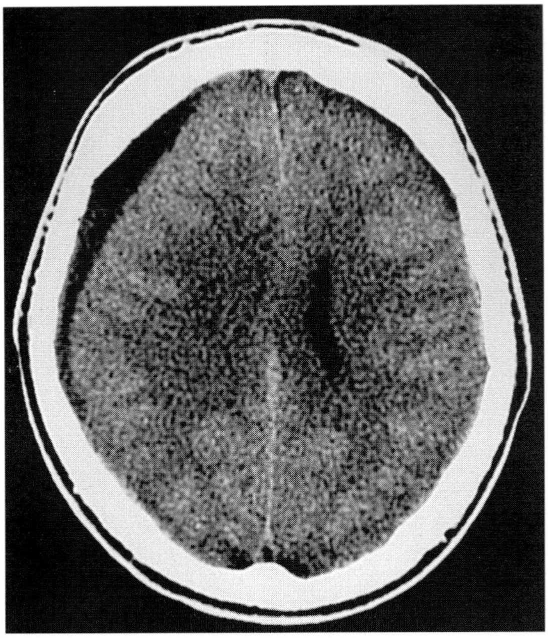

Figure 13–2 Axial CT scan shows chronic right subdural hemorrhage with mass effect in a 60-year-old man with a history of mild repeated head trauma. He experienced bifrontal headaches for 3 weeks that resolved after surgical drainage.

Blows to the head will cause both deformation of the head and acceleration (or deceleration, if the head was initially moving toward the object of impact). In general, if skull fracture does not occur, the effect of deformation can be disregarded, and the force of injury can be thought of as primarily accelerational in nature. Because the brain tends to lag behind the skull in acceleration ("inertial loading"), there is tissue compression next to the point of impact, and negative pressure develops at the lagging surface. Theoretically, head acceleration may be translational or rotational, but in practice it tends to involve both. Investigators have shown that pressures on the surface of the brain vary linearly with the magnitude of acceleration. Furthermore, the forces causing acceleration (and deceleration) sufficient to induce brain injury can be generated without any direct impact. Thus, patients may have severe brain injury without evident injury to the overlying skull or facial structures.

These theoretical physical principles allow an understanding of the pathological sequelae of traumatic brain injury. A contusion, for example, is an area of hemorrhagic necrosis of brain tissue and tends to occur at the crests of gyri rather than in the depths of sulci. It is the result of the movement of the brain against irregular bone and dural surfaces and tends to occur most frequently in the subfrontal and anterior temporal regions, which are in contact with the jagged surfaces of the orbital roof, petrous ridges, and floor of the middle cranial fossae. The injury occurring beneath the site of impact is referred to as the *coup injury,* and that which occurs on the opposite side of the brain (frequently occipital) is referred to as the *contrecoup injury.* Contrecoup injuries may occur more commonly when the individual's head is not held immobile at the time of impact. Although the etiology of contrecoup injuries is not entirely certain, it may reflect the presence of negative pressure developed as a result of the brain moving away from the skull surface.

An important development in the understanding of the pathophysiology of brain injury was the discovery by Strich in 1956[22] in patients with fatal brain injuries without skull fractures, intracranial hematomas, or brain lacerations, of widespread degeneration of white matter with small hemorrhages at the cortical–white matter interface, corpus callosum, and superior cerebellar peduncles (Fig. 13–3). Although the cortex appeared normal, there were reduced numbers of axons, "blobs" of axoplasm ("retraction balls"), and lipid-laden macrophages in the white matter of the corpus callosum, fornix, anterior commissure, and brainstem. These pathological changes are thought to represent the effects of shearing forces on axons and are referred to as DAI. Although DAI frequently is associated with substantial acceleration forces and often results in coma from onset of injury with little or no recovery, recent evidence suggests that there may be a spectrum of dysfunction, with less severe DAI allowing for recovery with sequelae of the post-traumatic syndrome.[23, 24] Obviously, the nonfatal outcome of the majority of these mildly head–injured patients hinders clinicopathological correlation. Less severely injured patients, moreover, may not have hemorrhage associated with their lesions, so even the use of very sensitive MRI techniques that detect hemorrhage may not identify these patients.

Vascular mechanisms may also contribute to the pathogenesis of head injury and post-traumatic headache. Hypoxia at the time of injury or during treatment in the hospital may result in ischemic brain injury. In addition, some investigators have found evidence of endothelial damage, perhaps induced by

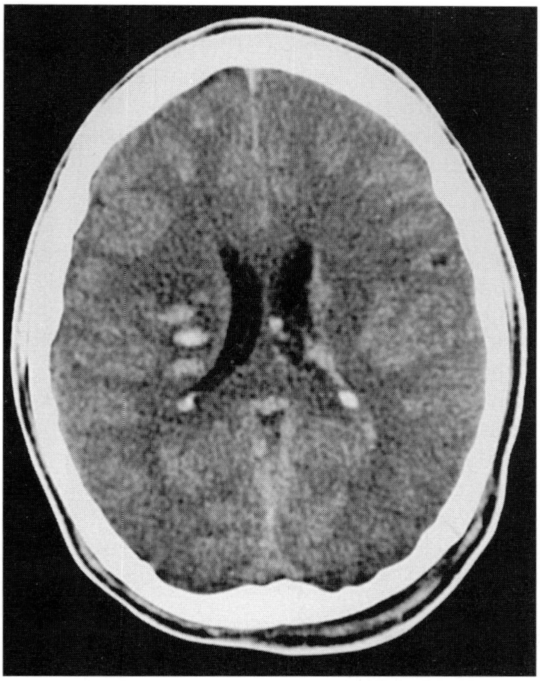

Figure 13–3 Axial CT scan shows punctate hemorrhages in the right corona radiata and corpus callosum of a 27-year-old man involved in a motor vehicle accident and thrown from his car several hours before the scan. These abnormalities are consistent with diffuse axonal injury.

prostaglandin release, after experimental brain injury.[25] This might result not only in ischemia but also in breakdown of the blood-brain barrier, allowing the entry of excitotoxic neurotransmitters and other toxins and contributing to brain injury. Excitatory amino acids such as glutamate, for instance, may cause depolarization of neurons, resulting in excessive calcium influx and cell dysfunction or death.[25]

There are several other mechanisms that may contribute to delayed symptomatology or neurological deterioration after head trauma. Hydrocephalus, both communicating and obstructive, may develop. Subarachnoid hemorrhage, a common accompaniment of traumatic brain injury, may cause a decrease in the resorptive capacity of arachnoidal granulations, resulting in normal pressure hydrocephalus, with its clinical triad of dementia, gait disorder, and incontinence. Headache, of note, is not a common feature of that disorder. Traumatic dissection of the internal carotid artery or vertebral artery may present with head pain, typically referred to the orbit, or neck pain; unrecognized, dissection may cause debilitating stroke due to artery-to-artery embolism. Similarly, traumatic carotid-cavernous fistula due to laceration of the intracavernous carotid artery may occur with painful exophthalmos.

Finally, neck injuries should not be overlooked as a cause of headache and morbidity after trauma. Whiplash injury is due to hyperextension of the neck when an individual, usually in a motor vehicle, is struck from behind. The resultant injuries are due to the relative velocities of the vehicles, as well as the use of restraints such as seat belts and head rests. The afferent fibers of the upper three cervical roots make synaptic connections with descending neurons of the trigeminal nucleus located in the cervical cord, so pain may be felt in the neck as well as in the trigeminal distribution.

Clinical Features

Although headache is the most common symptom after head trauma, it frequently coexists with one or many of the other symptoms comprising the post-traumatic syndrome.[26–28] The common symptoms include dizziness, fatigue, sleep disturbance, loss of memory and concentration, depression, anxiety, loss of appetite, and blurred vision (Table 13–2); however, many patients do not spontaneously report these symptoms. Packard et al[28] found that 65 of 100 patients with post-traumatic headache reported cognitive difficulties only when specifically asked.

The headache that develops after trauma may take many forms depending on its etiology, but it often mimics other primary headache disorders. There does not appear to be a particular type of headache associated with head trauma that is reliably distinguished from other headache disorders. Earlier studies of the categorization of headaches after

Table 13–2 Common Post-traumatic Symptoms

Headache	Hearing impairment
Dizziness	Diplopia
Fatigue	Blurred vision
Insomnia	Impaired taste and smell
Memory impairment	Photophobia
Concentration impairment	Sonophobia
Weakness	Irritability
Numbness	Depression
Tinnitus	Anxiety

head trauma are limited by selection bias, sample size, and an absence of standardized and generally accepted diagnostic criteria.[29–34] Despite these methodological problems, they suggest that chronic tension-type headache is the most common form of headache after trauma. One recent study,[35] which did use the International Headache Society diagnostic criteria,[36] found that almost all of the chronic post-traumatic headaches could be classified as chronic tension-type (75%) or migraine without aura (21%).

In our experience, pain may be localized to the site of injury but often is bilateral and generalized. It may be throbbing, aching, or squeezing, with sensitivity over the injured area, and it may be exacerbated by concentration or physical activity, including even limited movements of the head. It often radiates to the occipital, suboccipital, and nuchal regions. Pulsating pain may superimpose on a more steady baseline discomfort. The headache usually begins soon after injury but may be delayed for days, weeks, or, rarely, months. The pain may follow a variable course, with pain increasing, remitting, and recurring with greater severity at a later time.

Post-traumatic migraine[29, 34, 37] is perhaps best exemplified by *footballer's migraine*, in which soccer players experience recurrent bouts of migraine with repeated episodes of trauma. In addition to headache, other symptoms of migraine may be present, including nausea, vomiting, scintillating scotomas, photophobia, and phonophobia. Post-traumatic basilar artery migraine has been reported after uncomplicated neck injury of the whiplash type. Haas and Lourie[38] reviewed the literature on this subject and suggest that more severe episodes of transient post-traumatic derangement of brain function, including transient global amnesia, stupor, and hemiparesis, may be due to migraine, a syndrome they refer to as trauma-triggered migraine.

Cluster headache–like symptomatology may also occur.[39, 40] Two patients with bilateral sympathetic dysfunction and generalized throbbing headaches were reported by Khurana and Nirankari[41] after trauma. Vijayan[42] reported seven patients with post-traumatic vasodilator-type headaches in the frontotemporal area associated with ipsilateral mydriasis, facial hyperhidrosis, partial ptosis, and miosis. All patients had injury to the anterior neck, and the author suggested third neuronal sympathetic pathway damage in the neck was responsible. Evans[26] described a case of transient orgasmic cephalalgia occurring after mild head injury in a patient with no prior history of migraine; the symptoms resolved with the use of β-blockers and tricyclic antidepressants.

Differential Diagnosis

In addition to post-traumatic headaches that mimic primary headache disorders, there are many other conditions associated with trauma that may cause headache (Table 13–3). Some of these conditions are potentially life-threatening if not recognized early enough, and others are treatable with specific therapy. It is thus imperative to keep in mind the differential diagnosis of headache after trauma.

Pain may result from injury to extracranial structures. Superficial scalp, muscle, and subgaleal injuries may cause pain. Site of in-

Table 13–3 Differential Diagnosis of Post-traumatic Headache

Primary headache disorders
Tension-type headache
Migraine without aura
Migraine with aura
Cluster headache
Analgesic rebound headache
Trigeminal neuralgia
Occipital neuralgia
Unusual headache types
Headache with unilateral or bilateral sympathetic dysfunction
Site of injury headache
Supraorbital neuralgia
Previously subclinical Chiari malformation
Headaches associated with complications of trauma
Carotid artery dissection
Vertebral artery dissection
Carotid-cavernous fistula
Low-pressure headache
Epidural hematoma
Subdural hematoma
Subarachnoid hemorrhage
Delayed intraparenchymal hemorrhage (spat-apoplexie)
Hydrocephalus (communicating or noncommunicating)
Headache due to facial or skull fracture
Temporomandibular joint syndrome
Myofascial pain syndrome
Cervical subluxation or other neck injury
Other disorders
Depression
Anxiety disorder
Malingering

jury headache, first noted by Wolff in 1946,[43] was described in eight patients by Vijayan and Watson.[44] These patients experienced direct facial trauma with local soft tissue injury, such as laceration. They frequently had sensory loss in the distribution of the supraorbital nerve, tender scars, decreased sweating, and a neuralgic type of pain. Temporomandibular joint and facial bone injuries may also occur and cause tenderness. A myofascial pain syndrome may occur in patients with jaw injuries with stretching or tearing of the ligamentous structures of the jaw. Heyck[45] reported trigeminal neuralgia occurring after jaw and facial bone fractures.

Intracranial hematomas should be excluded in the presence of focal examination abnormalities. Delayed intraparenchymal hemorrhage, or *spat-apoplexie*, is an interesting and cryptic sequela of trauma that may present with focal findings. It may be more common than presently recognized.[46] Delayed subdural hematomas, which may particularly occur in elderly individuals in whom some degree of atrophy has already caused some stretching of the bridging cerebral veins, can cause a state of apathy or confusion without obvious focal abnormalities. Epidural hematoma with extension through an orbital roof fracture, causing headache and proptosis without change in consciousness, has also been described.[47]

Several other important conditions must be excluded in the appropriate setting. Headache with Horner's syndrome should raise suspicion of internal carotid dissection; sometimes patients will also note paresthesias in a trigeminal distribution or have 12th nerve palsy.[48] Vertebral artery dissection may also occur and is characterized by nuchal pain and symptoms of ischemia in the posterior fossa. T1-weighted MRI of the neck in the axial plane may exclude this condition. Progressive headache with gait difficulties, lethargy, incontinence, and visual symptoms may suggest obstructive hydrocephalus; normal pressure hydrocephalus generally does not present with head pain. Headache occurring primarily in the upright posture may suggest the possibility of intracranial hypotension, which has been reported after mild trauma and may be related to an occult cerebrospinal fluid leak.[49–51] Headache occurring with exertion after trauma may be due to a previously asymptomatic Chiari type I malformation.[52]

Cervical spine injury should be excluded in all patients because subluxation in this area can refer pain to the head and face. Occipital neuralgia may cause jabbing pains in the occipital region, sometimes superimposed on more chronic pain, and can be treated with local lidocaine injection.

Depression and other psychiatric disorders should also be considered. Patients with depression may present with many of the same features as post-traumatic patients, including headache, multiple somatic complaints, insomnia, anxiety, diminished concentration, and poor memory. The diagnosis of malingering must be considered in some cases, although this is an uncommon cause of post-traumatic headache.[53] If necessary, psychiatric consultation may be useful in the diagnosis of depression and malingering.

Symptoms may also be iatrogenic. Medications taken regularly to treat headache, including acetaminophen or nonsteroidal agents, may lead to a chronic daily headache syndrome, often associated with hypertension.[54] In a recent case series, Warner and Fenichel[54] reported that 9 of 11 patients referred to a headache clinic for evaluation of post-traumatic headache actually had analgesic rebound headaches, causing them to question the very notion of post-traumatic headache. In such cases, cessation of analgesic medications with substitution or more gradual tapering of antidepressant agents may be of benefit.

As in any headache syndrome, a sudden or significant change in the symptomatology warrants a fresh look at the patient and consideration of investigations to exclude new and unexpected pathology.

Evaluation

Although the management of the acutely head-injured patient is beyond the scope of this chapter, a few comments are worth making. Patients seen soon after the traumatic incident require particular attention. Pulmonary edema and cardiac irregularities may complicate head trauma, leading to hypoxia, worsening cerebral edema, and even sudden death. Signs of increased intracranial pressure, such as pupillary irregularity, sixth nerve palsies, vomiting, and obtundation, must be vigorously sought and excluded. Raccoon eyes or discoloration behind the ears (Battle's sign) and hemotympanum, indicators of basilar skull fracture, should be ruled out. Any indication of a fluctuating or declining mental status mandates close monitoring and prompt neurosurgical attention. Patients with a skull fracture or a history of loss of consciousness and amnesia, even with a normal neurological examination, probably benefit from CT scanning to exclude surgically treatable lesions.[55, 56]

Patients with post-traumatic headache will usually be seen at a later stage in the development of their symptoms, perhaps months later, when symptoms have failed to resolve. Patients seen with headache after head and neck trauma require a careful history regarding details of the accident as well as past medical history. Whenever possible, records of the initial emergency department visit and hospitalization should be reviewed for details of patient presentation, especially because amnesia may prevent the patient from providing all the necessary details. Important factors regarding the accident include the mechanism of injury; occurrence of loss of consciousness; associated facial, scalp, or bodily trauma; emergency measures taken; and initial evaluation, including neuroradiological studies and neurological examination findings. It is also important to inquire about a prior history of headache, head or neck trauma, or other neurological disease. A record of medications or other therapies already used and their effectiveness is helpful in guiding further recommendations. The headache itself should be carefully characterized with respect to quality of the pain, severity, location, duration, precipitating and mitigating factors, and associated symptoms. Often, patients will have more than one type of headache syndrome. In addition, the presence of additional symptoms of the post-traumatic syndrome should be specifically sought, as already described. A history of occupational and psychosocial dysfunction should also be sought because a significant premorbid psychiatric history may contribute to a patient's chronic disability.[13, 57]

Examination of the patient must be complete but should focus on the neurological examination and evaluation of the head and neck. Vital signs, including blood pressure, should be checked because the syndrome of chronic daily headache associated with analgesic abuse may include hypertension. The cranial nerves should be examined closely. The first cranial nerve, the olfactory, is frequently injured in head trauma due to its location beneath the orbitofrontal cortex and above the cribriform plate; the patient may be left with persistent and discouraging anosmia. Vision should be assessed because visual complaints are frequent and traumatic optic neuropathy may occur. Pupillary abnormalities may occur as the result of direct ocular trauma or sympathetic nerve injury and generally do not imply increased intracranial pressure in the alert chronic headache sufferer. Horner's syndrome, however, characterized by oculosympathetic palsy with or without anhidrosis, should raise the possibility of carotid or vertebral dissection as a sequela of trauma. Fifth and 12th nerve palsies can also occur after carotid dissection,[48] and a lateral medullary syndrome may occur with vertebral dissection. Fourth and sixth nerve palsies and, less commonly, third nerve palsies frequently occur after trauma and may cause disabling diplopia. Neuro-ophthalmological evaluation may be required to exclude carotid-cavernous fistula, the possibility of entrapped muscles in an injured orbit, or other unrelated causes. Positional vertigo with nystagmus may also occur. Lower cranial nerves are less often injured.

The presence of long tract signs such as increased reflexes, clonus, Babinski's signs, spasticity, weakness, diminished rectal tone, or loss of joint position and vibration sensation should suggest the possibility of spinal cord injury. This may occur over time with the development of, for example, a post-traumatic syrinx in the cervical region. The syndrome of the *man-in-the-barrel*, characterized by weakness and wasting of the proximal arms with sparing of the distal musculature should also raise the question of a syrinx. A *central cord* syndrome, characterized by weakness of the arms more than the legs with disassociated sensory loss, may occur after trauma. Mental status testing is imperative and may detect abnormalities in memory, concentration, or other focal areas of cognitive function.

CT scanning is the diagnostic modality of choice in the acute evaluation of the head-injured patient, but MRI often is of greater benefit in the evaluation of the chronic headache sufferer. Correlation of findings with clinical signs and symptoms is essential, however, because MRI may disclose abnormalities that bear no relation to the patient's syndrome. As Moore points out,[58] no study has demonstrated a correlation between MRI abnormalities and symptoms associated with mild head injury. *Unidentified bright objects*

(UBOs) may be detected in a large number of normal individuals and should not be misconstrued as representing pathology. On the other hand, important abnormalities to look for include evidence of epidural, subdural, and intraparenchymal hemorrhage. Although CT is useful to detect acute blood, MRI often is better at detecting chronic hematomas. Delayed subdural hemorrhage may occur, particularly in elderly individuals, as noted above. Subacute contusions may be detected with MRI, and areas of encephalomalacia will persist indefinitely, suggesting remote trauma. Diffuse axonal injury may appear on MRI as multiple punctate areas of hemorrhage, characterized by low signal intensity on T2-weighted images. Gradient echo MRI sequences, when available, may increase the sensitivity for such lesions. Despite these advantages of MRI, evaluation of the bony structures of the face, sinus, and orbit often will require CT. Routine skull radiography in a well-controlled study was found to be of low yield in head-injured patients.[59]

Although neuropsychological testing is not indicated in all patients with the post-traumatic syndrome, it may be useful when patients complain of persistent cognitive difficulties. Cognitive testing may provide useful information of several types; it may provide evidence of focal but subtle brain dysfunction, which may correlate with abnormalities, such as chronic contusions, on MRI. It may also help to distinguish malingerers from patients with organic brain injury. Patients with mild head injury may manifest diminished speed of cognitive processing, attentional problems, diminished reaction time, and memory impairment. Interpretation is required, however, because additional factors such as anxiety, depression, drugs (illicit and prescribed), and pain may affect results.

Additional neurodiagnostic studies such as electroencephalography, evoked potentials, and electronystagmography may have limited roles in particular situations. Routine and other more sophisticated laboratory investigations may be helpful when electrolyte or endocrinological abnormalities are suggested; for example, the syndrome of inappropriate anti-diuretic hormone (SIADH) and hypopituitarism may result after trauma.[60, 61]

Treatment

Several modalities of therapy, including pharmacological agents, physical and cognitive rehabilitation, and surgery, are available to treat the patient with post-traumatic headaches and other symptoms (Table 13–4). Many patients will require a combination of pharmacotherapy and physical modalities. The use of cognitive rehabilitation remains somewhat controversial, but preliminary studies suggest it may benefit certain patients.[62–65] Medina[65] reported the results of his experience using a multidisciplinary, individualized outpatient program to treat 20 patients with post-traumatic headache injured as long as 8 years in the past. Using a program centered on the physician-patient relationship, he was able to return 17 of the 20 patients to work after several weeks of combined pharmacological, biofeedback, physical, and stress management therapy. Although his results are anecdotal and uncontrolled, they suggest that dedicated physicians may be able to help

Table 13–4 Treatment Modalities

Pharmacological
Acute
Acetaminophen
Nonsteroidal anti-inflammatory drugs
Muscle relaxants
Ergotaminergic agents (e.g., Cafergot, dihydroergotamine mesylate)
Isometheptene
Sumatriptan
Combination products (e.g., Midrin)
Prophylactic
Tricyclic antidepressants
β-Blockers
Calcium channel blockers
Valproate
Methysergide
Corticosteroids
Phenytoin
Carbamazepine
Narcotics
Other
Local anesthetic injection (occipital neuralgia)
Physical Therapy
Thermal treatments
Transcutaneous electrical nerve stimulation (TENS)
Cervical collar
Surgical (when indicated)
Cervical stabilization
Occipital nerve section
Trigeminal rhizotomy
Other
Biofeedback training
Stress management techniques
Cognitive rehabilitation
Emotional support
Education
Multidisciplinary pain treatment program

many chronic patients recover and resume productive lives. Nevertheless, some patients will be refractory to multiple methods of treatment and require all the available resources of the treating physician, consultants, and other health care professionals.

Treatment must begin with as accurate a diagnosis as possible. Management of post-traumatic headaches mimicking primary headache disorders uses the same therapeutic agents. Tricyclic antidepressants are probably the most useful drugs for the treatment of post-traumatic headache and other symptoms.[66] Facial pain may also respond. Amitryptiline in a dosage range of 25 to 75 mg/day is often effective, although patients may discontinue it because of the side effects of fatigue, lightheadedness, xerostomia, or, particularly in older men, urinary difficulty. Other tricyclics, which may have a lower rate of adverse effects, include nortriptyline, protriptyline, and maprotiline. Patients should recognize that it may take as long as 2 to 3 weeks for symptoms to improve.

Nonsteroidal anti-inflammatory drugs and muscle relaxants may also be of use in patients with tension-type headache. In our experience, ibuprofen, naproxen sodium, fenoprofen, ketoprofen, and indomethacin are effective. They may also be effective in migraine and mixed headaches after trauma and have the additional advantage of reducing swelling and inflammation in areas of soft tissue injury. Ibuprofen in dosages of 400 to 800 mg up to four times daily may also abort migraines if taken early enough. Side effects are well known and include gastrointestinal distress, gastric ulceration, and renal insufficiency. Patients should not remain on these drugs indefinitely without monitoring.

Patients with migrainous headaches may also be treated with ergotamine-containing agents or sumatriptan for the acute episodes of headache. Ergotamine is available in forms suitable for oral use, rectal suppository, sublingual administration, and oral inhalation. Several preparations (e.g., Cafergot) also contain caffeine. Ergotamine should not be given in dosages that exceed 6 mg/day or 10 mg/week. Dihydroergotamine mesylate is also available for parenteral injection (IM or IV); an antiemetic is usually given, followed several minutes later by 0.75 mg dihydroergotamine mesylate slow IV. Contraindications to its use include peripheral or coronary artery disease, renal or hepatic disease, hypertension, and pregnancy. The abuse of ergotamine-containing compounds should be recognized promptly because this may result in withdrawal headaches. Isometheptene is another agent that may be slightly less useful than ergotamine, but it appears to have fewer side effects and contraindications. A combination product containing isometheptene, acetaminophen, and dichloralphenazone (Midrin) is available and may be taken at the onset of headache.

Sumatriptan, a selective 5-hydroxytryptamine$_1$ receptor agonist, is another medication for migraine. It is available for subcutaneous self-injection in 6-mg doses and for oral administration in a recommended dose of 25 to 100 mg. Like ergotamine-containing agents, sumatriptan should not be given to patients with ischemic heart disease or uncontrolled hypertension or in whom unrecognized heart disease is likely. It should not be used within 24 hours of the use of ergotamine-containing compounds.

Patients with frequent migraine or mixed-type headache may require a prophylactic agent. Tricyclics, β-blockers, calcium channel blockers, methysergide, and other agents have been used for this purpose. Propranol (10 to 40 mg TID or QID) or Inderal LA, a sustained-release preparation (60 to 240 mg/day) may be used. Dosages should begin with the minimal amount and be gradually titrated upward until therapeutic effect is achieved. Patients may complain of fatigue and depression, so these agents may be of limited value in patients with multiple other post-traumatic symptoms. Contraindications to the use of β-blockers include asthma, congestive heart failure, and bradycardia. Some patients may respond to a combination of β-blockers and tricyclics, although controlled studies of such combinations are lacking. Calcium channel blockers, particularly verapamil, may also be of benefit in some patients.

Methysergide is also approved for the short-term prophylaxis of migraine and may be effective after trauma. Because of the risk of retroperitoneal fibrosis, however, patients should not take this drug for more than 4 to 6 months continuously. Dosages are generally in the range of 4 to 6 mg/day in divided doses. Contraindications include peripheral and coronary artery disease, thrombophlebitis, hypertension, renal or hepatic disease, and pregnancy. Other agents that may prove useful in migrainous headaches include anticonvulsants such as phenytoin and valproate, cyproheptadine, and monoamine oxidase inhibitors.

Cluster headache after trauma may also respond to methysergide. Corticosteroids, calcium channel blockers, and lithium have also been used. Acute cluster episodes may respond to oxygen therapy and/or ergotamine agents.

Opiate analgesics may be prescribed for acute and subacute pain, but quantities should be limited. Close follow-up should be maintained, and any evidence of the development of dependence or chronic daily headache warrants a rapid taper. Hospitalization and detoxification may be necessary in individuals who abuse these medications.

Patients with neuralgic pains due to trigeminal or occipital neuralgia or other atypical facial pains may benefit from carbamazepine or phenytoin. Occipital neuralgia may also be treated with local injection of anesthetic with or without steroid. Vijayan and Watson[44] reported that anticonvulsants were also helpful in their patients with site of injury headache. Robbins[67] reported the use of phenytoin in a patient with post-traumatic headache and scintillating scotoma without seizures. It should be noted that most individuals with post-traumatic headache do not exhibit seizure activity.

Patients with head or neck injury and chronic pain may respond to thermal therapy, transcutaneous electrical nerve stimulation (TENS), biofeedback training, or other physical methods of therapy. A cervical collar may facilitate relief of pain in neck sprain. Cervical immobilization may be necessary in more severe injuries with subluxation, and surgical fixation may be indicated in some patients.

Prognosis

Studies on the prognosis of post-traumatic headache are limited. The 1944 study by Denker[12] estimated that 10% of patients had symptoms for less than 30 days, 65% for less than 1 year, 78% for less than 2 years, and 80% for less than 3 years. Edna[68] found rates as high as 24% at 4 years. Approximately 20% of patients, therefore, may have symptoms lasting 3 or more years and are generally thought to have "permanent" post-traumatic headache. Predictors of poor prognosis appear to include older age and possibly a vascular type of headache, although studies on this topic are lacking. Although many physicians feel that pending litigation is a deterrent to resolution of symptoms, many investigators in the field believe that this is not the case, as discussed below.

Legal Aspects

Because post-traumatic headache frequently is the result of accident or negligence, patients may become involved in litigation. Pain and suffering, as well as physical or cognitive disability, are compensable, and legal professionals may attempt to use the patient's complaints in the patient's interests. In the absence of objective signs of neurological injury on examination or other neurodiagnostic studies, the patient's attorney may have difficulty proving a causal relationship between the trauma, which often is slight, and the symptoms or disability. The physician may be called on as a medical authority to give credence to this relationship, even when an unequivocal causal connection does not exist. Adversarial legal counsel will also frequently be activated by insurance companies, corporations, and other individuals. Other physicians, acting as expert witnesses, may contradict the treating physician's opinions. The treating physician therefore may find himself or herself in the center of this struggle and grow frustrated with the patient, injuring the physician-patient relationship. The litigation itself may be viewed by the physician as the problem, and he or she may lose sight of the patient's symptoms.

This scenario undoubtedly occurs in some situations and has been the basis for some of the prejudice against the post-traumatic syndrome as a true nosologic entity. Evans[2] reports, for example, that nearly 25% of neurologists responding to a questionnaire about post-traumatic symptoms believe that patients' symptoms resolve quickly after settlement of litigation. Some support for the notion of a "compensation neurosis" came from Miller in 1961[69]; he claimed that a large proportion of 200 patients who claimed to have post-traumatic symptoms were obviously dramatizing and exaggerating their symptoms. His study, however, was clearly methodologically flawed: it used only patients referred for medicolegal consultation and used no blinded, objective, or valid criteria for diagnosis. Much evidence at present, in fact, suggests that the great majority of patients are not malingering or suffering from "compensation neurosis." Brenner et al[14] found no relationship between headache and litigation in their early study. Kelly[70] reported anecdotal evidence suggesting that 76% of patients with post-traumatic symptoms recover before legal settlement and that a large proportion of patients develop the syndrome without ever filing a claim. Guthkelch[53] studied 398 patients and found that fewer than 10% of patients exploited their condition for financial gain. In 1992, Packard[71] found that stable, chronic post-traumatic headache usually does not resolve after settlement of claims. In a large study of mildly head–injured patients in Virginia, Rimel[5] found that litigation was uncommon and did not predict return to work. Although such studies are methodologically imperfect, they do support the opinion of most experts in the field that there is an identifiable syndrome that occurs in a large number of individuals after head injury, is disabling, is directly related to the injury itself, and does not resolve with settlement of litigation. In addition, experimental evidence supports the notion that many post-traumatic symptoms may occur without evident neuroimaging or examination abnormalities.

As Evans points out,[26] the physician must be alert to the possibility of malingering and must judge each case on its own merits. In the setting of litigation, the physician should attempt to distinguish between factors that are objective, as determined by the results of examination and neurodiagnostic testing, and those that are subjective.

Conclusion

Although much controversy exists about the relative roles of functional and organic damage in post-traumatic symptomatology, advances in neuropathology, neuroimaging, and experimental neuroscience have helped identify and clarify mechanisms by which even mild head injury may lead to persistent symptoms. The precise way in which headache is generated is not entirely clear. The practicing physician must be prepared to handle patients with these common complaints, however, and in particular to offer effective therapy to those with distressing symptoms without becoming overly discouraged by the few whose symptoms may relate in part to litigation.

References

1. Trimble MR. Post-Traumatic Neurosis: From Railway Spine to the Whiplash. New York: John Wiley and Sons; 1981:5–34.
2. Evans RW. The postconcussion syndrome: 130 years of controversy. Semin Neurol 1994;14:32–39.
3. Teasdale G, Jennett B. Assessment of coma and impaired consciousness: A practical scale. Lancet 1974;2:81–84.
4. Klauber MR, Barrett-Connor E, Marshall LF, et al. The epidemiology of head injury: A prospective study of an entire community: San Diego County, CA 1978. Am J Epidemiol 1981;113:500–509.
5. Rimel RW, Giordani B, Barth JT, et al. Disability caused by minor head injury. Neurosurgery 1981;9:221–228.
6. Vasquez-Barquero A, Vasquez-Barquero JL, Austin O, et al. The epidemiology of head injury in Cantabria. Eur J Epidemiol 1992; 8:832–837.
7. Hesselink JR, Dowd CF, Healy ME, et al. MR imaging of brain contusions: A comparative study with CT. AJNR 1988;9:269–278.
8. Levin HS, Williams DH, Eisenberg HM, et al. Serial MRI and neurobehavioral findings after mild to moderate closed head injury. J Neurol Neurosurg Psychiatry 1992;55:255–262.
9. Kraus JF, McArthur DL, Silberman TA. Epidemiology of mild brain injury. Semin Neurol 1994;14:1–7.
10. Collins JG. Types of injuries by selected characteristics: United States, 1985–7. Natl Center Health Stat Vital Health Stat 1990;10(175).
11. Kraus JF, Nourjah P. The epidemiology of mild uncomplicated brain injury. J Trauma 1988;28:1637–1643.
12. Denker PG. The post-concussion syndrome: Prognosis and evaluation of the organic factors. NY State J Med 1944;44:379–384.
13. Rutherford WH, Merrett JD, McDonald JR. Symptoms at one year following concussion from minor head injuries. Injury 1978;10:225–230.
14. Brenner C, Friedman AP, Merritt HH, et al. Post-traumatic headache. J Neurosurg 1944; 1:379–392.
15. Casey R, Ludwig S, McCormick MC. Morbidity following minor head trauma in children. Pediatrics 1986;78:497–502.
16. Lanser JB, Jennekens-Schinkel A, Peters AC. Headache after closed head injury in children. Headache 1988;28:176–179.
17. Lanzi G, Balottin U, Borgatti R, et al. Late post-traumatic headache in pediatric age. Cephalalgia 1985;5:211–215.

18. Uomoto JM, Esselman PC. Traumatic brain injury and chronic pain: Differential types and rates by head injury severity. Arch Phys Med Rehab 1993;74:61–64.
19. Yamaguchi M. Incidence of headache and severity of head injury. Headache 1992;32:427–431.
20. Goodman JC. Pathologic changes in mild head injury. Semin Neurol 1994;14:19–24.
21. Elson LM, Ward CC. Mechanisms and pathophysiology of mild head injury. Semin Neurol 1994;14:8–18.
22. Strich SJ. Diffuse degeneration of the cerebral white matter in severe dementia following head injury. J Neurol Neurosurg Psychiatry 1956;19:163–185.
23. Blumbergs PC, Jones NR, North JB. Diffuse axonal injury in head trauma. J Neurol Neurosurg Psychiatry 1989;52:838–841.
24. Jane JA, Steward OS, Gennarelli T. Axonal degeneration induced by experimental noninvasive minor head injury. J Neurosurg 1985; 62:96–100.
25. Hayes RL, Dixon CE. Neurochemical changes in mild head injury. Semin Neurol 1994;14:25–31.
26. Evans RW. The postconcussion syndrome and the sequelae of mild head injury. Neurol Clin 1992;10:815–847.
27. Colohan ART, Dacey RG, Alves WM, et al. Neurologic and neurosurgical implications of mild head injury. J Head Trauma Rehab 1986;1:13–21.
28. Packard RC, Weaver RG, Ham LP. Cognitive symptoms in patients with post-traumatic headache. Headache 1993;33:365–368.
29. Behrman S. Migraine as a sequela of blunt head injury. Injury 1977;9:74–76.
30. Benoliel R, Eliav E, Elishoov H, et al. Diagnosis and treatment of persistent pain after trauma to the head and neck. J Oral Maxillofac Surg 1994;52:1138–1147.
31. De Benedittis G, De Santis A. Chronic post-traumatic headache: Clinical, psychopathological, features and outcome determinants. J Neurosurg Sci 1983;27:177–186.
32. Duckro PN, Greenberg M, Schultz KT, et al. Clinical features of chronic post-traumatic headache. Headache Q 1992;3:295–308.
33. Mandel S. Minor head injury may not be 'minor.' Postgrad Med 1989;85:213–225.
34. Weiss HD, Stern BJ, Goldberg J. Post-traumatic migraine: Chronic migraine precipitated by minor head or neck trauma. Headache 1991; 31:451–456.
35. Haas DC. Chronic post-traumatic headaches classified and compared with natural headaches. Cephalalgia 1996;16:486–493.
36. Headache Classification Committee of the International Headache Society. Classification and diagnostic criteria for headache disorders, cranial neuralgias and facial pain. Cephalalgia 1988;8(suppl 7):9–96.
37. Mathews WB. Footballer's migraine. BMJ 1972;2:326–327.
38. Haas DC, Lourie H. Trauma-triggered migraine: An explanation for common neurological attacks after mild head injury. J Neurosurg 1988;68:181–188.
39. Mathew NT, Rueveni V. Cluster-like headache following head trauma (abstract). Headache 1988;28:297.
40. Reik L. Cluster headache after head injury. Headache 1987;27:509–510.
41. Khurana RK, Nirankari VS. Bilateral sympathetic dysfunction in post-traumatic headaches. Headache 1986;26:183–188.
42. Vijayan N. A new post-traumatic headache syndrome: Clinical and therapeutic observations. Headache 1977;17:19–22.
43. Simons DJ, Wolff HG. Studies on headache: Mechanisms of chronic post-traumatic headache. Psychosom Med 1946;8:227–242.
44. Vijayan N, Watson C. Site of injury headache. Headache 1989;29:502–506.
45. Heyck H. Headache and Facial Pain: Differential Diagnosis, Pathogenesis, Treatment. Chicago: Year Book Medical Publishers; 1981:161.
46. Alvarez-Sabin J, Turon A, Lozano-Sanchez M, et al. Delayed post-traumatic hemorrhage. Stroke 1995;26:1531–1535.
47. Stewart CR, Salmon JF, Domingo Z, et al. Proptosis as a presenting sign of extradural hematoma. Br J Ophthalmol 1993;77:179–180.
48. Mokri B, Silbert PL, Schievink WI, et al. Cranial nerve palsy in spontaneous dissection of the extracranial internal carotid artery. Neurology 1996;46:356–359.
49. Mokri B, Krueger BR, Miller GM, et al. Meningeal gadolinium enhancement in low-pressure headaches. J Neuroimaging 1993;3:11–15.
50. Good DC, Ghobrial M. Pathologic changes associated with intracranial hypotension and meningeal enhancement on MRI. Neurology 1993;43:2698–2700.
51. Sable SG, Ramadan NM. Meningeal enhancement and low CSF pressure headache: An MRI study. Cephalalgia 1991;11:275–276.
52. Foletti PG, Regli F. Traumatisme cranio-cervical mineur, malformation cerebrale et cephalees chroniques. Rev Med Suisse Romande 1995;115:901–903.
53. Guthkelch AN. Post-traumatic amnesia, post-concussional symptoms and accident neurosis. Eur Neurol 1980;19:91–102.
54. Warner JS, Fenichel GM. Chronic post-traumatic headache: Often a myth? Neurology 1996;46:915–916.
55. Harad FT, Kerstein MD. Inadequacy of bedside clinical indicators in identifying significant intracranial injury in trauma patients. J Trauma 1992;32:359–363.
56. Stein SC, Ross SE. Mild head injury: A plea for routine early CT scanning. J Trauma 1992; 33:11–13.

57. Lishman WA. The psychiatric sequelae of head injury: A review. Psychol Med 1973;3:304–318.
58. Moore KL. Trauma and headaches. Headache Q 1996;7:21–29.
59. Masters SJ, McClean PM, Arcarese JS. Skull x-ray examinations after head trauma: Recommendations by a multi-disciplinary panel and validation study. N Engl J Med 1987;316:84–91.
60. Verier A, Wemeau J-L, Cappoen J-P, et al. Hyponatremie neurogene post-traumatique de revelation tardive. Rev Med Interne 1984; 5:114–121.
61. Edwards OM, Clark JDA. Post-traumatic hypopituitarism. Medicine 1986;65:281–290.
62. Berrol S. Issues in cognitive rehabilitation. Arch Neurol 1990;47:219–220.
63. Levin HS. Cognitive rehabilitation: Unproved but promising. Arch Neurol 1990;47:223–224.
64. Volpe BT, McDowell FH. The efficacy of cognitive rehabilitation in patients with traumatic brain injury. Arch Neurol 1990;47:220–222.
65. Medina JL. Efficacy of an individualized outpatient program in the treatment of chronic post-traumatic headache. Headache 1992; 32:180–183.
66. Label LS. Treatment of post-traumatic headaches: Maprotiline or amitriptyline? Neurology 1991;41(suppl 1):247. Abstract.
67. Robbins L. Post-traumatic headache with scintillating scotoma treated with phenytoin (Dilantin). Headache 1989;29:515–516.
68. Edna T-H, Cappelen J. Late post-concussional symptoms in traumatic head injury: An analysis of frequency and risk factors. Acta Neurochir (Wien) 1987;86:12–17.
69. Miller H. Accident neurosis. BMJ 1961;1:919–925.
70. Kelly R. The post-traumatic syndrome: An iatrogenic disease. Forens Sci 1975;6:17–24.
71. Packard RC. Post-traumatic headache: Permanency and relationship to legal settlement. Headache 1992;32:496–500.

14

Cerebrovascular Disease and Headache

Alan M. Rapoport, M.D.

Introduction

Although most patients who present with acute head pain have primary headache disorders such as migraine, tension-type, and cluster headache, about 10% of patients with headache who are seen in the emergency department have secondary headaches, the organic origin of which must be determined.

Secondary headaches, which can stem from intracranial masses such as brain tumors and abscesses as well as intracranial and extracranial vascular disorders, must be investigated to determine their origin. This chapter provides a review of the relationship between cerebrovascular disease and headache.

Most patients with primary headache disorders present with unilateral or bilateral head pain, usually unaccompanied by other neurological dysfunction, except for aura preceding or associated with migraine. These patients' headaches are likely to have begun before the age of 25 years. In contrast, patients who present with serious intracranial pathology usually have at least some neurological signs and symptoms and often are 45 years of age or older. Only very rarely do intracranial lesions cause headaches that exactly mirror those associated with primary headache disorders.[1]

If a patient has a negative history of headache and positive risk factors for cerebral thrombosis or embolus and develops a focal headache of unusual quality, workup for vascular disease is indicated.

Cerebrovascular Disorders That Cause Headache

Headache has been associated with intracranial hemorrhage, occlusive or embolic cerebrovascular disease, dissecting aneurysm of intracranial or extracranial arteries, arteritis/vasculitis, fibromuscular dysplasia, hypertensive encephalopathy, and post–carotid endarterectomy, as listed in Table 14–1.[2] Headache may occur concurrently with the neurological symptoms of a basilar artery transient ischemic attack (TIA) and is less likely to occur during a carotid artery distribution TIA. Headache also is unlikely to occur during a lacunar infarct; some patients experience a headache before a cerebral ischemic event.

Stroke-related headache is associated with factors such as age, sex, smoking history, and history of migraine but not with stroke severity or outcome.[3]

The onset of headache after the age of 35 years and a history of cardiac and/or peripheral vascular disease also may be clues that point to an impending cerebrovascular event. Physicians should be alert to older patients

Table 14–1 Types of Cerebrovascular Disorders That May Cause Headache

Headaches due to intracranial hemorrhage
Subarachnoid hemorrhage
Cerebral hemorrhage
Cerebellar hemorrhage
Subdural and epidural hematoma
Headaches due to occlusive cerebrovascular disease
Transient ischemic attacks
Internal carotid artery occlusion and stenosis
Occlusion of middle cerebral artery with infarction and brain swelling
Vertebrobasilar arterial occlusion and stenosis
Dissecting aneurysm of the carotid, vertebral, and middle cerebral arteries
Arteritis
Fibromuscular dysplasia
Hypertensive encephalopathy

From Kawamura J, Meyer JS. Headaches due to cerebrovascular disease. Med Clin North Am 1991;75:617–629.

who state they are having their *first* headache ever or their *worst* headache ever or who complain of *persistent* localization and *progressive* increase in pain or duration.

Prevalence of Headache Related to Cerebrovascular Disease

Overall, headache occurs in about one fourth of patients with acute stroke.[4] Headache occurs in 16% of patients who experience a TIA, 18% with reversible ischemic neurological deficit, 19% with minor strokes,[5] and 65% to 80% of patients with cerebellar hemorrhage.[6–8] Headache is less likely to occur in lacunar infarct and in small, deep basal ganglia stroke because the small intracerebral arterioles that nourish deep structures are not innervated.

A prospective study of 182 patients with ischemic stroke registered during a 1-year period in a hospital stroke data base established that 34% of patients complained of headache within 72 hours of stroke onset. Headache was more frequently reported by patients under the age of 70 years, nonsmokers, those with a history of migraine, and those who presented with transient loss of consciousness, nausea or vomiting, or visual field defects. Of these 182 patients, 57% with vertebrobasilar stroke reported headache compared with 20% of those with carotid territory stroke. Ninety percent of patients with posterior cerebral artery infarcts had headache, as did 80% of patients with cerebellar infarcts. Only 7% of patients with subcortical infarct and 9% of those with lacunae due to single perforator disease reported headache.[9]

Diagnostic Considerations

The clinical details of the headache pain may suggest locale and pathogenesis; thus, it is important that patients be encouraged to describe their *pain* accurately as intermittent, constant, variable, throbbing, steady, unilateral or bilateral, piercing, severe, moderate, or dull.

Timing of headache often has diagnostic value. The time of day at which a headache starts or worsens, the frequency with which headache occurs, and the patient's age at onset are all important.

Patients can have a headache before, during, or after a cerebral ischemic event. A late-onset headache, starting days or weeks after an acute cerebrovascular event, is not easily attributable to stroke or TIA. Clues that suggest that a headache is due to an impending or existing intracerebral vascular event include advancing age, increased blood pressure, bruits, and heart disease. *Sentinel headache,* a sudden, severe headache that disappears and may herald an impending hemorrhage, can occur days or weeks before subarachnoid hemorrhage (SAH).

Quality of headache may provide diagnostic clues. The abrupt onset of explosive, intense pain suggests SAH. Some patients describe ischemic headache as throbbing; others describe it as steady. Headache may be exertional after a cerebrovascular accident, worsening with coughing, jarring of the head, and Valsalva maneuver.

The site of pain may be an important localizing factor. Some pathological lesions are more likely than others to produce headache, and the location of a headache often provides clues as to its cause, as is discussed for each cerebrovascular disorder. Lesions in the anterior cerebral artery are least likely to produce headache; those of the carotid, middle cerebral, and basilar arteries commonly produce headache. Lesions in the posterior cerebral and vertebral arteries are most likely to be accompanied by head pain. Posterior circulation stroke is more likely to cause head pain than anterior circulation stroke. Vascular lesions that are commonly associated with headache may also occur without accompanying head pain.

Evaluation of Patients with Acute Headache

Painstaking evaluation of patients with acute headache may reveal an underlying condition responsible for the head pain; such evaluation includes taking a detailed headache history with specific inquiries about risk factors for vascular disease, family history, and medication history and performing careful physical and neurological examinations. Physical examination should be complete and include measurement of vital signs and of blood pressure in both arms and an evaluation to uncover sinus tenderness, evidence of trauma, or meningismus; palpation of the carotid and superficial temporal arteries; and auscultation of the cranium, eyes, and neck. Neurological evaluation should include mental status, cranial nerve function, muscle strength and tone, reflexes, sensation, coordination, and gait. Table 14–2 provides modifiable and nonmodifiable risk factors for stroke.

If indicated, tests to be performed include carotid Doppler, intracranial Doppler, computed tomography (CT), magnetic resonance imaging (MRI), lumbar puncture, cholesterol panel, sedimentation rate (ESR), and antinuclear antibody (ANA).

Overview of the Innervation of Intracranial and Extracranial Structures

The meninges and blood vessels that supply the meninges respond to electrical or mechanical stimulation by producing an intense boring or throbbing pain. The parenchyma of the cerebral hemispheres and cerebellum are relatively insensitive to pain. The brain, blood, and perivascular tissues may produce chemicals that provoke pain. Pain-sensitive intracranial structures include the proximal 2 cm of the middle cerebral arteries and the anterior cerebral arteries, vertebral arteries, basilar artery, intracranial portion of the internal carotid arteries, and vessels of the circle of Willis. The supratentorial region is innervated primarily by the first (ophthalmic) division of the trigeminal nerve; these bipolar neurons innervate the large cerebral arteries and dura mater. Branches of cranial nerves IX and X and some branches of the trigeminal nerve (V) plus the first three cervical nerves innervate the subtentorial regions. Branches of the trigeminal nerve synapse in the trigeminal nucleus caudalis in the medulla and interface with input from C2 and C3, which accounts for referred pain from the neck to the anterior head and vice versa.

The trigeminovascular system is defined by the relationship between the trigeminal nerve and adjacent blood vessels as well as central connections of the trigeminal nerve. The trigeminal ganglia contain pseudounipolar neurons that innervate the meninges and meningeal vessels peripherally by projecting small-caliber C fibers into these structures. After activation, C fibers transmit impulses centrally in the direction of the first synapse within lamina I and II_0 of the trigeminal nucleus caudalis in the medulla. The impulses then move caudally to the level of C2 or C3 and rostrally to the thalamus and cortex, creating the perception of pain.

This process is accompanied by the release of neuropeptide transmitters such as substance P, calcitonin gene–related peptide, and neurokinin A from the terminals of the widely branching perivascular axons. These neuropeptides mediate a neurogenic inflammatory process that appears to contribute to the pain of migraine.[10]

Table 14–2 Modifiable and Nonmodifiable Risk Factors for Stroke

Treatable/Modifiable Risk Factors	Nonmodifiable Risk Factors
Hypertension	Advancing age
Coronary artery disease	Race (African Americans)
Diabetes	Heredity
Elevated blood lipid levels	
Asymptomatic and symptomatic carotid artery stenosis	
History of transient ischemic attack (suggesting cardiac or carotid artery disease)	
Cigarette smoking	
Obesity	
Lack of exercise	

Medications, Foods, and Food Additives

Medications that may produce headache include *nitroglycerin,* which dilates the vascular system to produce headache and probably does so through the nitric oxide hypothesis; *ergotamine tartrate,* which constricts vessels to relieve headache and may cause headache via the rebound phenomenon when used too frequently; *propranolol,* which prevents dilation of cerebral vessels and occasionally produces headache when initiated; *triptans,* when used daily for an extended period; and *oral contraceptives,* which may cause headache by affecting receptors on neurons and blood vessels. Furthermore, certain food additives such as monosodium glutamate and aspartame (Nutra-Sweet) may cause headache on a chemical basis, as may some foods such as cheese, excessive caffeine, chocolate, hot dogs, liver, and alcohol. Note that glutamate, as in monosodium glutamate, is one of the excitatory amino acids and may trigger pain processes.

Intracranial Hemorrhage

Subarachnoid Hemorrhage

The most common causes of SAH are ruptured berry aneurysm, arteriovenous malformation, and trauma; other causes include saccular aneurysm, bleeding diathesis, arteritis, mycotic aneurysm, and amyloid angiopathy. Of these etiologies, however, ruptured aneurysm is responsible for 75% of SAH[2]; arteriovenous malformation is the second most common cause.[11]

SAH is associated with about 50% mortality; fewer than one third of surviving patients return to their premorbid neurological status.[12] Headache is present in almost all patients with ruptured aneurysm[13, 14] and in about 70% of all patients with SAH from any cause.[2] Headache associated with SAH may be the result of aneurysmal thrombosis, arterial wall expansion, meningeal inflammation, or blood vessel and cerebral tissue response to blood, or it may occur secondary to TIAs or stroke caused by the ruptured aneurysm.

The headache of aneurysmal rupture is characteristically bilateral, severe, and diffuse.[13, 15] About 30% of patients experience sentinel (warning) headache days or weeks before the aneurysmal rupture.[16] Unilateral onset of headache may predict ipsilateral pathology, although the pain rapidly becomes bilateral and severe. The headache may spread to the occipital region, neck, and lumbar region. *Thunderclap headache* (sudden and severe) may signal rapidly expanding but unruptured aneurysm, for which initial diagnostic tests (CT scan and lumbar puncture) will be negative for a subarachnoid bleed; angiography may be required for diagnosis.[17]

Nausea, vomiting, neck pain, and loss of consciousness are commonly associated with SAH.[14] Patients may cry out and lose consciousness; they often are transported to the emergency department by ambulance, and emergency personnel may note seizure activity and changes in vital signs. Although the headache presentation usually is dramatic, misdiagnosis may occur in patients whose headaches are less severe and/or appear to improve while under observation.[13] Gastroenteritis is a frequent misdiagnosis.

Before aneurysm rupture, patients may demonstrate a cranial neuropathy, often a third-nerve palsy; symptoms that suggest ischemia in the circulation distal to the aneurysm; or mass effect.[13]

On examination, patients may be sweating, obtunded, or unconscious and may exhibit elevated or diminished blood pressure, decreased respiration and pulse, electrocardiographic changes such as inverted T waves, or other signs of myocardial ischemia.[13]

Eighty percent of patients will have a stiff neck, and 15% will experience seizures. Five percent will have third-nerve palsy with ipsilateral large pupil, decreased ocular motility, and ptosis. On funduscopic examination, as many as 7% of patients will show subhyaloid hemorrhages.[13] Papilledema and meningeal signs may not be evident for 5 to 7 hours after SAH.

Subarachnoid blood will be evident in about 85% of cases on CT scan of the head (without contrast) if it is performed immediately after the event.[13] Sensitivity drops to 74% after 3 days.[18] If CT scan results are negative, then MRI or magnetic resonance angiography (MRA) may be indicated (Fig. 14–1).

Lumbar puncture is indicated in patients who do not undergo CT scan or when the CT results are negative and clinical suspicion of SAH is high. Owing to the distance from the site of hemorrhage, cerebrospinal fluid obtained from the lumbar subarachnoid space may be clear and colorless for as long as 3 hours after the event. A yellow-tinged supernate or xanthochromia caused by enzymatic breakdown of in vivo red blood cells always is present within 7 to 12 hours of SAH but not after a *traumatic tap*.[19]

Once SAH has been confirmed, four-vessel cerebral angiography should be per-

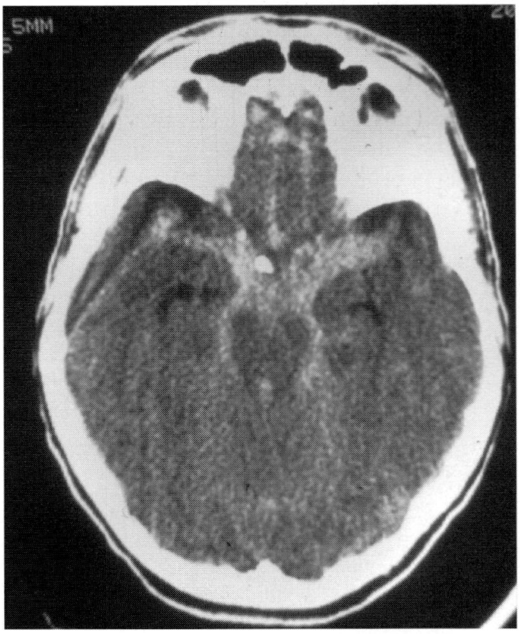

Figure 14–1 CT scan showing subarachnoid hemorrhage secondary to rupture of a right internal carotid artery aneurysm. (Courtesy of Rick Velaj, M.D., Greenwich Hospital Radiology, Greenwich, CT.)

formed to establish the location of an aneurysm or arteriovenous malformation. Because multiple aneurysms are present in 20% of patients, four-vessel angiography may reveal unruptured aneurysms as well as the one responsible for the SAH.[13] If the angiography is unrevealing, it may need to be repeated in 2 to 4 weeks when arterial spasm is decreased. Spasm should be treated vigorously because it can lead to widespread infarction.

Intracerebral Hemorrhage

Intracerebral hemorrhage is associated with headache in 23% to 57% of cases.[20–22] Headache is more likely to occur in large, lobar hemorrhages and may be ipsilateral to the bleed. The headache of frontal hemorrhage projects to forehead and eyes; that of occipital hemorrhage projects to occiput and neck; and all headaches associated with intracerebral hemorrhage can be diffuse with signs of meningeal irritation, including stiff neck, Kernig's and Brudzinski's signs, and obtundation if bleeding erupts into the ventricular system.

Patients with intracerebral hemorrhage may be alert or drowsy and typically present with sudden, severe headache accompanied

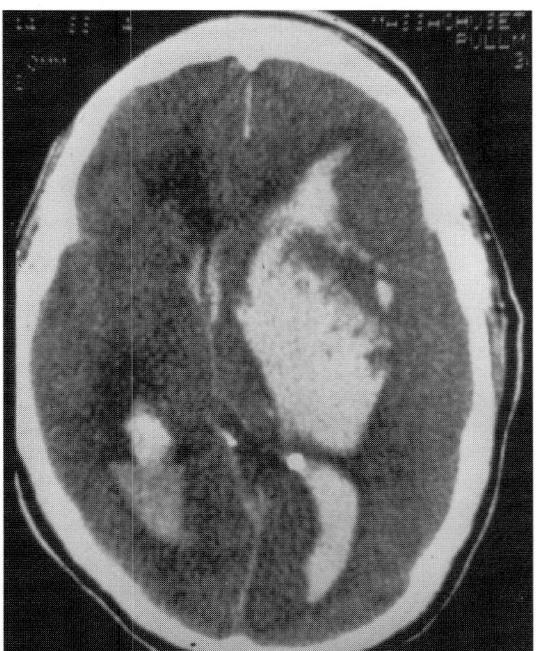

Figure 14–2 CT scan showing cerebral hemorrhage. (Courtesy of Rick Velaj, M.D., Greenwich Hospital Radiology, Greenwich, CT.)

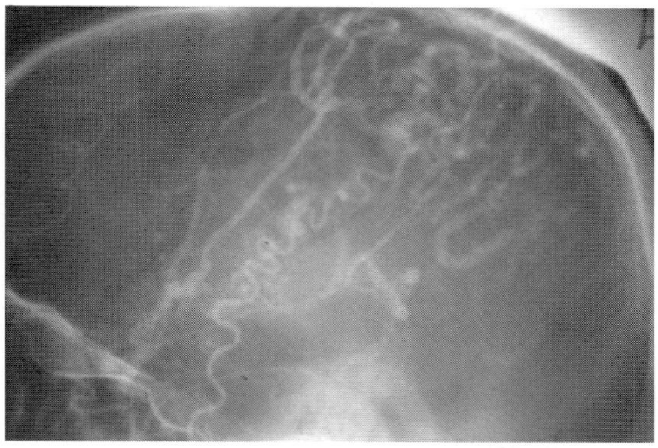

Figure 14–3 Angiogram showing unruptured arteriovenous malformation in the middle cerebral artery distribution. (Courtesy of Rick Velaj, M.D., Greenwich Hospital Radiology, Greenwich, CT.)

by nausea, vomiting, and focal neurological signs. On examination, patients may exhibit elevated blood pressure, slowed pulse, focal cerebral findings such as a visual field defect, hemiparesis, hemianesthesia, and aphasia as well as signs of meningeal irritation.

Workup should include emergency CT scan of the head. Lumbar puncture is indicated when CT results are negative, there are no signs of increased pressure, and the possibility of hemorrhage or infection persists. MRI scan of the head and cerebral angiography may be indicated later in the course (Fig. 14–2).

Causes of intracranial hemorrhage include arterial hypertension, atherosclerosis, arteriovenous malformation (which may be cryptic), brain tumor, bleeding diathesis, arteritis, amyloid angiopathy, and systemic bleeding disorders (Fig. 14–3).

The approach to treatment should include control of hypertension, reduction in cerebral edema and intracranial pressure, use of analgesics to control pain, and rarely surgery.

Cerebellar Hemorrhage

It is estimated that 65% to 80% of patients with cerebellar hemorrhage experience headache.[6–8] Although the headache usually is sudden, bilateral, and occipital, radiating to the neck and occasionally to the eyes, it also may be frontal. The headache usually is accompanied by nausea, vomiting, vertigo, dizziness, ataxia, and drowsiness.

On examination, patients may exhibit decreased level of consciousness, vomiting, nystagmus, ataxia, coordination difficulties, and breathing problems such as ataxic and Cheyne-Stokes respiration.

Some patients demonstrate conjugate deviation of the eyes to the side opposite the brainstem hemorrhage, with miosis and ataxia. The severity of clinical symptoms and signs is a function of the location of hemorrhage, its size, and the rate of expansion of the cerebellar hematoma.

All patients in whom cerebellar hemorrhage is suspected should have an emergency CT scan of the head. Lumbar puncture is contraindicated because it is associated with risk of cerebellar tonsilar herniation and death. Vertebral angiography may be useful to uncover a structural cause of bleeding (Fig. 14–4).

Idiopathic cerebellar hemorrhage should be differentiated from ruptured aneurysms of the vertebrobasilar arteries, brainstem infarction, and hemorrhage from arteriovenous malformation of the cerebellum and usually is caused by arterial hypertension, atherosclerosis, tumor, or bleeding diathesis. Surgery may be necessary.

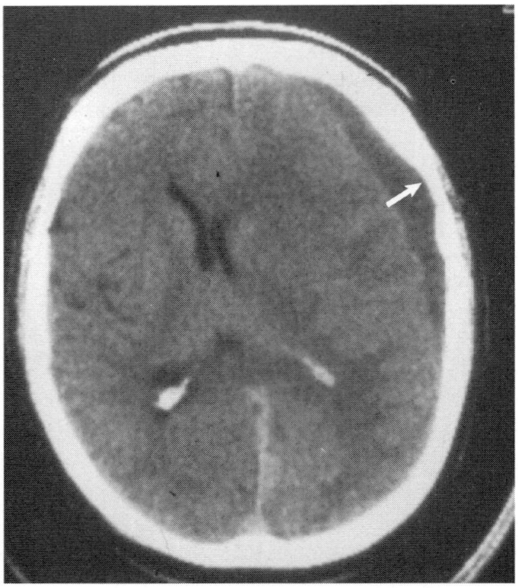

Figure 14–5 CT scan showing left frontal subdural hematoma with mass effect *(arrow)*. (Courtesy of Rick Velaj, M.D., Greenwich Hospital Radiology, Greenwich, CT.)

Subdural Hematoma

Mild-to-moderate headache is the most common presenting symptom of subdural hematoma. There often is a history of head trauma, but this may be absent in elderly patients. Elderly patients may have disturbance of consciousness, mental deterioration, and dementia, all of which may mask the symptoms of subdural hematoma and delay the diagnosis. The headache is steady and nonthrobbing, characterized by gradual worsening and diffuse location, sometimes ipsilateral to the hematoma. Occasionally, the headache is accompanied by nausea, which may be persistent and progressive and should be investigated. Nonlocalizing neurological signs are likely to occur when a hematoma is sufficiently large to compress the brain. Subdural hematoma occurs when veins that stretch across the subdural space are torn.

Patients may demonstrate waxing and waning of level of consciousness or slowly progressive focal neurological symptoms as well as nausea and visual problems (Fig. 14–5).

On examination, patients usually seem drowsy; papilledema and focal neurological signs may be present.

Appropriate workup for subdural hematoma includes CT scan of the head, with particular attention to the possible presence of

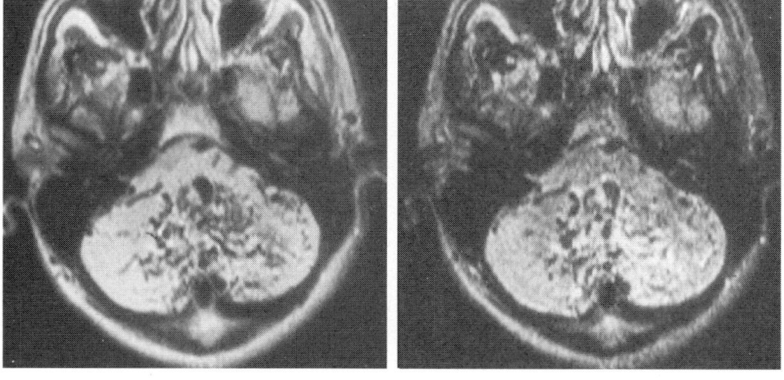

Figure 14–4 MRI of an unruptured cerebellar arteriovenous malformation. (Courtesy of Rick Velaj, M.D., Greenwich Hospital Radiology, Greenwich, CT.)

bilateral isodense subdural hematomas, which can occur about 2 weeks after injury. In this situation, the brain may appear normal on quick review of a noncontrast CT scan (Fig. 14–6). Treatment may be medical or surgical.

Epidural Hematoma

Epidural hematoma, which is particularly common in children, typically manifests as a diffuse, severe headache after significant head trauma; the headache often is ipsilateral to the bleeding. The hematoma results from a tear in the middle meningeal artery and often is associated with skull fracture.

Epidural hematoma is characterized by sudden loss of consciousness, followed by an asymptomatic lucid period, which in turn gives way to drowsiness and impaired consciousness. The headache results from separation of the dura from the skull, which has pain-sensitive vascular structures. As the hematoma volume increases, impairment of consciousness may worsen and, with it, the threat of early fatal outcome increases.

On examination, patients exhibit drowsiness, focal neurological signs such as hemiplegia, and papilledema, which is evident early in the course. Epidural hematoma should be surgically removed on an emergency basis.

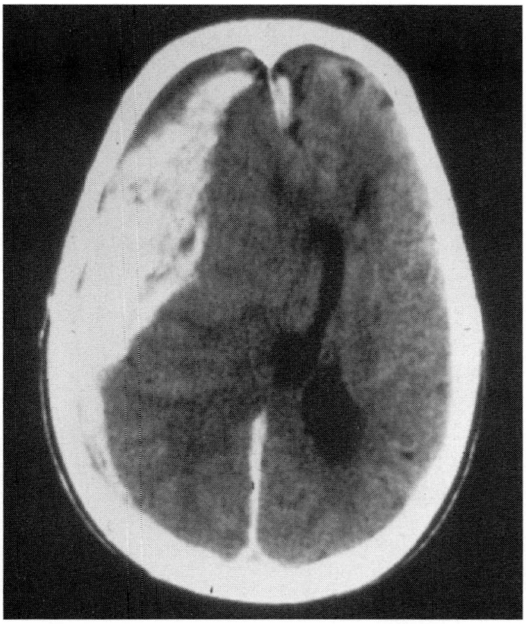

Figure 14–6 CT scan showing right frontal subdural and epidural hematoma. (Courtesy of Rick Velaj, M.D., Greenwich Hospital Radiology, Greenwich, CT.)

Occlusive Cerebrovascular Disease

Transient Ischemic Attack

Headache is associated with TIAs in 25% to 40% of patients.[2] When due to internal carotid artery disease, headache is characterized by throbbing or steady pain that may be unilateral or bilateral, orbital, frontal, temporal, parietal, or cervical. The majority of headaches due to internal carotid artery disease are mild to moderate in intensity. Middle-aged or elderly individuals with stroke risk factors such as hypertension, diabetes, smoking history, or history of heart disease are at risk for developing TIA. A history of neurological deficits and/or the finding of cervical bruits in a patient with transient neurological dysfunction suggests TIA.

Neurological symptoms such as *amaurosis fugax* (loss of vision in one eye as though a window sash has been pulled down) and transient numbness and weakness of one arm may occur before, during, or after the event. Headache that occurs as a result of carotid TIA is usually referred to the frontal areas and the eye ipsilateral to the involved vessel. Headache due to basilar artery TIA is usually referred to the occipital region.

A TIA is a 10- to 30-minute reversible, focal, neurological deficit that is often related to constrictive internal carotid artery disease at or near the carotid artery bifurcation. It is caused by stenosis (thrombosis and decreased blood flow), irregularity of the vessel wall (intimal plaque causing embolization), or cardiac disease (embolus or arrhythmia). All of the above result in decreased blood flow to the brain.

On examination, focal neurological signs such as blindness in one eye, ipsilateral carotid bruit high in the neck, and hemiparesis or monoparesis may be present. Eye examination reveals diminished visual acuity, a visual field defect in one eye, or a bright plaque of Hollenhorst in a branch of the central retinal artery, which represents a cholesterol fragment from a proximal atheromatous lesion, usually in the ipsilateral carotid artery. Some patients may, however, have a normal neurological examination.

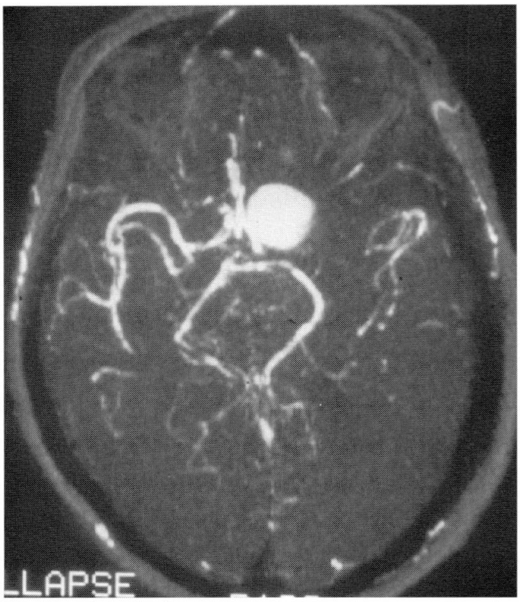

Figure 14–7 MRA showing unruptured aneurysm in the anterior portion of the circle of Willis. (Courtesy of Rick Velaj, M.D., Greenwich Hospital Radiology, Greenwich, CT.)

Because clinical details of the headache do not help to predict the cause of the TIA, investigation should always include Doppler flow study of both carotid arteries. Transcranial Doppler study may reveal an atheromatous lesion of the distal intracranial portion of the internal carotid artery. CT scan of the head (with contrast) or MRI of the head should be performed to rule out space-occupying and other vascular lesions. An echocardiogram may be indicated to uncover a cardiac source of emboli; arch and carotid angiography may be required to view the origins of the great vessels and the carotid bifurcations and complete the diagnostic picture (Fig. 14–7).

Patients can take oral aspirin (one 325-mg tablet daily) plus acetaminophen as needed for pain; endarterectomy to prevent further ischemic episodes may be appropriate for some patients.

Anterior and Middle Cerebral Artery Disease

None of a series of nine patients with anterior cerebral artery disease described headache.[20] In another series, 1 of 10 patients with isolated left anterior cerebral artery territory infarction experienced bifrontal, severe headache before hemiparesis.[23] The same authors[24] later reported headache at the onset of TIA or infarction in the anterior cerebral artery territory in 5 of 27 patients. Two of these patients experienced bifrontal headache, 2 experienced unilateral-frontal headache, and 1 experienced bioccipital headache. Fisher[20] reported an overall incidence of headache of 17% in patients with middle cerebral artery occlusion. Similarly, Silverstein and Hollin[25] reported headache in 5 of 50 patients with angiographically demonstrable middle cerebral artery occlusion, and Caplan and colleagues[26] noted that 39% of patients with middle cerebral artery occlusive disease had experienced headache at the onset of neurological deficits.

Thus, the incidence of headache in patients with anterior and middle cerebral artery disease ranges from 10% to 39%. The headache is characteristically steady and nonthrobbing and may involve the eye ipsilateral to the involved vessel. It tends to occur before or during the ischemic period. When middle cerebral artery occlusion is due to embolism, the headache is ipsilateral to the involved vessel and is perceived above the temple. The diagnosis of middle cerebral artery occlusion can be confirmed with CT scan, MRI, and cerebral angiography. With the pain relieved with acetaminophen, the headache subsides after 7 to 10 days when no cerebral edema is present (Fig. 14–8).

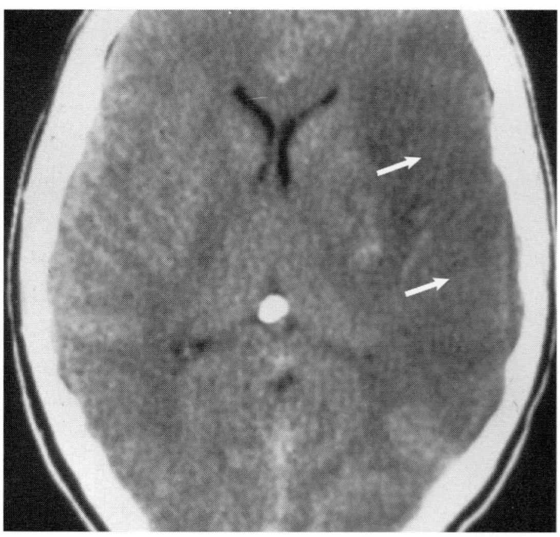

Figure 14–8 CT scan showing cerebrovascular accident in the left middle cerebral artery distribution *(arrows)*. (Courtesy of Rick Velaj, M.D., Greenwich Hospital Radiology, Greenwich, CT.)

Internal Carotid Artery Disease

Headache due to internal carotid artery disease is discussed in the section on TIAs.

Posterior Cerebral Artery Occlusion

Headache associated with posterior cerebral artery occlusion is steady and associated with either a homonymous field defect or temporal lobe symptoms and occurs in 71% of patients.[20] Emboli are less likely than thrombi to cause headache.

Vertebrobasilar Artery Occlusion and Stenosis

Throbbing pain that is aggravated by a change in position and associated with occipital tenderness and neck stiffness characterizes headache due to vertebrobasilar artery occlusion. Occurring in 37% of patients,[27] the headache is experienced in the eye, nose, and cheek and may or may not be referred to the occipital area. The headache may be followed by numbness of the face.

Neurological examination may reveal visual field defects, blurred vision, dysphagia, ataxia, and alternating hemiparesis or hemisensory loss (one side of the face and the opposite side of the body) (Fig. 14–9).

Vertebral angiography or intravenous subtraction angiography may be indicated when vertebrobasilar artery occlusion and stenosis are suspected if the MRA is unrevealing.

Stenosis of the basilar artery *without* occlusion *does not* usually produce headache.

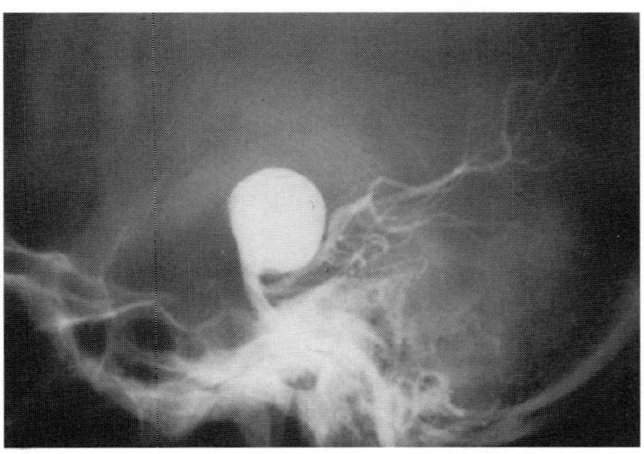

Figure 14–9 Angiogram showing unruptured aneurysm at the head of the basilar artery. (Courtesy of Rick Velaj, M.D., Greenwich Hospital Radiology, Greenwich, CT.)

Dural Sinus and Cerebral Venous Thrombosis

Thrombotic occlusions of the dural sinus and cerebral veins can produce severe headache. Patients with cerebral venous thrombosis tend to be younger than those with arteriosclerotic disease.

Severe, diffuse headache, papilledema, and obtundation occur as a result of thrombosis of the superior sagittal sinus over the top of the brain. The thrombus may spread from the sagittal sinus into the cerebral veins, progressing to hemorrhagic infarction and resulting in bilateral weakness and focal seizures. Otitic hydrocephalus occurs as a result of lateral sinus thrombosis that increases intracranial pressure without focal neurological deficits.

Cavernous sinus thrombosis is associated with periorbital and frontal pain, congestion of the conjunctiva, proptosis, facial edema, and ophthalmoplegia. The initial complaint, however, may be only retro-orbital headache. The headache of cavernous sinus thrombosis is distinguished from a primary headache on examination by neurological deficits attributable to cranial nerves III, IV, and the first two divisions of V, all of which pass through the cavernous sinus.

CT scan with contrast, MRI with gadolinium contrast, angiography, and venography are all useful in making the diagnosis of cerebral venous thrombosis (Fig. 14–10).

Treatment includes control of seizures and reduction in intracranial pressure, as well as the administration of anticoagulants and fibrinolytics. If sinus or mastoid infection is an underlying condition, antibiotics should be added to the treatment regimen.

Other sources of cavernous sinus disease include trauma, thrombus, granulomatous disease (Tolosa-Hunt syndrome), fungal infections such as aspergillosis (particularly in diabetics), herpes zoster, tumor, and vascular malformation. MRI with gadolinium enhancement is the current state-of-the-art diagnostic procedure; treatment must be targeted to the cause of disease.

Dissecting Aneurysm of Intracranial or Extracranial Arteries

Patients with dissecting aneurysm of the intracranial or extracranial arteries may experi-

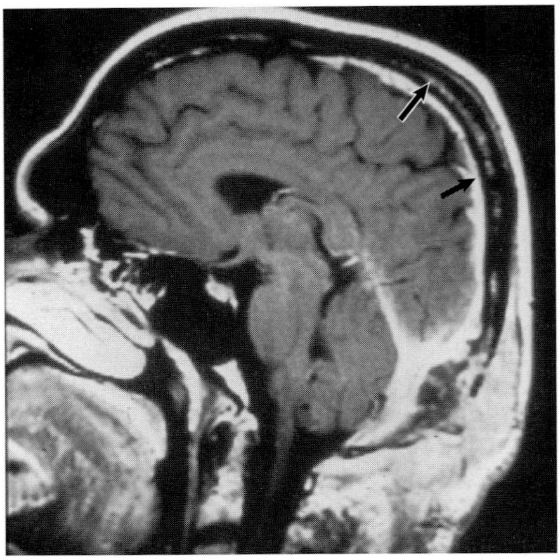

Figure 14–10 MRI showing superior sagittal sinus thrombosis *(arrows)*. (Courtesy of Rick Velaj, M.D., Greenwich Hospital Radiology, Greenwich, CT.)

ence head and/or neck pain before the onset of neurological deficits. In many cases, the pain is similar to that of cluster headache but is continuous and long lasting rather than intermittent and brief.

The headache associated with carotid artery dissection is characteristically moderate to severe and frontal or in the eye; visual acuity in the ipsilateral eye may be diminished. In most patients, the pain persists for less than 3 months.[13]

Patients with dissecting aneurysm of the carotid artery may experience neck pain and tenderness in the upper part of the common carotid artery (Fig. 14–11). The headache and neck pain may be accompanied by neurological symptoms such as Horner's syndrome (ipsilateral ptosis and miosis), bruit, and visual disturbances. Such patients may also have TIAs and strokes in the distribution of the involved vessel or vessels.

Ultrasound, angiography, and MRI/MRA are helpful in confirming the diagnosis. Treatment with analgesics to relieve pain is indicated. Patients with arterial occlusion due to carotid dissection may undergo external carotid–internal carotid bypass surgery (see Fig. 14–11). Some patients' occlusions may partially or completely resolve without surgical intervention.

Dissection of the vertebral arteries is accompanied by a similar headache that is experienced in the occipital region; patients may develop symptoms of vertebrobasilar arterial insufficiency. The patient's history may reveal prior trauma and rotation injuries to the neck and head; such injury may occur rarely in the course of chiropractic manipulation. Differential diagnosis includes Raeder's syndrome and migraine with pupillary dysfunction. In most patients, neck pain is accompanied by severe occipital pain that may radiate anteriorly to the forehead, periorbital region, or temple.

Initially sharp and severe, the pain gradually improves over a period of 1 to 3 weeks. In common with dissection of the carotid artery, TIA and/or stroke may occur as a result of emboli or decreased perfusion distal to the stenosed region.

Onset of pain may not be accompanied immediately by neurological deficit, which may occur after hours or as long as 3 weeks. Symptoms due to diminished blood flow secondary to the dissection include diminished consciousness, vertigo, vomiting, facial and

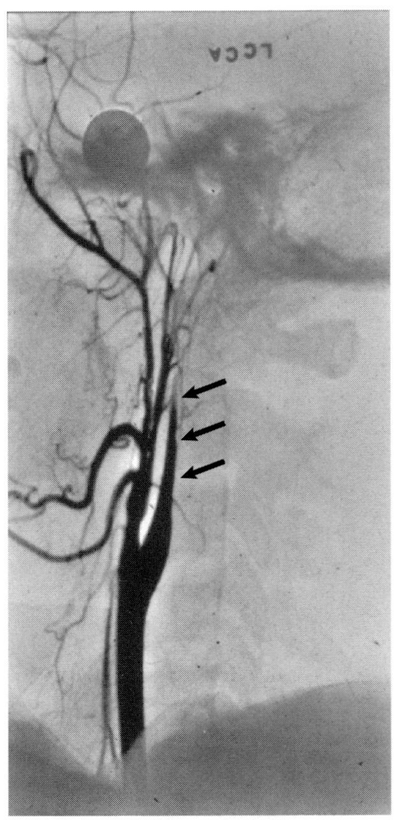

Figure 14–11 Angiogram showing internal carotid artery dissection *(arrows)*. LCCA, left common carotid artery. (Courtesy of Rick Velaj, M.D., Greenwich Hospital Radiology, Greenwich, CT.)

bilateral limb paresthesias and motor deficits, diplopia, and hemianopia.

Ultrasound, MRI/MRA, and cerebral angiography can be used to confirm the diagnosis. Conservative treatment (heparin initially, followed by coumadin) is usually sufficient.

Postcarotid Endarterectomy

More than 50% of patients who undergo carotid endarterectomy may experience throbbing, ipsilateral headache; most such headaches occur within 5 days after surgery. The onset of headaches may, however, begin within minutes or up to 3 weeks after surgery. Although throbbing headache is most common, the pain may be steady, continuous or variable, and focal or diffuse and may mimic migraine or cluster or any other headache type. In rare cases, the headache can be accompanied by seizures and cerebral hemorrhage.[13]

Postcarotid endarterectomy headache must be differentiated from postoperative vascular occlusion and dissection of the vessel. Such postsurgical headache may be the result of increased cerebral blood flow and disorganized cerebral autoregulation, but the headache cannot be explained on the basis of blood flow alone.[13]

Fibromuscular Dysplasia

Fibromuscular dysplasia (FMD) often is an incidental finding in patients who undergo angiography for other reasons. It may affect any of the major cerebral and cervical arteries in addition to arteries that supply other organs. It often occurs in the common carotid artery.

Patients with FMD present with a history of multiple, recurrent neurovascular symptoms, among which headache is the most prominent. In addition to headache, FMD is associated with neck pain, vertigo, tinnitus, TIAs, and syncope as well as with symptoms from lesions throughout the arterial system.

The diagnosis is usually confirmed with carotid angiography, which typically reveals multiple, irregularly spaced concentric constrictions with normal or dilated intervening segments (the *string of beads* pattern).

Arteritis and Vasculitis

The arteritides include temporal arteritis (giant cell arteritis), a multifocal panarteritis that may involve the superficial temporal and other arteries; periarteritis nodosa; Takayasu's disease; Wegener's granulomatosis; and systemic lupus erythematosus, all of which may cause headache as a result of inflammation of adjacent meninges, irritation of blood vessels, and cerebral infarction and microhemorrhages in the brain substance. Temporal arteritis is the most common of the arteritides.

Temporal arteritis, a granulomatous vasculitis, typically affects women over the age of 50 years; about 90% of patients with temporal arteritis have an elevated sedimentation rate.[13] Its characteristic signs are tenderness and irregular swelling of the superficial temporal and occipital arteries. Headache, which occurs in approximately 90% of patients,[13] is highly variable and may be throbbing, boring, dull, sharp, continuous, or intermittent; it also may be severe. The headache may be experienced at the temple only, or it may involve the temple and other areas of the head, including frontal, vertex, or occipital regions as well as the face and neck. Patients also may have symptoms of polymyalgia rheumatica with proximal leg pain and weakness and/or jaw claudication. Diagnosis may be confirmed with temporal artery biopsy.

Untreated, temporal arteritis may result in blindness and stroke. Treatment with glucocorticoids should be begin as soon as the diagnosis has been made. The dosage is 25 to 100 mg of prednisone daily, which is given over 6 to 12 months and then slowly tapered. Symptoms, including the headache, tend to improve rapidly, often within 24 hours after treatment has been instituted.

Migraine and Stroke

The association between migraine and stroke has been well established. Stroke may present as a complication of migraine, raising a number of intriguing questions, as posed by Welch[28]: Does stroke occur in the course of the migraine attack, causing true migraine-induced cerebral infarction? Does migraine cause stroke because similar risk factors are present? Can stroke present as a migraine syndrome, that is, symptomatic migraine?

Few epidemiological studies have addressed the relationship between migraine and stroke, and results to date have been inconclusive. There are, however, data to suggest that migraine and stroke are strongly associated. The National Health and Nutrition Examination Survey,[29] a large-scale study of men and women in the United States, showed a strong association between migraine and stroke in both men and women. The study controlled for such stroke risk factors as hypertension, diabetes, heart disease, and sex. The Physicians' Health Survey[30] also noted an elevated risk of ischemic and hemorrhagic stroke of all types in men with migraine compared with men without migraine.

It has been estimated that each year stroke affects 3.36 of 100,000 adults with migraine.[31] According to Bougousslavsky and colleagues,[32] women with migraine are far more likely to develop stroke. Symptoms develop more slowly in this group of patients, whose strokes are more frequently in the distribution of the posterior cerebral artery. These patients' angiograms and echocardiograms exhibited significantly more abnormalities than did those of control subjects.

Rothrock et al,[33] however, noted no significant differences in sex ratio or the frequency of smoking, estrogen use, hypertension, mitral valve prolapse, or family history in evaluating epidemiological and clinical data from 310 patients with migraine and 30 with acute migrainous stroke.

Aura symptoms of migraine may resemble those of TIA in some patients; both may be characterized by monocular or homonymous hemianopic visual loss, diplopia, somatosensory disturbances, memory loss, aphasia, and focal weakness. Although the neurological deficit of TIA is likely to be fully developed and negative (loss of vision, loss of sensation) at onset, the symptoms of aura tend to increase in intensity over time and often are characterized by positive somesthetic phenomena such as scintillation and moving, bright, zig-zag lines (*fortification*).[34]

Migrainous cerebral infarction has been characterized as a typical aura symptom that does not fully disappear within 7 days in a patient who has migraine with aura; Welch[28] has suggested naming this condition *migraine-induced stroke.*

When determining whether a stroke may be related to migraine, consider that (1) transient focal neurological symptoms accompanied by headache do not always satisfy the criteria for migraine, (2) migraine is not always associated with headache, and (3) a patient with migraine may have a stroke that is related to a condition other than migraine.[34] Table 14–3 presents the differential diagnosis of transient focal deficits with headache.

Table 14–3 Differential Diagnosis of Transient Focal Deficits with Headache

Migraine with aura
Cerebral ischemia
Neoplasm (transient tumor attacks)
Seizure
Arteriovenous malformation
Demyelinating disease
Panic attacks
Hypoglycemia
Subdural hematoma
Vasculitis / focal encephalitis

Adapted from Ramadan NM, Merikangas KR. Comorbidity of migraine and stroke. Semin Headache Mgmt 1996;1:7–9.

To meet the criteria for migraine-induced stroke, the neurological deficit must be identical to the symptoms of the patient's stereotypical migraine attacks, stroke must occur during the course of a migraine attack, and other causes of stroke must be excluded although risk factors for stroke can be present. Classification of migraine-related stroke is shown in Table 14–4.

In response to Welch's well pointed questions, migraine can indeed coexist with stroke. Furthermore, stroke *with clinical features of migraine that are not related to migraine* has been described.

Coexisting stroke and migraine requires a clearly defined clinical stroke syndrome that occurs remotely in time from a typical migraine attack. Stroke with clinical features of migraine suggests a structural lesion that is not related to migraine pathogenesis that presents with the clinical features of a migraine attack; it may be characterized as symptomatic migraine or migraine mimic.

Table 14–4 Classification of Migraine-Related Stroke

Category	Feature
I	Coexisting stroke with migraine
II	Stroke with clinical features of migraine
	a. Symptomatic migraine
	b. Migraine mimic
III	Migraine-induced stroke
	a. Without risk factors
	b. With risk factors
IV	Uncertain (such as drug interactions)

This may occur in cases of arteriovenous malformation, in which neurological symptoms masquerade as migraine.

Migraine-induced stroke begins with primary neural phenomena in the brain, after which cerebral hemodynamic and metabolic consequences ensue. These events may be associated with low cerebral blood flow, coagulopathy, and platelet changes that can lead to thrombosis.

A migrainous infarction is a stroke that occurs during a migraine aura. The International Headache Society criteria for a migrainous infarction are (1) previously fulfilled diagnostic criteria for migraine with aura, (2) an attack under consideration for migrainous infarction that is typical of previous attacks but with neurological deficits that are not completely reversible within 7 days and/or neuroimaging that demonstrates ischemic changes in relevant brain area, and (3) other causes of infarction are ruled out.[35] Few patients who have had a migraine-induced stroke have a recurrence.[34]

The International Headache Society definitions of migraine-induced stroke do not permit diagnosis of migraine-related stroke in patients with migraine without aura. Further study of the migraine-stroke relationship will, however, eventually yield information about stroke in patients with migraine without aura.

The differential diagnosis of migrainous infarction[36] is shown in Table 14–5.

Mitochondrial encephalomyopathies are characterized by recurrent headaches accompanied by vomiting, proximal weakness due to myopathy, and stroke-like episodes that involve hemiparesis, hemianopia, cortical blindness, and seizures. Abnormalities on CT may include focal encephalomalacia. Although many migraineurs note weakness during aura or migraine attacks, few develop myopathy.

Internal carotid and basilar artery dissection should be ruled out, as should marantic endocarditis, intracranial arterial vasculitis, and atherosclerotically related artery-to-artery embolism.

Table 14–5 Differential Diagnosis of Migrainous Infarction

Mitochondrial encephalomyopathies
Intracranial artery dissection
Basilar artery dissection
Intracranial arterial vasculitis
Atherosclerotic occlusion secondary to artery-to-artery embolus

Adapted from Schuaib A. Stroke from other etiologies masquerading as migraine-stroke. Stroke 1991;22:1068–1074.

Antiphospholipid antibodies (anticardiolipin antibodies, lupus anticoagulants, or both) have been studied in patients with migraine, stroke, and both. Migraine is about twice as prevalent among patients with stroke and antiphospholipid antibodies than in the general population.[37] Similarly, antiphospholipid antibodies are found about twice as frequently in patients who meet criteria for migraine with aura than they are in those with migraine without aura. Approximately one third of patients with migrainous cerebral infarction have been found to have either anticardiolipin antibodies or antilupus antibodies in the absence of other risk factors for stroke.[38] These studies suggest that antiphospholipid antibodies may be associated with migraine-induced stroke, but further study is required, because direct evidence for this phenomenon has not been found, and several negative studies have been reported.

Hypertensive Encephalopathy

Although formerly commonplace, hypertensive encephalopathy seldom occurs because hypertension is treated early and aggressively. Patients whose blood pressure is higher than 240/120 mm Hg for extended periods may develop headache and other symptoms. Headache accompanies hypertensive encephalopathy in 85% of patients,[20] is characterized as diffuse or occipital, and usually occurs on awakening in the morning. The headache is followed by symptoms such as blurred vision, vomiting, vertigo, generalized weakness, irritability, seizures, and disturbances of consciousness. Papilledema and retinal vasospasm or bleeding occur due to increased intracranial pressure in the majority of cases.

Workup should rule out cerebral hemorrhage and seek a cause for the elevation in blood pressure. Untreated hypertensive encephalopathy is a medical emergency because the lack of treatment can result in cerebral hemorrhage, seizure, and death. Hypertensive encephalopathy should be treated promptly and aggressively with one or a combination of antihypertensive medications, diet, exercise, and relaxation techniques.

Conclusion

Most types of cerebrovascular disease can cause headache. Hemorrhagic lesions are more likely to produce headache than are nonhemorrhagic lesions. Posterior cerebral artery disease is more likely to produce headache than is anterior and middle cerebral artery disease. Headache in older persons with risk factors for cardiac and vascular disease may signal an impending stroke.

All patients who present with their first headache after the age of 35 years, worst headache ever, a persistent or consistently worsening headache, or a change in established headache pattern should be worked up aggressively to rule out intracranial and extracranial vascular lesions.

The cause of headache in cerebrovascular disease probably is related to neurogenic inflammation in the trigeminovascular system at the interface of the dural arteries and the terminal branches of the fifth cranial nerve in the meninges.

Migraine-associated stroke is a complex association between two illnesses that may share risk factors and can be difficult to distinguish clinically.

References

1. Edmeads JG. Headache as a symptom of organic diseases. Curr Opin Neurol 1995;8:233–236.
2. Kawamura J, Meyer JS. Headaches due to cerebrovascular disease. Med Clin North Am 1991;75:617–629.
3. Jorgensen HS, Jespersen HF, Nakayama H, et al. Comment. Neurology 1995;45:1427–1428.
4. Vestergaard K, Andersen G, Nielsen MI, et al. Headache in stroke. Stroke 1993;24:1621–1624.
5. Koudstaal PJ, van Gijn J, Kappelle LJ, et al. Headache in transient or permanent cerebral ischemia. Stroke 1991;22:754–759.
6. Rosenberg GA, Kaufman DM. Cerebellar hemorrhage: Reliability of clinical evaluation. Stroke 1976;7:332–336.
7. Scotti G, Spinnler H, Sterzi R, et al. Cerebellar softening. Ann Neurol 1980;8:133–140.
8. van der Hoop RG, Vermeulen M, van Gijn J. Cerebellar hemorrhage: Diagnosis and treatment. Surg Neurol 1988;20:6–10.
9. Ferro JM, Melo TP, Oliveira V, et al. A multivariate study of headache associated with ischemic stroke. Headache 1995;35:315–319.
10. Moskowitz MA, Cutrer FM. Trigeminovascular system and migraine. Semin Headache Mgmt 1996;1:7–9.
11. Sahs AL: Subarachnoid hemorrhage. *In* Harrison MJG, Dyken ML, eds. Cerebral Vascular Disease. London: Butterworths; 1983:354–402.
12. Solomon RA, Rink ME. Current strategies for the management of aneurysmal subarachnoid hemorrhage. Arch Neurol 1987;144:L769–L774.
13. Ward TN. Headache in cerebrovascular disease. *In* Samuels MA, Feske S, eds. Office Practice of Neurology. New York: Churchill Livingstone; 1996:1141–1144.
14. Perkins AT, Ondo W. When to worry about headache: Head pain as a clue to intracranial disease. Postgrad Med 1005;96:107–208.
15. Fontanarosa PB. Recognition of subarachnoid hemorrhage. Ann Emerg Med 1989;81:1199–1205.
16. Gorelick PB, Hier DB, Caplan LR, et al: Headache in acute cerebrovascular disease. Neurology 1986;36:1445–1450.
17. Day JW, Raskin NH. Thunderclap headache: Symptom of unruptured cerebral aneurysm. Lancet 1985;2:1247–1248.
18. Adams HP Jr, Kassel NF, Torner JC, et al. CT and clinical correlations in recent aneurysmal subarachnoid hemorrhage: A preliminary report of the Cooperative Aneurysm Study. Neurology 1983;33:98–108.
19. Fishman RA. Cerebrospinal Fluid in Diseases of the Nervous System, 2nd ed. Philadelphia: WB Saunders; 1992:183–188.
20. Fisher CM. Headache in cerebrovascular diseases. *In* Vinken PJ, Bruyn GW, eds. Handbook of Clinical Neurology, Vol V. Headache. Amsterdam: North-Holland Publishing Company; 1968:124–156.
21. Mohr JP, Caplan LR, Melski JW, et al. The Harvard Cooperative Stroke Registry: A prospective study. Neurology 1978;28:754–762.
22. Portenoy RK, Abissi CJ, Lipton RB, et al. Headache in cerebrovascular disease. Stroke 1984; 15:1009–1012.
23. Bougousslavsky J, Regli F. Infarctus du territoire de l'artière cérèbrale antérieur gauche. Rev Neurol 1987;143:21–31.
24. Bougousslavsky J, Regli F. Anterior cerebral artery territory infarction in the Lausanne Stroke Registry. Arch Neurol 1990;47:144–150.
25. Silverstein A, Hollin S. Internal carotid vs. middle cerebral artery occlusions. Clinical differences. Arch Neurol 1964;12:468–471.
26. Caplan L, Babikian V, Helgason C, et al. Occlusive disease of the middle cerebral artery. Neurology 1985;35:975–982.
27. Jorgensen HS, Jespersen HF, Nakayama H, et al. Headache in stroke: The Copenhagen Stroke Study. Neurology 1994;44:1793–1797.
28. Welch KMA. Relationship of stroke and migraine. Neurology 1994;44(suppl 7):S33–S36.
29. Merikangas KR, Fenton BT, Cheng SH, et al. Association between migraine and stroke in a large-scale epidemiological study of the United States. Arch Neurol 1995;54:362–368.
30. Buring JE, Herbert P, Romero J, et al. Migraine

and the subsequent risk of stroke in the Physician's Health Study. Arch Neurol 1995;52:129–134.
31. Henrich JB, Sandercock PAG, Warlow CP, et al. Stroke and migraine in the Oxfordshire Community Stroke Project. J Neurol 1986;223:257–262.
32. Bougousslavsky J, Regli F, Van Melle G, et al. Migraine stroke. Neurology 1988;39:223–227.
33. Rothrock J, North J, Madden K, et al. Migraine and migrainous stroke: Risk factors and prognosis. Neurology 1993;43:2473–2476.
34. Ramadan, NM, Merikangas KR. Comorbidity of migraine and stroke. Semin Headache Mgmt 1996;1:7–9.
35. International Headache Society. Classification and diagnostic criteria for headache disorders, cranial neuralgias, and facial pain. Cephalalgia 1988;suppl 7:1–96.
36. Schuaib A. Stroke from other etiologies masquerading as migraine-stroke. Stroke 1991; 22:1068–1074.
37. Tietjen GE, Levine SR, Welch KMA. Migraine and antiphospholipid antibodies. *In* Appel SH, ed. Current Neurology. Vol 12. Chicago: Mosby–Year Book; 1992:201–213.
38. Silvestrini M, Cupini LM, Matteis M, et al. Migraine in patients with stroke and antiphospholipid antibodies. Headache 1993;33:421–426.

15

Headaches of Ocular Origin

Robert L. Tomsak, M.D., Ph.D.

Introduction

The differential diagnosis of headache should include primary disease of the eye and its surrounding structures. The sensory innervation of the eye and periocular region is from the first and second divisions of the fifth cranial nerve. Recurrent branches of the trigeminal nerve also supply the intracranial dura, venous sinuses, and cerebral vessels. Headache of nonocular cause is often referred to the eye and orbit, and pain of primary ocular origin commonly radiates to other parts of the head and face.

With few exceptions, ocular causes of pain tend to be associated with a red eye.

Eyestrain (Asthenopia)

Asthenopia (literally *sight without strength*) has been defined by Duke-Elder[1] as "the symptoms experienced in the conscious striving of the visual apparatus to clarify vision by ineffectual adjustments." The symptoms of eyestrain have been documented since the time of ancient Greece, but the American neurologist S. Weir Mitchell is credited with first considering eyestrain to be a legitimate cause of headache. Those who have become presbyopic will attest to the periocular discomfort that can accompany this condition and lead to headache. Others have been more skeptical. Derby[2] suggested that eyestrain was a functional disturbance, or "ocular neurosis," and stated "eyestrain is a terrible and serious bugbear to the public; would that the word had never been coined." Donders,[3] a famous nineteenth-century ophthalmologist, pronounced that "asthenopics sometimes have a sad past and a gloomy future."

The symptoms of eyestrain commonly include mild, dull, aching pain around or behind the eyes and a sensation that the eyes are tired, hot, uncomfortable, sore, or strained. The pain may spread to the forehead and temples, and tearing and mild conjunctival injection occasionally occur.

Causes of eyestrain include uncorrected refractive errors as well as minor disturbances of ocular alignment (*heterophoria*); however, when confronted with a patient with headache who has had one or more changes in eyeglasses prescriptions in the recent past, the chance that the cephalalgia is due to an optical error is unlikely. Asthenopic discomfort is thought to be generated from fatigue of the ciliary muscle, which is responsible for the process of accommodation. Eyestrain is always directly related to use of the eyes and is relieved through rest from visual tasks; it is never associated with other symptoms, such as nausea, photophobia, or visual aura.

Eye muscle imbalances often lead to asthenopic symptoms. Convergence insufficiency[4] is frequently seen in the age group of 20 to 40 years as an idiopathic condition. It may also occur after head trauma and other states of debility. Ocular discomfort, tearing, heaviness of the eyelids, sleepiness on reading, and blurred vision characterize this condition. Individuals with this condition often arise very early to do their studying as opposed to reading late in the evening. Fatigue of the normal mechanism for near vision—consisting of convergence of the eyes, accommodation of the physiological lenses, and pupillary miosis—leads to drifting of the eyes away from one another during prolonged close work. Diagnosis requires ophthalmological testing of the power of the convergence system. Treatment involves eye exercises to strengthen convergence ability.

Spasm of the near reflex is another cause for asthenopia; it can be thought of as the exact opposite of convergence insufficiency. With this condition, the near synkinesis is hyperactive, leading to intermittent, usually painful bouts of convergence, accommodation, and pupillary miosis. Episodic brow ache, variable diplopia, and blurred vision at distance are common symptoms.

Spasm of the near reflex is thought to be a functional visual disturbance in the majority of cases, and only rarely is it linked with structural brain disease.[5] It may be falsely diagnosed as bilateral sixth nerve palsy, thus provoking an extensive, expensive, and futile evaluation.[6] The diagnosis of accommodative spasm is made on the basis of the symptoms just noted and the telltale combination of intermittently crossed eyes accompanied by pupillary constriction. Treatment of this condition is frustrating, but fortunately the problem is self-limited. Cycloplegic eye drops, like homatropine, can be used to paralyze the near response. Bifocals, prisms, and various other optical aids have been tried with little success.

Corneal and Conjunctival Disease

The cornea and conjunctiva are two of the most pain-sensitive ocular structures. Discomfort arising from these areas ranges from a well-localized mild foreign-body sensation to extremely severe pain. Conjunctival redness, tearing, and blepharospasm are invariably present with conjunctival and corneal disease and aid the examiner in diagnosis. Ordinarily, this discomfort is not confused with headache; however, there are two types of corneal irritation that may have confusing symptoms. Patients who have a recurrent erosion syndrome affecting the corneal epithelium and its basement membrane may complain of intense pain on opening their eyes in the morning; this pain is associated with blurred vision. Presumably, eyelid movement over a poorly adherent epithelium gives rise to these symptoms. Diagnosis is made by observing telltale abnormalities in the basement membrane of the corneal epithelium with the slit-lamp.

Patients with tear-film abnormalities, or dry eyes (*keratoconjunctivitis sicca*), commonly complain of a sandy feeling in their eyes. On occasion, a severe lightning-like pain, lasting less than 1 or 2 seconds, is perceived. This is sometimes described as an electric shock or as if a hot pin were jabbed into the eye. The pain is similar to what has been called "ice-pick-like pain"[7] or *ophthalmodynia periodica*.[8]

Both of these types of corneal irritation are symptomatically treated with ocular lubricants.

Glaucoma

Intraocular pressure is maintained by a balance between production of aqueous humor by the ciliary body and drainage of this fluid through the trabecular meshwork of the eye located at the angle formed by the junction of the peripheral cornea with the iris.[9] If drainage of aqueous humor is impeded, intraocular pressure (IOP) rises, resulting in the disease called *glaucoma*. If elevated IOP is sustained or repetitive, characteristic abnormalities develop in the optic disc and visual field. Although multiple subtypes of glaucoma are delineated by ophthalmologists, categorization centers about whether the anterior chamber filtration angle is open or closed. The gravamen for pain production is not so much the absolute degree of elevated pressure but rather the rate of rise of IOP.

Acute (Narrow-Angle) Glaucoma

Angle-closure glaucoma, with its attendant rapid rise in IOP, is often associated with acute pain and headache. The pain is frequently confused with migraine or intracranial aneurysm. In its fulminant form, angle-closure glaucoma presents with excruciating, prostrating pain that is centered around the eye and orbit and often associated with nausea, vomiting, and lethargy. At this stage, the eye is red, the cornea may be cloudy, and the pupil is often fixed to light and mid-dilated secondary to iris ischemia. This latter finding often leads the nonophthalmologist to incorrectly consider an aneurysmal cause. However, if the eye is gently ballotted, it is usually rock hard compared with its fellow and ptosis and ophthalmoplegia are not present, thus excluding third cranial nerve dysfunction. Acute angle-closure glaucoma is an ophthalmological emergency.

A subacute form of angle-closure glaucoma exists in which the symptoms are transient pain and blurred vision, sometimes associated with the appearance of halos around lights due to corneal edema. These attacks may be self-limited and can occur after a prolonged time in darkness (e.g., in a movie theater) or after emotional upset or in other circumstances in which the pupil dilates and mechanically obstructs aqueous drainage from the eye.

Neovascular Glaucoma

The growth of abnormal new vessels in the filtration angle can obstruct aqueous outflow, resulting in a secondary form of glaucoma that is often painful. This condition is often associated with severe, persistent, throbbing ocular and orbital discomfort. Common predisposing factors for neovascular glaucoma are diabetic retinopathy and central retinal vein occlusion. Neovascular glaucoma also occurs in eyes with chronic uveitis and ipsilateral to occluded carotid arteries or carotid-cavernous fistulas. The mechanism for neovascularization is ocular ischemia with production of angiogenesis factors, and much of the discomfort with neovascular glaucoma may be due to ischemia rather than to increased IOP. To confirm the diagnosis, ophthalmological examination is needed, sometimes combined with fluorescein angiography of the iris (Figs. 15–1 and 15–2).

Ocular Ischemic Syndrome (Ischemic Ocular Inflammation)

Signs and symptoms of ocular inflammation can result from ocular ischemia of local (e.g., ophthalmic artery occlusion) or more proximal (e.g., carotid occlusion) causes.[10] A few cells and aqueous flare are sometimes seen on slit-lamp examination of the anterior chamber of the eye and presumably are related to hypoxic alterations in iris and ciliary

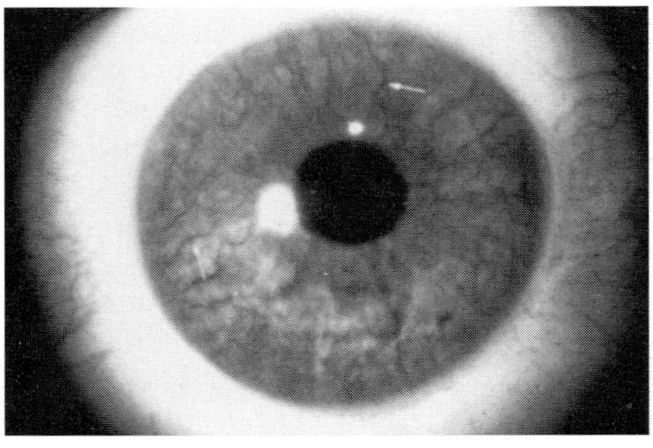

Figure 15–1 Iris neovascularization. Note multiple new vessels on surface of the iris (*arrow*).

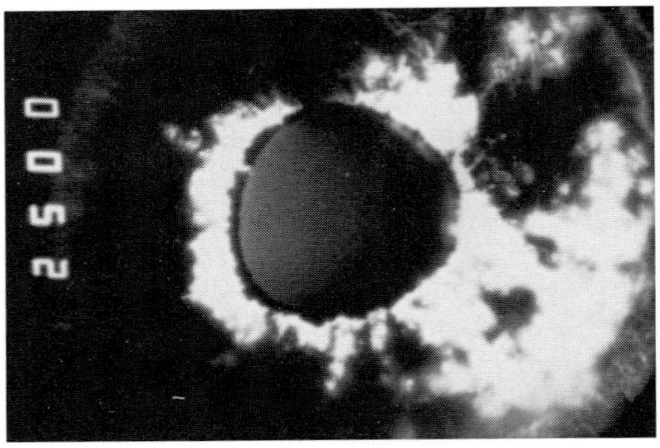

Figure 15–2 Iris fluorescein angiogram. Bright areas represent leakage of fluorescein dye from neovascularization.

body vascular permeability. Often, there are characteristic changes seen in the ocular fundus termed *venous stasis retinopathy*. Ophthalmoscopic findings include intraretinal, or *blot*, hemorrhages in the retinal midperiphery and posterior pole, venous dilation, nerve fiber layer infarcts (*cotton-wool spots*), and areas of retinal neovascularization (Figs. 15–3 and 15–4). These changes are similar to those of diabetic retinopathy but are unilateral and ipsilateral to the involved carotid artery. Venous stasis retinopathy occurs in about 30% of patients with carotid occlusions.

Ischemic ocular pain from carotid occlusion is constant and aching and localized to the brow area, upper part of the face, and temple. It is often worse when the patient is standing and improves when supine, presumably due to gravitational effects on orbital

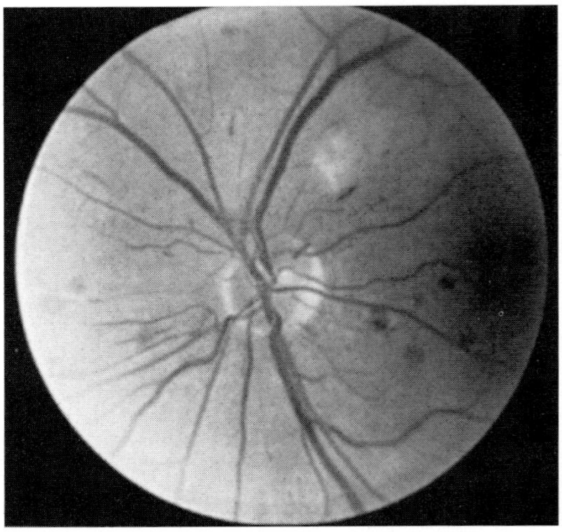

Figure 15–3 Venous stasis retinopathy. Multiple hemorrhages and one nerve fiber layer infarct around optic disc.

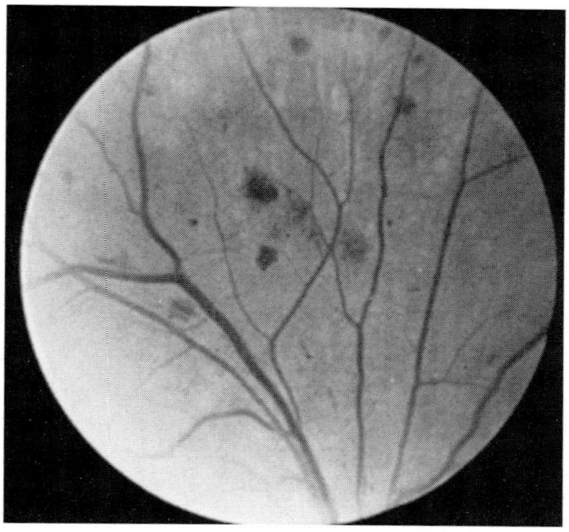

Figure 15–4 Venous stasis retinopathy. Multiple "blot" hemorrhages in retinal midperiphery.

perfusion. At times, flow to the orbit comes from external carotid artery collaterals. The pain may also be due in part to dilation of these collateral vessels, such as the superficial temporal artery. Ischemic ocular pain occurs in 5% to 40% of patients with carotid artery occlusion. Symptoms and signs may regress after cerebral revascularization surgery.[11]

A useful test to perform when venous stasis retinopathy is suspected is *finger ophthalmodynamometry* to estimate retinal artery pressure. With the direct ophthalmoscope, the central retinal artery and vein are visualized on the surface of the optic disc. Gentle pressure is then placed on the lower eyelid with a finger. Normally, the central retinal vein will collapse with minimal pressure on the eye, but more force is required to elicit arterial pulsations. In patients with true venous stasis retinopathy, the central retinal artery will collapse at about the same finger pressure needed to collapse the central retinal vein.

Uveitis

Uveitis is a generic term used to describe intraocular inflammation affecting the uvea (iris, ciliary body, and choroid) and sometimes contiguous structures such as the retina and vitreous.[12] One classification of uveitis is based on the anatomic site of inflammation in the eye, such as *uveitis involving the anterior segment of the eye* (iritis, iridocyclitis) or *uveitis involving the posterior segment of the eye* (choroiditis).[12]

Uveitis affecting the anterior segment of the eye tends to be the most painful. The pain is often severe, aching, or throbbing and is commonly associated with light sensitivity or photophobia. At times, the pain may be referred to the ear, teeth, and sinuses. Tearing, *floaters* (vitreous opacities), and blurred vision are common complaints. Examination reveals redness of the eye, especially at the junction of the cornea and sclera. The pupil may be small and poorly reactive due to iris sphincter muscle spasm. Inflammatory cells in the anterior chamber and vitreous and aqueous flare are present in variable amounts depending on the severity and cause of the uveitis (Fig. 15–5).

There are numerous causes for intraocular inflammation, including sarcoidosis, histoplasmosis, toxoplasmosis, syphilis, herpes simplex, and ankylosing spondylitis. Patients with acquired immune deficiency syndrome are often affected by cytomegalovirus retinitis and *Pneumocystis carinii* as well as the other infectious agents just mentioned; however, very often no cause is found. Uveitis of noninfectious etiology is primarily treated with topical or periocular steroids and atropine-like drops to paralyze the pain-sensitive iris and ciliary muscles.

Infectious causes of uveitis, termed *endophthalmitis*, may be especially devastating to the eye. The symptoms and signs include lid swelling, pain, conjunctival edema, redness, and loss of vision. The most common setting for bacterial endophthalmitis is after eye surgery or penetrating eye trauma, and it usually occurs within the first few days or weeks after surgery or injury. However, en-

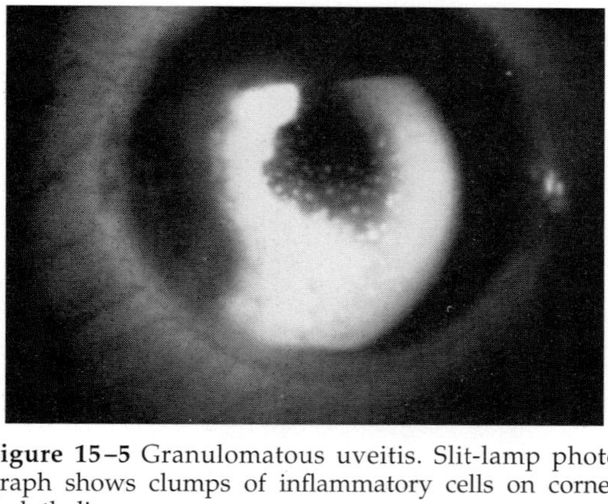

Figure 15–5 Granulomatous uveitis. Slit-lamp photograph shows clumps of inflammatory cells on corneal endothelium.

dophthalmitis may occur months or years after cataract or glaucoma surgery and can be of metastatic origin in virgin eyes of septic patients. Eye pain in any patient with a history of prior ophthalmic surgery or injury, in association with the signs just noted, requires immediate evaluation by an ophthalmologist.

Retrobulbar Optic Neuritis

Patients with acute inflammation of the retrobulbar optic nerve may complain of mild to severe discomfort in the orbital and supraorbital areas that is worsened by eye movement and pressure on the globe. Approximately 90% of patients with acute retrobulbar neuritis have discomfort beginning at the time of visual loss or within hours to days later.[13] The pain resolves as the acute inflammatory process abates and rarely requires treatment, although systemic steroids have a salutary effect on the discomfort. The pain accompanying optic neuritis is thought to be due to irritation of the meninges surrounding the optic nerve (Fig. 15–6). The presence or absence of pain seems to have no relation to the severity of visual loss or ultimate visual prognosis.

Orbital Disease

Distressingly severe discomfort may accompany orbital disorders. Krohel and colleagues[14] emphasized that evaluation of orbital signs and symptoms can be reduced to six Ps: pain, progression, proptosis, palpation (for masses and resistance to retrodisplacement), pulsation (thrills and bruits), and periocular changes. Orbital cellulitis, inflammatory orbital pseudotumor, posterior scleritis, lacrimal gland malignancies, and metastatic cancer to the orbit are the most painful orbital diseases. The diagnosis of these conditions is greatly aided by high-resolution computed tomography scanning of the orbit, orbital ultrasonography, and magnetic resonance angiography.

Orbital cellulitis is usually bacterial in nature and presents with the rapid onset of pain, ophthalmoplegia, proptosis, conjunctival chemosis, and visual loss over a period of days (Fig. 15–7). It is most common in children, and contiguous sinusitis is often present. *Haemophilus influenzae, Staphylococcus aureus, Streptococcus pyogenes,* and *Streptococcus pneumoniae* are the common pathogens.

Inflammatory orbital pseudotumor (*idiopathic orbital inflammation*) seems to be an immune complex–mediated disease that may diffusely affect the orbit or eye muscles (*orbital myositis*) (Fig. 15–8). It may be recurrent and related to other allergic phenomena or

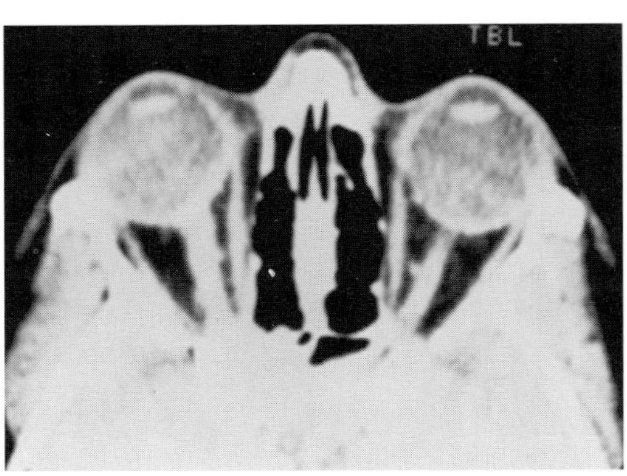

Figure 15–6 Retrobulbar optic neuritis. High-resolution CT shows thickening of optic nerve (*left*).

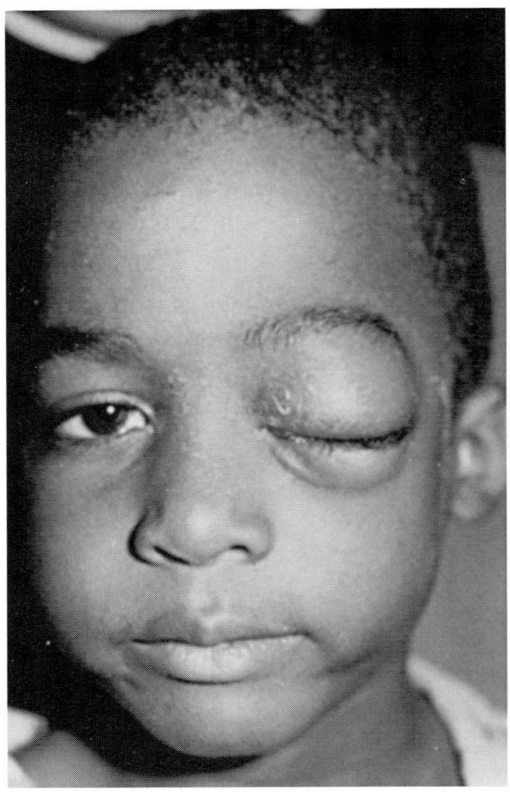

Figure 15–7 Orbital cellulitis. Note marked periocular swelling and ptosis.

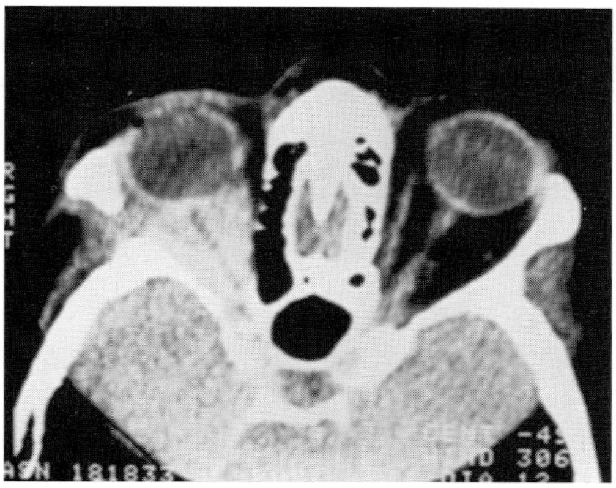

Figure 15–8 Inflammatory orbital pseudotumor. High-resolution CT shows diffuse infiltration of orbit (*left*).

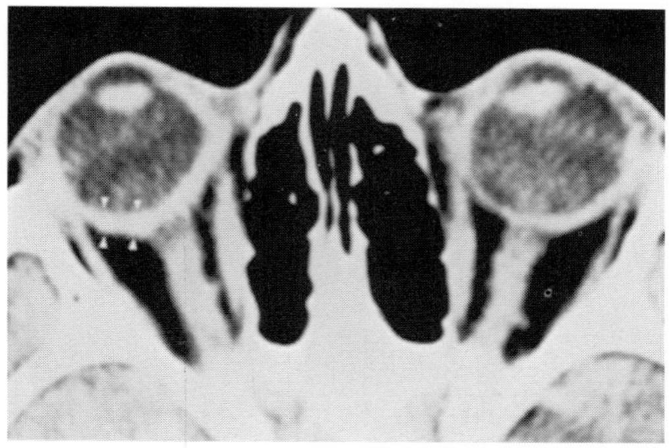

Figure 15–10 Posterior scleritis. Contrast-enhanced high-resolution CT shows thickening of sclera (*left*).

upper respiratory tract problems.[15] Unilateral pain, diplopia, proptosis, adnexal erythema, edema, and visual loss occur over a period of days (Fig. 15–9). Short-term, high-dose oral corticosteroids or, sometimes, orbital irradiation is needed to resolve the inflammatory process. Serious systemic illnesses are rarely present, with the exception of Wegener's granulomatosis, in which orbital involvement occurs in about 40% of cases.

Posterior scleritis is a related condition that is characterized by deep orbital pain often referred to the temple (Fig. 15–10). Systemic rheumatic diseases, such as rheumatoid arthritis or other collagen vascular disorders, are present in at least 25% of patients. Treatment is accomplished with systemic and topical corticosteroids, nonsteroidal anti-inflammatory drugs, or immunosuppressants.

Malignant lacrimal gland tumors, especially adenoid cystic carcinoma, cause deep-seated, boring orbital pain from periosteal and perineural invasion. The onset of this condition is usually insidious over a period of months.

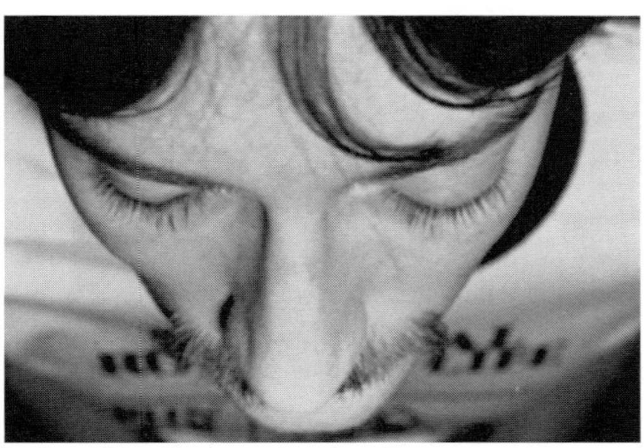

Figure 15–9 Inflammatory orbital pseudotumor. Proptosis of left eye is evident when patient is viewed from above.

Metastases to the orbit present with pain in about 20% of cases. Common tumors include breast cancer in women and lung or prostate cancer in men. Pain seems to be correlated with periosteal involvement. Enophthalmos, as opposed to exophthalmos, is sometimes seen when scirrhous carcinoma of the breast metastasizes to the orbit. New onset of cluster headache has been reported after orbital exenteration for invasive basal cell carcinoma. Whether this is a chance association or a cause-and-effect relationship is not known.[16]

Miscellaneous Problems

Preherpetic Neuralgia

Neuritic pain in the brow and temple area may precede the appearance of the classic vesicular eruption (Fig. 15–11) on the skin supplied by the first division of the trigeminal nerve by 4 to 5 days. The appearance of the vesicles confirms the diagnosis.[17]

Photophobia

Photophobia is defined as an abnormal intolerance to light, usually combined with eye pain. The neural pathway that subserves this sensation is not clearly defined but certainly includes the trigeminal nerve.

Miller[18] notes four different types of light sensitivity: (1) photophobia occurring with disease of the anterior segment of the eye (e.g., corneal disease, iritis), (2) photophobia

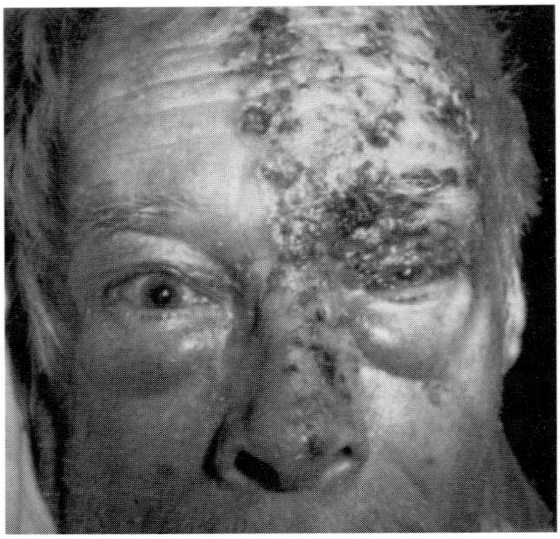

Figure 15–11 Herpes zoster ophthalmicus.

associated with vitreoretinal disease (e.g., vitreous opacities, albinism, achromatopsia), (3) photophobia with acquired optic neuropathies, and (4) photophobia after intracranial trauma, surgery, infection, or inflammation. Photophobia also occurs as an idiopathic phenomenon and certainly as concomitant with migraine.*

The first category seems to be related to the exquisite pain sensitivity of the iris and to pupillary constriction in response to light; the second type is not understood, although it is known that the electroretinogram is supranormal in ocular albinism. In the third category, the observation is correct, but the explanation is not apparent. Photophobia after some form of head trauma is well recognized, and the thalamus may play a role in these "central" cases.[19, 20] Naturally light-sensitive persons sometimes are considered to be neurotic, but this is not always the case.

Tables 15–1 through 15–3 provide examples of headache with diplopia, headache with pupillary abnormalities, and headache with visual loss.

* I used the β-blocker nadolol to successfully treat a middle-aged woman with episodic photophobia without headache or other ocular or intracranial causes.

Table 15–1 Headache with Diplopia

Painful isolated third nerve palsy
  Ischemic (microvascular)
  Compressive (aneurysm or tumor)
  Ophthalmoplegic migraine
Painful isolated sixth nerve palsy
  Ischemic (microvascular)
  Gradenigo's syndrome (mastoiditis and petrositis)
Painful isolated fourth nerve palsy
  Ischemic (microvascular)
  Trochleitis
Painful multiple cranial nerve palsies or eye muscle dysfunction
  Tolosa-Hunt syndrome (cavernous sinusitis)
  Carotid cavernous fistula/dural shunt syndrome
  Cavernous sinus tumor (primary or metastatic)
  Orbital cellulitis
Orbital inflammatory syndrome

Data from Tomsak RL. Ophthalmologic aspects of headache. Med Clin North Am 1991;75:693–706.

Table 15–2 Headache with Pupillary Abnormalities

Adie's tonic pupil
Episodic pupillary dilation with migraine
Raeder's syndrome (painful Horner's syndrome)

Data from Tomsak RL. Ophthalmologic aspects of headache. Med Clin North Am 1991;75:693–706.

Summary

Pain around the eye can be caused by local ophthalmic disorders or disease of other structures sharing trigeminal nerve sensory innervation. In general, most ocular causes for pain also cause the eye to be red, thus alerting the examiner to the focality of the problem. However, conditions such as eyestrain, intermittent angle-closure or neovascular glaucoma, and low-grade intraocular inflammation can be painful and not associated with obvious redness.

Ocular signs and symptoms also occur with numerous other causes of headache. Double vision in association with periocular pain can result from orbital lesions, isolated cranial neuropathies, and cavernous sinus lesions. Pupillary abnormalities like Horner's syndrome (Fig. 15–12) may result from a variety of painful conditions, including cluster headache, parasellar neoplasms or aneu-

Table 15–3 Headache with Visual Loss

Migraine with aura (classic migraine)
Retinal migraine
Optic neuritis
Giant cell arteritis
Pseudotumor cerebri

Data from Tomsak RL. Ophthalmologic aspects of headache. Med Clin North Am 1991;75:693–706.

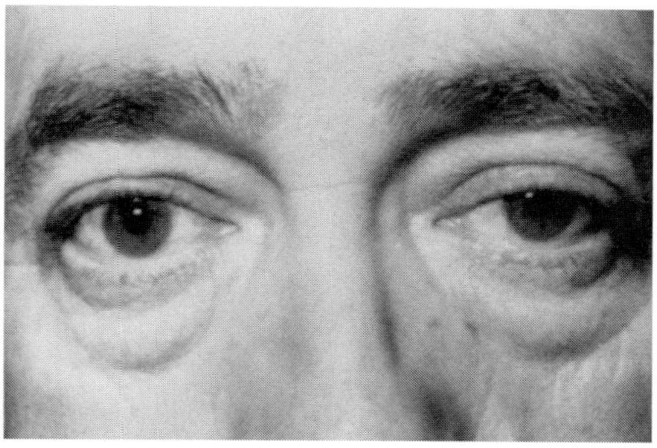

Figure 15–12 Horner's syndrome. Note ptosis and miosis (*left*).

rysms, internal carotid dissection or occlusion, and Tolosa-Hunt syndrome. Pain with a dilated and unreactive pupil may reflect a benign condition like Adie's syndrome or ophthalmoplegic migraine, or it may herald the presence of a life-threatening posterior communicating artery aneurysm. Headache and transient visual loss can be manifestations of classic migraine or symptoms of ocular hypoperfusion from ipsilateral internal carotid occlusion or increased IOP from pseudotumor cerebri. In a young patient, head pain with a fixed visual deficit may result from optic neuritis; in an older adult, temporal arteritis may be the culprit.

Ophthalmological aspects of headache encompass problems that range from simple and benign to complex and formidable.

References

1. Duke-Elder S, ed. Eye-strain and visual hygiene. *In* System of Ophthalmology: Ophthalmic Optics and Refraction, Vol 5. St. Louis: Mosby; 1970:559.
2. Derby GS. Ocular neuroses: An important cause of so-called eyestrain. JAMA 1930; 95:913–916.
3. Donders GC. Accommodation and Refraction of the Eye. London: The New Sydenham Society; 1864.
4. Masow ML. The convergence insufficiency syndrome. J Pediatr Ophthalmol 1971; 8:243–247.
5. Dagi LR, Choursos GA, Cogan DG. Spasm of the near reflex associated with organic disease. Am J Ophthalmol 1987;103:582–585.
6. Griffin JF, Wray SH, Anderson DP. Misdiagnosis of spasm of the near reflex. Neurology 1976;26:1018–1020.
7. Raskin NH, Schwartz RK. Icepick-like pain. Neurology 1980;30:203–205.
8. Lansche RK. Ophthalmodynia periodica. Headache 1964;4:247–250.
9. Shields MB. Textbook of Glaucoma, 2nd ed. Baltimore: Williams & Wilkins; 1987.
10. Brown GC, Magargal LE. The ocular ischemic syndrome: Clinical, fluorescein angiographic and carotid angiographic features. Int Ophthalmol 1988;11:239–248.
11. Standefer M, Little JR, Tomsak RL, et al. Improvement in retinal circulation following superficial temporal to middle cerebral artery bypass. Neurosurgery 1985;16:525–529.
12. Bloch-Michel E, Nussenblatt RB. International Uveitis Study Group recommendations for the evaluation of intraocular inflammatory disease. Am J Ophthalmol 1987;103:234–238.
13. Optic Neuritis Study Group. The clinical profile of optic neuritis. Arch Ophthalmol 1991; 109:1673–1678.
14. Krohel GB, Stewart WB, Chavis RM. Orbital Disease: A Practical Approach. New York: Grune & Stratton; 1981.
15. Ludwig I, Tomsak RL. Acute recurrent orbital myositis. J Clin Neurol Ophthalmol 1983; 3:41–47.
16. Bond JB, Wesley RE. Cluster headache after orbital exenteration. Ann Ophthalmol 1987; 19:438–443.
17. Gilden DH, Dueland AN, Cohrs R, et al. Preherpetic neuralgia. Neurology 1991;41:1215–1220.
18. Miller NR. Facial pain and neuralgia. *In* Walsh and Hoyt's Clinical Neuro-ophthalmology, 4th ed, Vol 2. Baltimore: Williams & Wilkins; 1985:1071–1097.
19. Cummings JL, Gittenger JW. Central dazzle: A thalamic syndrome? Arch Neurol 1981;38:372–374.
20. Gutrecht JA, Lessell IM, Zamani AA. Central dazzle in trigeminal sensory neuropathy. Neurology 1990;40:722–725.
21. Tomsak RL. Ophthalmologic aspects of headache. Med Clin North Am 1991;75:693–706.

16

Otorhinolaryngological Causes of Head and Facial Pain

Robert E. Ryan, Jr., M.D.

Introduction

The otolaryngological causes of head and facial pain represent medical conditions with which patients frequently present to primary care physicians. Although these conditions do not frequently cause headaches or facial pain, they can be etiological factors in pain.

In this chapter, I list possible causes of pain and discuss in significant detail a few common and a few uncommonly seen and usually unrecognized causes. A good ear, nose, and throat examination is always important in the diagnosis of patients with facial pain.

Rhinological Causes of Facial Pain

Nasal Septal Deviation

Nasal septal deviation occurs frequently in the normal population. The patient most often, but not always, presents to the physician with a complaint of difficulty breathing.

There are different degrees of nasal septal deformity. The first is septal deviation with the cartilage or bony portion of the nasal septum off the midline and causing blockage of one or both nasal cavities (Fig. 16–1). It is not uncommon to have septal deviation to such a degree that the airways on each side are altered. A second degree of septal deviation is called a *septal spur*, or protrusion of the septum off to one side. This is a bony growth of the septum that protrudes from the cartilage or bony portion of the septum. It often does not cause significant blockage of the airway. The third and most important degree of septal deviation is *septal impaction*, or when a septal spur compresses the lateral wall of the nose, or one of the turbinates. These patients present with facial pain.

Most septal deviations are traumatic in origin, but they can be congenital.

Spurs and ridges are believed to form on the nasal septum due to the presence of a thin, flexible septum in childhood; the septum will not have room to grow because of the hard palate below and the strong roof above.

When the spur comes in contact with the lateral wall of the nose or with the inferior or middle turbinate, pressure can be precipitated. This pressure can be a constant or intermittent sensation, depending on the amount of swelling that occurs concurrently. The nose naturally undergoes a nasal cycle, in which one side of the nose periodically swells in the region of the inferior and middle turbinate while the opposite side rests. In a patient with a septal spur, when this side of the nose is at rest with minimal edema present, there will be no impaction. However, when this nasal cycle changes and edema occurs, there will be impaction. This is why pain can be intermittent. With a more severe impaction, there is constant pressure on the lateral wall of the nose; this pain should be constant. A patient with compression of the middle meatus and blockage of the natural ostea is predisposed to chronic sinus problems, which can lead to facial pain. If the septal deformity is in a location to block the natural ostea of the sinuses, the patient will be predisposed to infection due to improper drainage as well as the expected decrease in breathing.

Extensive studies have shown pressure on different areas of the lateral wall of the nose and turbinates to refer pain to various areas of the face and head. Williams stated that pressure of the septum against the mid-

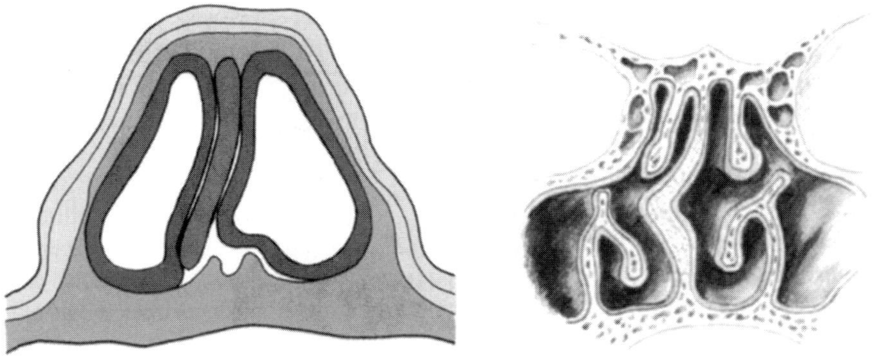

Figure 16–1 *A*, Septal dislocation. *B*, Deviated nasal septum. (From Ryan RE Sr, Ryan RE Jr. Headache and Pain. St. Louis: Mosby; 1978, p. 270.)

dle turbinate can produce pain in the mid-forehead or eye. He also stated that septal spur or contact in the sphenopalatine ganglion region can cause pain in the temporal or malar region.

The patient with a septal deformity who is experiencing facial pain should be examined while in the headache state. I examine the patient's nose and apply liquid cocaine to the area of the impaction with a cotton-tipped applicator or a cotton pledget. Depending on the severity of the impaction, it may be difficult to fit the applicator between the impaction and the lateral wall of the nose. The cocaine should remain in contact with the nose for 15 minutes. A second application may be done if the results are equivocal. If the headache pain is relieved, the diagnosis of facial pain secondary to the septal deviation should be considered. I suggest examining the patient when he or she is in the headache state again, on a second visit. At this time, I reproduce the technique described but apply a placebo solution instead of cocaine. If the pain is relieved, surgical success is doubtful.

I am reluctant to operate on a patient for this type of problem unless I can demonstrate on multiple occasions that anesthesia of the area of involvement provides relief of the pain. Surgery has been advocated for this problem, but it is appropriate for a small minority of patients and should not become commonplace therapy for headache pain. For many patients who undergo surgery, after the probable placebo effect wears off, facial pain persists.

"Sinus Headaches"

A significant number of patients present to an ear, nose, and throat specialist with the main complaint of sinus headaches. After an evaluation and thorough examination and history, the involvement of the sinuses in the patient's headache can be determined.

Paranasal sinusitis usually can be classified as acute or chronic; often, a transition period occurs between the two categories. *Acute sinusitis* denotes inflammation of the nasal mucosa and sinuses. The patient may have involvement of a single sinus or multiple sinuses. The problem can be unilateral or bilateral. An acute problem often occurs after a severe upper respiratory tract infection. When a significant degree of inflammation and edema occurs, there is decreased movement of the nasal cilia, which can lead to improper drainage of the nose. Usually, only acute nasal sinus disease causes facial pain. One diagnostic sign of acute sinusitis in the maxillary region is a patient who presents with pain in the teeth for whom the pain in the facial region increases when the head is bent down.

Computed tomography (CT) scanning provides a wonderful view of the sinuses and demonstrates sinus disease remarkably well. It is also quite helpful in viewing the natural ostea. This is a very important area in acute sinus disease, with blockage of the ostea predisposing one to chronic sinusitis. On physical examination of a patient with acute sinus disease, there may be tenderness to palpation or percussion over the affected teeth or the sinuses. Intranasal examination may show mucus coming from the middle meatus.

Endoscopic visualization can be performed in the office. Sinusitis should be treated with antibiotics; once the diagnosis has been made, the proper antibiotic can be prescribed. A good general guideline is 1-month course of antibiotics plus treatment of nasal congestion before surgical intervention is considered.

All of the sinuses can be involved in causing facial pain; those most commonly involved are the maxillary and ethmoid. Patients often present with headaches they think are sinus related and point to the frontal region as the area involved. On review of the patient's CT scans, only a small percentage are found to have sinus disease. A patient may complain of frontal sinus headache and on review of the CT scan be found to lack the frontal sinus itself.

In the discussion of sinus disease, conservatism should be emphasized. The proper diagnosis is of utmost importance. Acute sinusitis is a very common finding in the everyday population; pain is not always a symptom. Often, a patient will complain of pressure rather than pain, but many experience neither condition. If sinus disease is identified on CT and the patient does not respond to proper medical therapy, then surgical intervention becomes necessary to relieve the problem, but only a small minority of patients should progress to this point.

Sphenopalatine Ganglion Neuralgia

This uncommon condition should be considered in the refractory patient. It is attributed to involvement of the sphenopalatine ganglion, which lies beneath the maxillary division of the trigeminal nerve in the lateral bony wall of the nose. This ganglion gives nerve supply to the orbit, sphenoidal, and ethmoidal air cells along with the nose, hard and soft palates, tonsils, nasal pharynx, and gums. The nerve supply is diffuse and widespread. The cause of this condition is unknown; often, an infection seems to be a precipitating factor. Some patients have a septal deformity in this area, which is thought to play a role in the pain through the septum pressing on the small branches of the sphenopalatine ganglion that supply the middle turbinate.

Symptoms consist of pain in and around the nose; pain can spread to the ipsilateral cheek, upper teeth, and retroorbital and frontal temporal areas and posteriorly to the mastoid region. It is important to keep in mind that the pain is unilateral. The pain may last for several hours to many weeks; severe attacks can last 1 year. The pain is aching and burning. If the patient is examined during an attack, he or she is usually edematous on the involved side and may experience clear rhinorrhea and nasal obstruction on the involved side. A study at the Mayo Clinic showed that approximately half the patients were found to have deviation of the nasal septum. No patient had pressure on the sphenopalatine ganglion. The patient may also present with conjunctivitis or lacrimation, but this is not a strict criterion for the diagnosis. These patients are very hard to diagnose; by the time a diagnosis is made, they often have had dental extractions or sinus surgery. In the series at the Mayo Clinic, women outnumbered men by a ratio of 2:1, and the onset of symptoms occurs in the fourth through sixth decades of life.

Sphenopalatine ganglion is often misdiagnosed as a migraine or trigeminal neuralgia, but the entity that is closest is a cluster headache, the lower class type of cluster headache. Pain is located in the orbital region and radiated into the interorbital area over the cheek and into the upper teeth. The pain is unilateral. However, pain with cluster headache lasts only an average of 2 hours and pain with sphenopalatine ganglion lasts for a few weeks to months. In patients with lower half cluster headaches, men predominate with a ratio of 4:1.

The treatment of sphenopalatine ganglion consists of first making the correct diagnosis, which involves the same approach used in patients with nasal septal impaction. I apply topical cocaine to the sphenopalatine ganglion area when the patient is experiencing the pain. It is necessary to repeat this on multiple occasions to confirm that symptoms are reproducible before considering further treatment, including the use of a placebo on one of the visits to be sure the patient is not a placebo responder. If a severely deviated nasal septum is involved, a nasal septal reconstruction should be performed. In addition to this, constrict the nasal mucosa in the area of the ganglion itself and treat the ganglion with silver nitrate or use an electrocautery probe to cauterize the area. This produces a traumatic injury to the ganglion and interferes with the ganglion pain impulses. In a series of 20 cases treated in this manner, each patient had a prolonged symptom-free interval, with each patient achieving a longer symptom-free period than he or she experienced previously. The pain did recur, but the procedure can be repeated with the same results.

Sphenopalatine ganglion is a very uncommon finding; once suspected, the patient should be referred to an otolaryngologist for a thorough examination.

Otological Causes of Head Pain

Numerous conditions within and around the ear can cause head pain (Tables 16–1 and 16–2). Most causes of ear pain are obvious, such as an acute otitis media or acute external otitis. The following entity is often overlooked, and treatment depends on correct diagnosis.

Postherpetic Neuralgia

This condition is also referred to as Ramsay-Hunt syndrome. This involves an infection of the neurons of the geniculate ganglion by the herpes zoster virus, which is usually followed by the appearance of cutaneous vesicles in the area of the sensory distribution of the intermedions nerve. The edema of the ganglion itself puts pressure on the facial nerve and facial canal, causing facial paralysis.

Postherpetic neuralgia is often precipitated by an upper respiratory infection. The ganglion is usually involved, and the initial complaint is pain over the pinna in the external auditory meatus, which can be from deep

Table 16–1 Causes of Primary Otalgia

External ear
- External otitis
- Perichondritis
- Auricular abscess
- Furunculosis
- Injury
- Malignant external otitis
- Malignant or benign growth
- Fungal infection
- Foreign body
- Impacted cerumen
- Ballous myringitis
- Frostbite

Middle ear and mastoid
- Acute otitis media
- Acute mastoiditis
- Barotrauma
- Malignant or benign growth
- Acute petrositis
- Gradenigo's syndrome

From Ryan RE Sr, Ryan RE Jr. Headache and Pain. St. Louis: Mosby; 1978.

Table 16–2 Causes of Referred Otalgia

Oral cavity
- Acute glossitis
- Stomatitis
- Carcinoma of tongue

Pharynx
- After tonsillectomy or adenoidectomy
- Acute pharyngitis
- Peritonsillar abscess
- Malignant growth
- Ulceration
- Elongated styloid process
- Nasopharyngeal angiofibroma

Larynx
- Malignancy
- Ulceration
- Arthritis of cricoarytenoid joint
- Perichondritis

Esophagus
- Foreign body
- Inflammation
- Malignant or benign growth

Neuralgias
- Idiopathic geniculate
- Postherpetic
- Trigeminal
- Tympanic
- Glossopharyngeal
- Sphenopalatine ganglion
- Dental

Miscellaneous
- Thyroiditis
- Thyroid cancer
- Temporomandibular arthritis
- Mumps
- Acoustic neuroma
- Tumor of gasserian ganglion
- Injury or inflammation of C1 to C3

From Ryan RE Sr, Ryan RE Jr, Headache and Pain. St. Louis: Mosby; 1978.

in the ear or throat. This is followed by the development of typical herpetic vessels in the painful areas. This is accompanied by facial paralysis if the facial nerve is involved. The patient may also have loss of taste in the anterior two thirds of the tongue on the affected side. Pain is usually deep seated, and eruption of the skin on the external ear is frequently found on the anterior surface of the auricle. This usually follows the terminal branches of the auriculotemporal nerve. Because this nerve does not supply the posterior surface of the auricle, it is rare to find a herpes eruption in this area. If the skin eruption is situated in the external auditory canal, it may extend to the tympanic membrane and also involve this structure.

The eruption is initially papular and then vesicular. There usually is clear serum in the eruption, but this can become purulent. The vesicles usually remain present for 3 to 4 days before they dry up, leaving a crust or an ulcer. The lesions usually clear in time. They do remain painful after the onset.

Proper treatment consists of symptomatic therapy consisting of analgesics and ointment to keep the skin from crusting. Local topical anesthetic can be applied to the area for pain relief.

Laryngological Causes of Head and Facial Pain

I discuss a few uncommon disease entities to possibly help in the diagnosis of a difficult patient.

Elongated Styloid Process

This condition is also referred to as Eagle's syndrome. The elongated styloid process can produce two syndromes characterized by a painful sensation in the pharynx along with painful deglutition. The pain may spread to the ear; this is usually, but not always, seen after a tonsillectomy. The pain may be present for years.

The symptoms vary from a slight sore throat to severe pain that radiates to the ear and the sensation of a foreign body in the throat. The patient will often say they feel something in their throat. Eagle noted that most of the patients had undergone a tonsillectomy, and scar tissue had possibly stretched the sensory nerve ending. However, others have reported that only a few patients had pain due to tonsillectomy. One patient who had her tonsils had complaints of pain in the left tonsillar region; her pain was produced by an elongated styloid process.

The diagnosis is confirmed when the palpating finger meets a firm bony resistance in the tonsillar fossa and the patient confirms this is the pain. A CT scan of this area will usually confirm the diagnosis. It is important to note that some patients with an elongated styloid process found on routine radiographic procedures are asymptomatic.

The treatment depends on the severity of the patient's symptoms. Transpharyngeal styloidectomy with the patient under general anesthesia has been the treatment of choice. Removal of the entire process is not necessary; it is contraindicated because of the proximity of the process to the facial nerve.

Glossopharyngeal Neuralgia

This disorder is characterized by symptoms of pain in the tonsil region and throat. Usually, it is an idiopathic condition, but other etiologies include elongation of the styloid process, atheromatous plaque of the vertebral artery, tuberculous laryngitis, ossification of the stylohyoid ligament, and nasopharyngeal and intracranial tumors.

Patients present with pain precipitated by chewing, swallowing, or yawning. It is a sudden pain that increases in intensity and radiates from the throat to the deeper portion of the ipsilateral ear. The pain can last from 20 to 30 seconds and is often followed by an intense burning sensation that can last a couple minutes. Men seem to be affected more frequently than women.

A differential diagnosis must include other diseases of the ear, nose, and throat such as inflammatory or neoplastic conditions. The only condition that strongly enters into the differential diagnosis is trigeminal neuralgia. Proper questioning will help determine the radiation of the pain confined to the distribution of the ninth nerve. Unlike patients with trigeminal neuralgia, those with this condition should have the trigger zone in the glossopharyngeal region. It is very important to rule out any local musculoskeletal neoplasm or bony or soft tissue abnormality.

Once a proper diagnosis of this condition has been made, treatment is conservative. Therapy with carbamazepine at the lowest possible dosage is recommended; the dosage should begin at 200 mg/day and increase only as necessary. It should be kept to a minimum because of possible side effects. If the carbamazepine is effective, then the medication may be withdrawn during a pain-free interval. If the pain recurs after the drug has been stopped, it may be restarted. Medical therapy of this condition is not as rewarding as the treatment of trigeminal neuralgia. When medical therapy is not successful, surgical intervention is necessary. Extracranial block of the glossopharyngeal nerve is not recommended because of the proximity to the 10th, 11th, and 12th nerves. The most satisfactory treatment consists of intracranial section of the ninth nerve if both glossopharyngeal pain and ear pain are present. The auricular branches of the vagus nerve are also active in the process. Cephalic fibers of the vagus nerve should be cut.

In all cases, surgical intervention should

be a last resort. The most important contribution clinicians can make to their patients with these types of problems is the proper diagnosis; often, this requires consultation with a head and neck specialist for a thorough ear, nose, and throat examination.

Bibliography

Eagle WW. Elongated styloid process: Report of two cases. Arch Otolaryngol 1937;25:584–587.

Hunt JRH. Herpetic inflammations of the geniculate ganglion: A new syndrome and its complications. J Nerv Ment Dis 1907;34:73–96.

Ryan RE Jr. Otologic and laryngologic etiologies of headache and facial pain. Consultant 1978;17:90–105.

Ryan RE Jr, Facer GW. Sphenopalatine ganglion neuralgia and cluster headache: Comparisons, contrasts, and treatment. Headache 1977;17:7–9.

Ryan RE Jr, Kern EB. Rhinologic causes of facial pain. Headache 1978;18:44–50.

Ryan RE Sr, Ryan RE Jr. Headache and Head Pain. St. Louis: Mosby; 1978.

Ryan RE Sr, Ryan RE Jr. Headache of nasal origin. Headache 1979;19:173–179.

Williams HL. Headache from the standpoint of the otolaryngologist. J Iowa Med Soc 1947;37:45.

17

Headache Syndromes in Children and Adolescents: Diagnosis and Management

A. David Rothner, M.D.

Merle L. Diamond, M.D.

Glen D. Solomon, M.D.

Introduction

Headache is a common problem in children and adolescents. It may be an incidental symptom related to a systemic illness with fever or a significant symptom in a child with acute or chronic central nervous system disease. In dealing with headache in children, physicians must consider both physical and emotional factors in determining the correct diagnosis and selecting the proper treatment. Parents must be reassured that in the vast majority of children and adolescents, serious neurological disease is an uncommon cause of headache. In a survey of 100 children (aged 3 to 17) with headache histories of 3 or more months, the patients reported what they wanted from the physician.[1] Three issues were voiced by the majority: What was the cause of the headache? What would make the headache better? Can the physician provide reassurance that the patient does not have a life-threatening illness? Twenty percent of the adolescents depicted themselves as dead, dying, or about to be killed by their headaches.

The frequency with which headache occurs in the pediatric and adolescent population is surprising to many. In a classic study from Scandinavia, it was shown that headaches of all kinds increase in a stepwise fashion between ages 7 and 15. Indeed, by age 15, 5% of all children have had a migraine attack, and another 15% have a significant problem with daily or almost-daily tension headaches.[2] In a 40-year follow-up study, in girls from the age of 11 years, there was a gradual increase in migraine headache.[3] A subgroup of 73 children from the original group experienced migraine. By the age of 25 years, 23% were migraine free—the males more significantly than the females.[3] In an epidemiological study of headaches in Washington County, Maryland, 56% of boys and 74% of girls between the ages of 12 and 17 reported having a headache within the past month.[4]

Classification of Headaches

The existing methods of classifying headaches have been reviewed, as has the pathophysiology of the various headache disorders.[5] However, some authors believe that the criteria established by the International Headache Society has poor sensitivity to those issues faced in a pediatric headache population.[6]

Clinically, we find it useful to classify headaches in two additional ways. The first is a simple, location-based classification, such as (1) extracranial, meaning the structure surrounding the brain, including the eyes, the sinuses, the ears, and so forth; (2) intracranial structures, the brain itself; (3) vascular structures, as might be implicated in migraine; and (4) psychological factors, as in chronic "muscle contraction" headaches.[7] The second useful method of classification is based on the temporal profile of the headache and includes the following five groups of headaches (Fig. 17–1).

Acute headaches comprise the first group. They are defined as a single event with no history of a previous similar event. If this event is associated with neurological symptoms or signs, an accurate diagnosis may be life saving. The differential diagnosis of the acute headache syndromes involves many disorders, such as systemic infection, central nervous system infection, hypertension, and subarachnoid hemorrhage. An acute headache may be related to structures outside the brain, to the brain itself, or to vascular structures. In a recent study of 288 children (aged 2 to 18 years) presenting with headache to an emergency department, the range of etiologies included viral illness (39.2%), sinusitis (16.0%), migraine (15.6%), and tension-type headache (4.5%).[8] No cases of brain tumor or bacterial meningitis were identified in this population, although 5.2% were found to have viral meningitis.

The second group is made up of acute recurrent headaches. Acute recurrent headaches are events that recur periodically and are separated by pain-free intervals. The best example of this acute recurrent type of headache is the migraine headache. Less common examples of acute recurrent headaches include cluster headaches, which are uncommon in children; chronic paroxysmal hemicrania, which also is uncommon in children; and exertional headaches.

The third classification is that of chronic progressive headaches. These headaches increase in severity and frequency over a period of several months. Other neurological symptoms and signs usually are present at the time the patient is seen. Additional neurological symptoms that are worrisome include balance difficulty, lethargy, personality change, focal weakness, loss of consciousness, and visual disturbances. The neurological examination may reveal abnormalities such as papilledema, focal hyperreflexia, or a sixth nerve palsy. In this instance, one must suspect hydrocephalus or a brain tumor.

The fourth type of headache is chronic and nonprogressive. This is a headache that occurs daily or several times weekly and usually does not change significantly in severity over time. There usually are few associated symptoms and no associated neurological abnormalities. This type of headache is most frequently associated with emotional factors relating to school or depression.

The fifth type of headache is a mixed headache; this is composed of recurrent, severe headaches associated with nausea and vomiting, superimposed on daily milder headaches. This probably represents a combination of migraine and stress-related headaches.

The history is the most valuable tool in evaluating the patient with headache. The questions that aid in properly categorizing the majority of headaches include

1. Do you have a single or several types of headache?

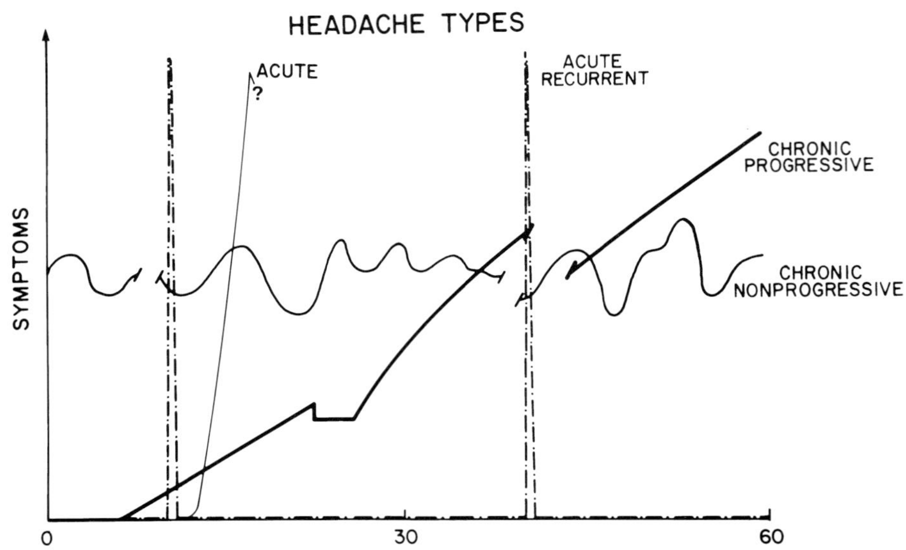

Figure 17–1 Headache types.

2. How did the headache begin? Was it initiated by trauma?

3. How long has each headache type been present?

4. Are the headaches worsening in severity or staying the same?

5. How frequently do the headaches occur? Are they becoming increasingly frequent?

6. Do they occur under any special conditions? Any special time?

7. Are they related to specific foods?

8. Are they preceded by warning symptoms? Describe them.

9. Where is the pain located?

10. What is the quality of the pain? Pounding? Squeezing? Sharp?

11. Are there associated symptoms during the headache, such as nausea, vomiting, speech arrest, or weakness?

12. What do you do during the headache? Do you stop playing? Do you have to lie down?

13. How long does the headache last? Seconds? Minutes? Hours?

14. What medications do you use or which maneuvers do you attempt that make the headache better? Does sleep relieve the pain?

15. Does anything you do make the headache worse?

16. Between headaches, are there problems with balance, weakness, vision, lethargy, or personality change?

17. Are you being treated for, or do you have any other, chronic medical problems such as sinusitis? Asthma? Hypertension?

18. Do you take medication for any other problems on a regular basis?

19. Does anyone else in your family have headaches? Daily or intermittent?

20. Can you tell me what you think is causing your headaches?

A complete history includes details concerning the mother's pregnancy, labor and delivery of the patient, growth and development, and any encephalopathic events, such as concussion or meningitis. Information regarding academic achievements and school absences may point to a school-related stressful situation. The family history may shed light on both environmental causes of headache and genetic causes. In the 40-year follow-up study of school children with migraine,[3] 52% reported recurrent headache, probably migraine, in one or more of their children. The review of systems provides information about medications, aberrant social situations, or the presence of a systemic illness contributing to the headache problem. The general physical examination must include vital signs. Occult hypertension may be a problem in an adolescent. Examination of the skin may give a hint to underlying neurological problems, such as neurofibromatosis. Keep in mind that headache may be a nonspecific symptom of almost any systemic disorder. The neurological examination includes measurement of the head circumference, searching for occult hydrocephalus and auscultation of the head, searching for intracranial bruits, and arteriovenous malformations. Any abnormality on the standard neurological examination is unexpected and must be explained. It must be assumed that it is related to the patient's headache until proved otherwise.

The choice of laboratory tests rests on the differential diagnosis formulated after the history and physical examination. In an otherwise uncomplicated patient with migraine, no laboratory tests may be indicated. In a retrospective chart review conducted at a pediatric neurology clinic, 133 cases were considered in determining the value of brain imaging in children with headaches.[9] Brain imaging was performed in 59% (magnetic resonance imaging [MRI] in 45, computed tomography [CT] in 27, and both in 6). The tests were performed due to atypical headache patterns, the presence of neurological abnormalities associated with the headaches, and parents' or physicians' concerns about brain tumors. Although cerebral abnormalities were found in four patients, none of those findings were related to the headache. The authors' conclusion suggested that brain imaging studies were of very limited value in pediatric patients with headache without clinical evidence of an underlying structural lesion. In a patient with chronic, nonprogressive headaches, CT or MRI of the sinuses and head may be indicated. However, in another study of the value of MRI in pediatric migraine, sinus findings on the MRI were not necessarily related to the child's headache complaints.[10] If the patient, however, has neurological symptoms or neurologic signs, an underlying organic process must be suspected and neuroimaging is necessary. The MRI may be more valuable in looking for abnormalities in the vicinity of the sella turcica and posterior fossa, as well as the cervical medullary junction. Electroencephalography is of little value and may be misleading.

Children experience pain as strongly as adults. They describe their pain reliably and accurately. Attempts should be made to relieve the pain with the judicious use of analgesics. Dosing should be computed by weight and not by age and should be sufficient to relieve pain. Both the child and the family should be educated regarding possible medication-related side effects and coping with pain and thereby avoiding its emotional consequences. Chronic pain can lead to regression, depression, withdrawal, sleep disorders, eating disorders, and aberrant psychological behavior. Participation of the patient and family in the management of the pain leads to successful management.

Specific Headache Syndromes

An isolated, acute headache may represent a difficult diagnostic problem. Many children with systemic illnesses associated with fever have a generalized nonspecific headache. In these patients, the diagnosis of the illness usually is straightforward, such as the flu, and the headache resolves with resolution of the underlying process. If, however, the patient has lethargy, nuchal rigidity, or any other central nervous system symptom or sign, underlying encephalitis or meningitis must be suspected. If the problem is of acute onset and the patient has nuchal rigidity and retinal hemorrhages, a subarachnoid hemorrhage should be considered.

In children and adolescents, acute headache related to exertion may occur as a single event or in a recurrent fashion. It most frequently occurs in athletes such as weightlifters and runners. Their generalized, severe, throbbing headaches may last from minutes to hours but are not usually associated with abnormalities on the neurological examination. If a transient neurological deficit occurs, further workup is indicated. If these headaches are recurrent and severe, indomethacin is useful as prophylactic therapy.[11] The laboratory evaluation of the patient with acute headache depends on the suspected diagnosis. Analgesics and especially sedatives should be avoided until a specific diagnosis is made.

Astigmatism, refractive errors, eyestrain, and squint are frequently thought of as causing headaches in children but rarely do. If the headache is localized to the frontal area and precipitated by watching television, reading, or doing school work and relieved by stopping that activity, eyestrain should be considered. An ophthalmological examination is required.[12]

Headaches are a prominent symptom in up to 13% of patients with acute or chronic sinusitis. Sinusitis is frequently found in association with upper respiratory tract symptoms and allergies. Acute sinusitis is heralded by fever, focal tenderness over the affected sinus, an elevated white blood count, and an elevated sedimentation rate. Subacute or chronic sinusitis may or may not be associated with respiratory symptoms. Fever and signs of an active infection are usually absent. The diagnosis is made by a simple CT scan of the sinus.[13] Complications may include brain abscess, orbital cellulitis, and meningitis. Although these complications are rare, sinusitis should be treated with antibiotics and decongestants and, if necessary, surgical drainage.

Case 1

A 5-year-old boy presented with headaches of 5 months' duration. The headaches were occasionally associated with nausea. Initially, the headaches occurred several times per week, but they evolved into a daily and then constant headache type. The headaches were localized to the frontal area and were occasionally pounding in nature and occasionally awakened the child from sleep. There was a positive family history of migraine, and an excessive number of school absences were noted. Allergies and chronic rhinitis had been noted in the past. Previous evaluations, including CT scan of the head and lumbar puncture, were negative. Previous treatment with cyproheptadine, propranolol, and amitriptyline was unsuccessful. The patient's general physical and neurological examinations were normal. CT scanning of his sinuses was abnormal (Fig. 17–2). Conservative management with antibiotics over a period of 3 weeks was unsuccessful, and surgical decompression was necessary to resolve the patient's symptoms.

Dental disorders usually cause localized pain in the jaw or teeth. The diagnosis is suggested by localized pain. Temporomandibular joint dysfunction is uncommon in children and adolescents. Psychological fac-

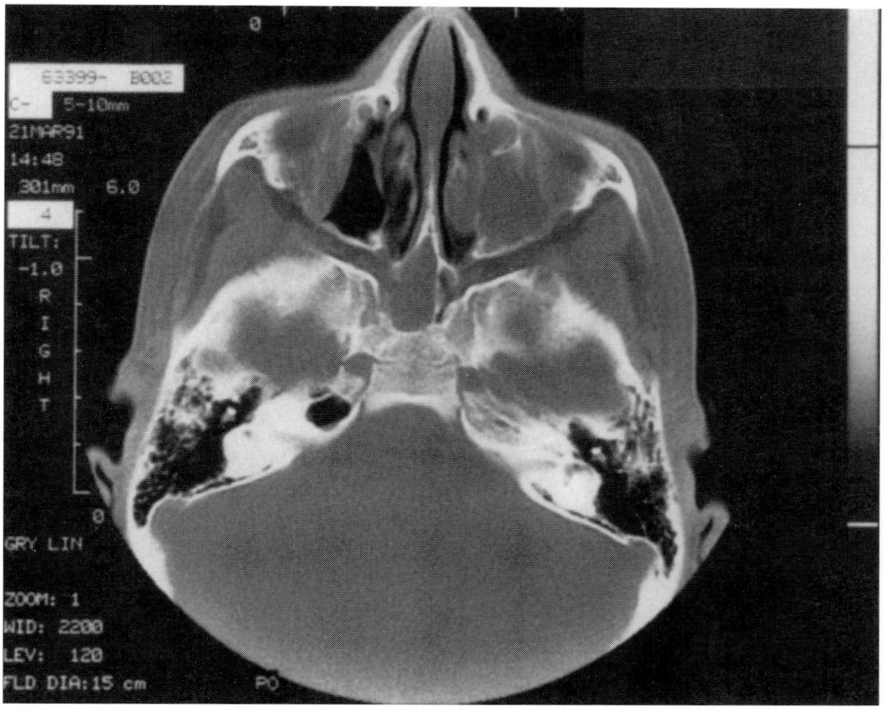

Figure 17–2 Sector CT scan of a 5-year-old boy showing pansinusitis.

tors are important, and referral to both a dentist and a psychologist may be indicated.[14] The author has seen this disorder in children who chew gum excessively and in others who constantly bite their lips. Behavioral modification techniques may lead to disappearance of the symptoms.

Headache associated with trauma frequently is related to the specific area of trauma and resolves within a few days. If the headache is protracted over months and the neurological evaluation, including neuroimaging, is negative, reassurance and analgesics usually improve the situation. If symptoms change, however, re-evaluation is necessary. If symptoms become protracted, psychological factors may be implicated.

Acute Recurrent Headaches

Migraine is the most common type of acute recurrent headache in both children and adolescents that leads to medical evaluation. In a series of patients, more than one third of patients presented before the age of 10 and more than half were not appropriately diagnosed until their symptoms had been present for about 3 years.[15] It is an autosomal dominant disorder with greater penetrance in females, characterized by paroxysmal attacks of vasoconstriction and vasodilation.

Prensky[16] suggested that the diagnosis of migraine should be based on recurrent headache with symptom-free intervals plus three of the following six symptoms: (1) abdominal pain, nausea, or vomiting; (2) hemicrania; (3) throbbing, pulsatile pain; (4) complete relief after a period of rest; (5) an aura, either visual, sensory, or motor; and (6) history of migraine in one or more family members.[16] These criteria are generally useful, but exceptions occur because common migraine is more frequent than classic migraine in children and usually does not manifest a visual aura and hemicrania. Five percent of children will have experienced migraine by the age of 15. Boys are affected more frequently than girls in early childhood, but after puberty, girls are affected more frequently than boys. The clinical features of children with migraine include paroxysmal headaches in 100%; relief after asleep in 94%; nausea, vomiting, and abdominal pain in 90%; a positive family history of migraine in 69%; a throbbing, pounding quality to the pain in 58%; a unilateral headache in 36%; and an aura in 17%.[15] Episodes may be triggered by anxiety, minor head trauma, exercise, menses, and travel. In a minority of patients, dietary factors such as chocolate, cola drinks, preserved meats, and monosodium glutamate may play a role.[7]

Migraine may be classified into four groups: classic, common, complex, and variant forms. The most common form of migraine in children is common migraine, or migraine without aura.[3] Premonitory symptoms usually consist of pallor, malaise, fatigue, and irritability. These symptoms are followed by frontal headache, nausea, and vomiting. Children frequently go to their rooms, are bothered by light and noise, and want to sleep. The usual attack resolves in 2 to 6 hours. In classic migraine (migraine with aura), the attack is heralded by a visual aura, and the headache is unilateral. The remainder of the symptoms are similar to those of common migraine.

Case 2

A 9-year-old girl was evaluated for recurrent headaches. Twice monthly, usually after school, she would come home appearing pale and with rings under her eyes. She was increasingly irritable on those occasions and complained of bifrontal headache. She would go to her room, turn off the lights, and avoid noise. She then developed abdominal pain, nausea, and vomiting followed by sleep. Four hours later, the patient would awaken and feel refreshed. Cyproheptadine (4 mg BID) was prescribed, and during the next 4 months, the patient was headache free. The medication was gradually discontinued, and no recurrence was noted.

Treatment of migraine is individualized depending on the age of the patient and the severity and frequency of attacks.[7] In younger children, especially those younger than age 14, with infrequent attacks, analgesics, antiemetics, and sedatives are useful. A recent study evaluated the use of subcutaneous sumatriptan in 50 children, aged 6 to 18 years, with severe migraine.[17] The patients received 0.06 mg/kg SC. A global rating of good to excellent response was reported by 84%, and the recurrence rate was only 6%. Mild and transient side effects were reported by 80%, and the author concluded that sumatriptan SC was effective and safe in childhood migraine. In children older than age 14, if an aura is present, the use of a combination agent (isometheptene, acetaminophen, and dichloralphenazone) or an ergotamine preparation is prescribed, as for adults. Studies have been undertaken on the use of dihydroergotamine mesylate in the treatment of acute headache in children.[18] The dose ranged from 0.1 to 0.5 mg IV with oral metoclopramide given thirty minutes earlier. Eighty percent of the subjects responded to this therapy with minimal side effects. Although the results were promising, the author suggested that this type of therapy should be undertaken only by a physician familiar with the evaluation and treatment of pediatric headache and only on an inpatient basis. Currently, both the oral and nasal routes of administering the "triptans" are undergoing trials in adolescents, aged 12 to 17.

In children with frequent attacks, prophylactic medications, including cyproheptadine or propranolol, are indicated. The usual dose of cyproheptadine is 8 to 12 mg divided into two or three doses daily. The major side effects are sedation and increased appetite. This author does not recommend the use of this medication in obese children. Propranolol has been used successfully in the prophylaxis of migraine in children and adolescents.[19] There seems to be fewer side effects in children and adolescents than in adults. Propranolol is contraindicated in patients with asthma. The usual dosage is 80 to 160 mg per day. The medication is used prophylactically for 4 to 6 months, and then attempts are made to discontinue it. Patients on propranolol should be observed for depression, and the medication should be discontinued if significant depression occurs.

Complex migraine includes patients presenting with recurrent headaches in association with neurological signs. Any child presenting with objective neurological signs should be suspected of having an arteriovenous malformation, tumor, or aneurysm. Only after the diagnostic workup proves negative should the diagnosis of complex migraine be suspected. Hemiplegic migraine, a form of complex migraine, is defined by hemiparesis, which may precede, accompany, or follow the headache. The disorder may be familial. Neuroimaging (utilizing both magnetic resonance imaging [MRI] and magnetic resonance arteriography [MRA]) is indicated in every patient. If the attacks are frequent, prophylactic medications are indicated.[20] If the usual agents are unsuccessful, calcium channel blockers or anticonvulsants should be tried.

Ophthalmoplegic migraine involves eye

pain and an incomplete or complete third nerve palsy. Pupillary dilation, outward deviation of the eye, and ptosis are most common. Concern regarding an intracranial process mandates neuroimaging. If attacks are recurrent and frequent, prophylactic medication should be considered. Corticosteroids during the acute attack are useful.[21]

The migraine variants actually are more common in children and adolescents than in adults; they include confusional migraine, basilar artery migraine, paroxysmal vertigo, and the periodic syndrome, also known as cyclic vomiting.

Confusional migraines are episodes of altered consciousness, agitation, and a receptive or expressive aphasia. Adolescent patients presenting with this disorder are frequently suspected of using street drugs. Before making the diagnosis of confusional migraine, drug ingestion and aseptic meningitis must be ruled out. Patients presenting with headache, disorientation, difficulty in speaking, and confusion are usually better within 6 hours. The patients may have experienced a prior migraine attack, or migraine attacks may occur after the confusional episode. Prophylactic medication may be used if the attacks are frequent and recurrent, but no data are available regarding its efficacy.[22]

Basilar artery migraine refers to recurrent attacks of neurological dysfunction referable to the brainstem and cerebellum. Episodes usually clear completely. Symptoms include occipital headache, nausea, vomiting, vertigo, tinnitus, and facial weakness; uncommonly, loss of consciousness occurs. Again, recurrent attacks can be treated with prophylactic medication, although data regarding the response to medication are not clear.[23]

Paroxysmal vertigo occurs in young children between the ages of 2 and 6 years. Episodes are brief and sudden and cause vertigo with difficulty maintaining posture. Consciousness is retained. Children are frightened and sit down because they cannot walk. They appear to hold on tightly because of their severe vertigo. An astute observer may note nystagmus. The attacks are over in a matter of minutes but may be recurrent. The use of cyproheptadine, diphenhydramine, or both has been suggested.[24]

Episodes of vomiting with abdominal pain that are paroxysmal and cyclic and result in acidosis and dehydration may represent a migraine variant. After structural gastrointestinal etiologies of recurrent vomiting and abdominal pain have been ruled out, a trial of antimigrainous medication may be initiated, even in the absence of headache. Metabolic causes of cyclic vomiting are rare.

There has been much confusion in the literature regarding the relationship of epilepsy to migraine.[25] In our series of patients, epileptiform discharges on the electroencephalogram occurred in 9% of children with migraine.[15] Differentiating epilepsy from migraine usually is not difficult. If the episodes of headache, nausea, and vomiting are associated with loss of consciousness or tonic-clonic activity, epilepsy should be considered, and anticonvulsants may be indicated. If, however, the episodes of headache, nausea, and vomiting are not associated with loss of consciousness and are simply associated with an incidental electroencephalographic abnormality such as benign focal or rolandic spikes, the diagnosis is migraine and not epilepsy. The usual forms of treatment for migraine are effective.

Chronic Progressive Headaches

When a patient presents with a headache that is chronic and progressive, worsening in severity and frequency over time, consideration must be given to a pathological process within the cranial vault. The rapidity with which the process progresses determines the speed of the evaluation. Symptoms of increased intracranial pressure include nausea, vomiting, weakness, ataxia, lethargy, personality change, visual disturbances, and seizures, and these symptoms, if present, necessitate a rapid evaluation. The physical examination usually shows abnormalities such as focal neurological deficits, a sixth nerve palsy, or papilledema. If a structural abnormality of the central nervous system is suspected, neuroimaging with MRI or CT is the diagnostic test of choice.

Headaches caused by brain tumors may be caused by the mass itself or by hydrocephalus secondary to cerebrospinal fluid obstruction.[26] The headache may be nonspecific in location. Exertion and changes in position frequently exacerbate the headache. The headache often is more severe in the morning and may be associated with vomiting. Diagnosis usually is made by MRI or CT scanning. Treatment depends on the type and location of the tumor.

Case 3

A 7-year-old boy developed headaches approximately 1 month before admission. Initially, the headaches occurred intermittently, but then they became more frequent, occurring every other day. They were frontal in location. On several occasions, vomiting occurred in the morning with the headaches. On several occasions, he awakened in the middle of the night with head pain. Physical examination showed a head tilt, early papilledema, bilateral finger-to-nose dysmetria, and slight ataxia on tandem gait. Scanning showed a large posterior fossa tumor that proved to be a cerebellar astrocytoma. Total resection of the mass was carried out, and the patient has done well postoperatively.

Pseudotumor cerebri is increased intracranial pressure without evidence of infection, mass, lesion, or hydrocephalus. The usual symptoms are headache, papilledema, and a sixth nerve palsy. Visual field testing may show an enlarged blind spot. Neuroimaging is normal and should precede a lumbar puncture. The lumbar puncture will show increased pressure with normal cerebrospinal fluid constituents. Menstrual irregularity, obesity, chronic otitis, and medications such as steroids may cause this disorder. Treatment consists of repeated lumbar punctures, each time removing sufficient cerebrospinal fluid to return the pressure to normal. Diuretics, steroids, or both also may be useful.[27]

A subdural hematoma is secondary to head trauma, child abuse, blood dyscrasia, or rupture of an arteriovenous malformation or aneurysm. The signs and symptoms are those of increased intracranial pressure. Neuroimaging confirms the diagnosis, and therapy includes surgical drainage. A brain abscess is a rare disorder in a child or adolescent but may be found in association with cyanotic congenital heart disease or chronic sinusitis or otitis or in an immunosuppressed child. The abscess may be single or multiple. The usual symptoms include fever, focal neurological symptoms, and symptoms of increased intracranial pressure. Neuroimaging is diagnostic. Antibiotics and surgical drainage are the treatments of choice.

Hydrocephalus implies ventricular enlargement secondary to obstruction in the cerebrospinal fluid flow. Congenital anomalies such as compensated aqueductal stenosis may not be apparent until adolescence. Patients present with symptoms of increased intracranial pressure. The physical examination usually shows macrocephaly, papilledema, and a sixth nerve palsy. Neuroimaging is diagnostic, and a shunting procedure is almost always necessary.

Chronic Nonprogressive Headaches

Chronic nonprogressive headaches are common in adolescents.[28, 29] They are less common in children younger than 10 years. They are associated with or precipitated by stress and usually have no organic substrate. The vast majority of these patients have daily headaches that last all day. A smaller percentage may have headaches several times a week or have several smaller headaches per day. The character of the pain and its location are variable. The patient usually describes the symptoms nonspecifically. Associated symptoms such as nausea and vomiting are not common. Symptoms in these patients have been present for weeks to months. Frequent school absences are supportive of the diagnosis. At this point, it is important to ask about headaches in other family members, divorce, parental absence from the home, alcoholism, overachievement, and underachievement. Previous emotional problems in the patient are supportive of an emotionally based disorder. In general, higher levels of impairment are associated with chronic daily headaches.[29]

Data concerning the pathophysiology of the disorder are sparse. Numerous studies have been conducted in an effort to delineate the psychological issues. Blaming others and wishful thinking were frequently cited coping mechanisms.[29] No significant differences have been demonstrated in externalizing and internalizing behaviors, type A behaviors, disability, pain severity, days missed from school, and number of coping skills used.[30] Data concerning the treatment of this disorder and prolonged follow-up are not available. A combined medical, psychological, and pharmacological approach is necessary. In families in which medication use is avoided, the use of biofeedback and counseling is suggested.[31, 32] At times, biofeedback combined with the use of amitriptyline has been helpful. Serum levels of the medication should be determined periodically because adolescents frequently are noncompliant.

Case 4

An 18-year-old woman was evaluated for headaches. The onset occurred 4 years previously. Initially, they were intermittent, but after about 6 months, the headaches occurred daily and were present from awakening until bedtime. They were generalized in location and of moderate severity. There were no associated symptoms or signs. The headaches did not interfere with her sleep. She had missed 43 days of school. A detailed neurological examination revealed no abnormality. Of interest was the fact that her father was disabled by severe daily headaches. Previous treatments with a butalbital-combination analgesic, pentazocine, propoxyphene, phenytoin, and phenobarbital had not been helpful. Family counseling and amitriptyline led to an improvement in her headache status.

In this type of headache, the general and neurological examinations, as well as laboratory tests, are negative. Psychosocial information usually is supportive of the diagnosis. The use of the Minnesota Multiphasic Personality Index may be valuable in older children. If there are difficulties in school, intelligence and achievement testing is necessary. Projective testing may offer additional information. Once the diagnosis is suspected, it should be discussed openly with the parents and child. Treatment modalities include family counseling, individual counseling, biofeedback, and antidepressants. A pharmacological approach alone is rarely helpful.

Mixed Headaches

Mixed headaches represent a combination of acute recurrent headache superimposed on chronic nonprogressive headaches. The acute recurrent headaches or migraine usually precede the onset of the daily headaches and are associated with nausea and vomiting. These patients also have daily mild headaches from morning until evening without other symptoms. The patient has no difficulty differentiating between the milder daily headaches and the intermittent severe headaches. These patients usually have no symptoms of increased extracranial pressure and normal general physical examination. Laboratory testing is generally unrevealing. Psychosocial evaluation may be valuable. Several authors have suggested an evolution from intermittent migraine to daily headaches, but to date this has not been well documented in children and adolescents.[33]

Case 5

A 17-year-old girl was evaluated for headaches. At the age of 12, she began to experience once-monthly headaches with nausea and vomiting. These headaches disappeared within 2 years. The patient then was headache free for an additional 2 years. Next, she developed intermittent headaches associated with visual disturbances, nausea, and vomiting. Eight months after the recurrence of these intermittent headaches, she began to experience daily headaches that would not awaken her from sleep but would be present in the morning and last the entire day. The patient was able to differentiate the milder headaches from the more severe headaches. Family history was positive for migraine. A general physical examination and a detailed neurological examination were normal. Psychological evaluation revealed no abnormality. The patient was a straight-A student and admitted to being stressed by the need to maintain her straight-A average. A combination of biofeedback therapy and amitriptyline led to the successful resolution of the headache syndrome within several months.

In this type of headache, the general and neurological examinations and laboratory testing are negative. Psychosocial information may be supportive of the diagnosis. Treatment modalities include counseling, biofeedback, and pharmacotherapy. Frequent and prolonged follow-up is necessary.

Summary

The diagnosis and management of children and adolescents with headaches are reviewed. The cause of the patient's headache usually can be discovered after a thorough history, physical examination, and selected laboratory tests. The treatment of the various headache syndromes is discussed.

References

1. Lewis DW, Middlebrook MT, Mehallick L, et al. Pediatric headaches: What do the children want? Headache 1996;36:224–230.

2. Bille BS. Migraine in school children. Acta Paediatr Scand 1962;1(suppl 136):1–151.
3. Bille BS. A 40-year follow-up of school children with migraine. Cephalalgia 1997;17:488–491.
4. Linet MS, Stewart WF, Celentano DD, Ziegler D, Sprecher M. An epidemiologic study of headache among adolescents and young adults. JAMA 1989;261:2211–2216.
5. International Headache Society. Proposed classification and diagnostic criteria for headache disorders, cranial neuralgias and facial pain. Cephalalgia 1988;8(suppl 7):1–96.
6. Maytal J, Young M, Shechter A, Lipton RB. Pediatric migraine and the International Headache Society (IHS) criteria. Neurology 1997; 48:602–607.
7. Rothner AD. Headaches in adolescents: Diagnosis and management. Med Clin North Am 1991;75:653–660.
8. Burton LJ, Quinn B, Pratt-Cheney JL, Pourani M. Headache etiology in a pediatric emergency department. Pediatr Emerg Care 1997;13:1–4.
9. Maytal J, Bienkowski RS, Patel M, Eviatar L. The value of brain imaging in children with headaches. Pediatrics 1995;96:413–416.
10. McAbee GN, Siegel SE, Kadakia S, Cantos E. Value of MRI in pediatric migraine. Headache 1993;33:143–144.
11. Diamond S. Prolonged benign exertional headache: Its clinical characteristics and response to indomethacin. Headache 1982;22:96–98.
12. Behrens MM. Headaches associated with disorders of the eye. Med Clin North Am 1978; 62:507–512.
13. Faleck H, Rothner AD, Erenberg G, Cruse RP. Headache and subacute sinusitis in children and adolescents. Headache 1988;28:96–98.
14. Belfer ML, Kaban LB. Temporomandibular joint dysfunction. Pediatrics 1982;69:564–567.
15. Kinast M, Lueders H, Rothner AD, Erenberg G. Benign focal epileptiform discharges in childhood migraine (BFEDC). Neurology 1982;32:1309–1311.
16. Prensky AL. Migraine and migrainous variants in pediatric patients. Pediatr Clin North Am 1976;23:1–71.
17. Linder SL. Subcutaneous sumatriptan in the clinic setting: The first 50 consecutive patients with acute migraine in a pediatric neurology office practice. Headache 1996;36:419–422.
18. Linder SL. Treatment of childhood headache with dihydroergotamine mesylate. Headache 1994;34:578–580.
19. Judvigsson J. Propranolol used in prophylaxis of migraine in children. Acta Neurol Scand 1974;50:109–115.
20. Lai CW, Ziegler DK, Lansky LL, et al. Hemiplegic migraine in childhood: Diagnostic and therapeutic aspects. J Pediatr 1982;101:696–699.
21. Robertson WC Jr, Schnitzler ER. Ophthalmoplegic migraine in infancy. Pediatrics 1978; 61:886–888.
22. Gascon G, Barlow C. Juvenile migraine presenting as an acute confusional state. Pediatrics 1970;45:628–635.
23. Lapkin ML, Golden GS. Basilar artery migraine: A review of 30 cases. Am J Dis Child 1978;132:278–281.
24. Fenichel GM. Migraine as a cause of benign paroxysmal vertigo in childhood. J Pediatr 1968;71:114–115.
25. Basser LS. The relation of migraine and epilepsy. Brain 1969;92:285–300.
26. Honig PJ, Charney EG. Children with brain tumor headaches. Am J Dis Child 1982;136:99–100.
27. Rothner AD, Brust JCM. Pseudotumor cerebri: Report of familial occurrence. Arch Neurol 1974;30:110–111.
28. Rothner AD. Diagnosis and management of headache in children and adolescents. Neurol Clin 1983;1:511–516.
29. Holden EW, Gladstein J, Trulsen M, Wall B. Chronic daily headache in children and adolescents. Headache 1994;34:508–514.
30. Gladstein J, Holden EW. Chronic daily headache in children and adolescents: A 2-year prospective study. Headache 1996;36:349–351.
31. Kain ZN, Rimar S. Management of chronic pain in children. Pediatr Rev 1995;16:218–222.
32. Fentress DW, Masek BJ, Mehegan JE, et al. Biofeedback and relaxation response training in treatment of pediatric migraine. Dev Med Child Neurol 1986;28:139–146.
33. Mathew NT, Stubits E, Nigam M. Transformational migraine into daily headache: Analysis of factors. Headache 1981;21:125–129.

18

Psychiatric Management of the Headache Patient

Russell C. Packard, M.D.

Introduction

In the era of sophisticated technology, headache is often discussed as if it were an abstraction existing outside a person. Discussion may center on impaired serotonin receptors, trigeminal vascular pathways, and intriguing new brain imaging techniques. It is important to remember, however, that actual diagnosis and treatment of headache disorders still require a careful interview, examination, and interaction with the patient. Emotional issues often play a primary role in precipitating headache, aggravating a headache, or influencing a reaction to headache. The recognition and management of emotional distress are a vital part of the treatment of headache, particularly in chronic cases.

Historical Note

For hundreds of years, the relationship between psychological factors and headaches has been observed. The ancient Greeks and Romans were aware that emotional distress often triggered headaches. Hippocrates described patients with migraine and wrote, "In order to cure the human body, it is necessary to have a knowledge of the whole of things."[1] Breuer and Freud[2] reported in the 1880s that many patients' complaints of headache disappeared after a cathartic experience or a state of improved emotional equilibrium had been reached.

The term *psychogenic* headache was introduced in the 1930s with the developing field of psychosomatic medicine. Similarly, Weiss and English[3] stated that psychogenic headaches were "reflex headaches" in that they were caused by conscious or unconscious emotional stress and were improved after emotional releases. In a summary of his research on psychological factors in headache, Wolff[4] wrote, "Since the human animal prides himself on 'using his head,' it is perhaps not without meaning that his head should be the source of so much discomfort . . . the vast majority of discomforts and pains of the head . . . are accompaniments of resentments and dissatisfactions." Because the head is commonly regarded as the portion of the body controlling consciousness, memory, talent, intellectual activity, cognition, and judgment, we begin to understand how the patient may use the complaint of *head*ache as a means of expressing anxiety.

Personality Factors

It has often been theorized that certain personality traits are characteristic of headache sufferers. Wolff[5] proposed that patients with migraine were perfectionistic, ambitious, angry (usually repressed), and rigid. Friedman[6] suggested personality manifestations in migraine embraced a variety of primarily unconscious emotional factors, including hostility, identification with a family figure, a wish to remain in a position of dependency, or a means to gain love, affection, or attention. The notion that pathological personality traits cause headache, however, is controversial. Obviously, no single personality type can be applied to all patients with headache, and not all patients with headache (namely, migraine) are compulsive, perfectionistic, or rigid.

Psychopathology in patients with different headache types has also been examined.

Some studies indicate that patients with muscle contraction headache (*tension-type headache*) were more neurotic than migraineurs.[7, 8] Kudrow and Sutkus[8] examined 258 untreated headache patients diagnosed with post-traumatic headache, migraine, tension, combination (migraine and tension), cluster, or conversion by using the Minnesota Multiphasic Personality Inventory (MMPI). Patients with post-traumatic and conversion headache displayed the most neurotic symptoms (extreme depression and anxiety, somatization, reliance on hysteroid mechanisms) compared with patients with combination and tension headaches (depression, repression, moderate somatization) and those with migraine or cluster headache (not significantly different from control subjects). Other studies report little support in relating headache diagnostic categories with personality profiles.[9–11] Instead, increased psychopathology was proposed as primarily related to headache frequency[10] or individual coping skills[11] rather than to specific personality types.

A study was conducted in which the association between migraine and personality was thoroughly examined[1] in a community-based sample. A significant association was found with neuroticism, even when a history of concurrent psychiatric disorders was controlled.[12] More specifically, more than 25% of persons with migraine uncomplicated by psychiatric comorbidity scored in the highest quartile of neuroticism.[12] It may be concluded that some migraine sufferers are more vulnerable to psychopathology and poor adjustment, whereas others cope well and handle their disorder with minimal psychological difficulties.

Affective Disorders

Frequently, affective disorders (i.e., depression and anxiety) are associated with chronic headache. These may range from mild cases of depression to very severe cases that require hospitalization. Although depression has a broad range of presentations, one of the most common appears to be that of a state of pain.[13] In a chronic pain state, there are often neurovegetative signs, sleep and appetite disorders, irritability, psychomotor retardation, social withdrawal, lowered pain tolerance, and somatic preoccupation.[14] The most common type of depression seen in the patient with chronic headache consists of a discouraged, anxious, or unhappy mood with sleep disturbance, irritability, and a sense of being caught in a trap and oppressed by unrelenting pain (termed *dysthymic pain disorder* by Blumer and Heilbronn).[15] In many instances, the major depression in headache patients, particularly young adults, is atypical.[13] Anxiety is often as common as depression and is typically characterized by a worried, apprehensive state.[16] The anxiety is often focused on the pain and increases when the pain persists for increasingly longer periods.

Rarely, patients with chronic headache present with manic attacks or bipolar II disorder (DSM IV).[17] Manic states usually assume a hypomanic form and are manifested as euphoria, reduced sleep, social affability, overtalkativeness, and overinvolvement with others.[16] These states can progress to a full-blown manic state with flight of ideas, grandiose delusions, hallucinations, overactivity, and excessive impulsiveness and poor judgment. Mania or hypomania can rarely occur as a side effect of medications used in headache treatment, such as antidepressants. If the manic state is secondary to medication, the adjustments in dosage or medications should bring the condition under control within a few days. If not, it is likely that mania was part of a primary bipolar disorder. In such cases, the patient should be treated with a drug for mania, such as lithium, while antidepressants are used to control the headache. In most instances, however, there is a mutually inhibiting relationship between mania and chronic pain; chronic pain seems to have the same neurovegetative pattern as depression, so chronic headache sufferers usually have too little energy or euphoria to be hypomanic.[18]

Although increased incidence of mood disturbance in patients with headache has been described for decades, much of the research has been criticized for its clinical nature. Critics argue that clinical samples might reflect a tendency on the part of those who seek treatment to have multiple disorders. They also contend it is difficult to determine whether depression or anxiety is a result of pain or the cause of pain. To guard against this potential bias, several studies examined the general population to determine psychiatric disturbances in chronic headache. Investigations by Breslau and colleagues[19, 20] revealed a high lifetime prevalence of affective disorders in subjects with migraine. Lifetime histories of dysthymia, major depression, manic episode, and bipolar II were more common in persons with migraine than in persons without migraine.[20] Similarly, the vast majority of subjects with migraine and depression also had a history of at least one anxiety disorder. Major depression was by far the most common and most consistent affective disorder in migraineurs.[20] The authors concluded that major depression was not simply a psychological response to migraine attacks because each influenced the other. These studies indicate rather convincingly that the association between migraine and depression is likely bidirectional (i.e., each disorder increases the risk for development of the other disorder). Future studies should address these issues in other headache types.

In a similar population-based study, Stewart et al[21] found a higher incidence of panic attacks in patients with migraine. More specifically, individuals with a history of panic attacks were at greater risk of having headaches in the week preceding the interview. The relationship was higher among patients with migraine than among those with tension-type headache or strictly forehead pain.

Post-traumatic Headache

Patients who have sustained trauma or injury to the head or neck frequently develop headaches (post-traumatic headaches [PTHs]) that require special attention. This is particularly important in situations in which headaches are chronic (longer than 6 months).[22] PTH may be exacerbated by the attitude of many physicians, attorneys, insurance companies, and laypersons. Because substantial organic causes for the headache are rarely identified, patients are often suspected or even accused of having functional neuroses or secondary gain issues or of outright malingering. Most clinical studies show the vast majority of patients have legitimate complaints, despite medicolegal circumstances or aggravation by psychological factors.[23, 24]

A variety of symptoms accompany PTH. In our experience, the psychiatric symptoms typically fall into one or more of three categories: neuropsychiatric symptoms (impaired memory, difficulty concentrating, decreased attention span), personality changes (increased irritability, reserved and withdrawn behavior, less open and communicative with spouse or family), and mood changes (depression, labile mood, anxiety).[24] To some extent, these may be a reaction to the pain, but they often present even when the patient is headache free. Many of these individuals are successfully treated with medication, biofeedback, limited psychotherapy, and pacing and coping skills (see "Management").

Certain patients with PTH exhibit more pronounced psychopathology. A study by Ham et al[25] found that a subgroup of chronic PTH sufferers showed higher elevations on psychological measures than did subjects with back pain or mixed migraine/tension headache. Clinicians often find that patients with severe psychological difficulties have a preexisting "vulnerability" to psychopathology; typically, such patients require psychiatric referral. Some PTH sufferers may be more impaired due to the presence of coexisting post-traumatic stress disorder. Although it is common for patients with PTH to be anxious, at least initially, when driving (assuming that the headaches were triggered by an automobile accident), some may have a profound fear of driving.[26, 27] The driving phobia may become so severe that activities of daily living are significantly limited. In such cases, patients must be treated similar to individuals who have experienced traumatic experiences in other areas (e.g., rape or combat situations).

Somatoform Disorders

Headaches can also appear as part of a somatoform disorder, which is characterized by physical symptoms suggesting a physical disorder for which no known organic findings or physiological mechanisms can be identified and for which there is a strong presumption that the symptoms are linked to psychological factors.[18] Somatoform disorders primarily include somatization disorder, hypochondriasis, and conversion disorder.

Somatization disorder is characterized by somatic complaints attributed to numerous organ systems. Such patients have been treated for a variety of illnesses of different systems (gastrointestinal symptoms are often a hallmark) and often have had multiple surgeries. Many are invalids. Unfortunately, treatment for chronic headache patients with an underlying somatization disorder is usually unsuccessful.

Hypochondriasis is manifested by preoccupation with or the belief that one has a serious disease, despite repeated evidence to the contrary. These patients with chronic headache are convinced they have a brain tumor or aneurysm despite the results of numerous imaging studies, such as computed tomography or magnetic resonance imaging. They often have little success with headache treatment and are more appropriately referred to a psychiatrist or psychologist, with whom treatment is still very limited. Perhaps the best management for hypochondriasis is to schedule regular follow-up visits with the patient.

Conversion disorder indicates a loss of physical functioning that suggests a physical disorder but for which no physical disorder can be found. Conversion headache has traditionally been considered the most pathological headache type. Most of the literature suggests a central process with little significant local change. In some instances, close observation has indicated suggestive evidence for a local focus around which symbolic tension has elaborated.[28] A key mechanism in the development of conversion headache may be the patient's identification with symptoms of a person with whom he or she has a close relationship[29]; this identification is commonly with a person who has recently died.

There often is a delay in the diagnosis of conversion headache. Clinicians may have a feeling that emotional factors are playing a role in headaches, but conversion headaches initially do not stand out in any remarkable way from other headache types. Patients will often deny any disturbing emotional relationships or events in their lives and will show a calm indifference to the pain. This denial and affective indifference is often a valuable clue in diagnosis.[29] It is important, however, to allow the patient to tell his or her own story, at his or her own rate. As in most other somatoform disorders, conversion headaches typically require long-term, often ongoing, dynamic psychotherapy. Some cases of conversion headache have been observed to spontaneously resolve after the patient makes the connection to the unrecognized stressful event. For example, a young military pilot developed continuous daily headaches after his wife became pregnant; when he realized his fears of flying "as a family man," the headache resolved, and he continued flying.

Drug Dependency

Occasionally, patients with chronic headache become dependent on pain medications. Some of these individuals will have had prior psychiatric disorders, although some drug-dependent patients have no history of psychopathology. Headache medications that are frequently overused include opioids, analgesics, benzodiazepines, butalbital compounds or barbiturates, and ergot derivatives. The withdrawal symptoms in headache medications involve a return of pain that had been masked by the medication.[17] Thus, the patient may begin taking the medication daily or several times daily and then follow with a pattern of gradually increasing doses as tolerance grows.[30] When the overuse of pain medication is minor and the clinician believes the patient is trustworthy and basically compliant, treatment may be done on an outpatient basis. Often, a 3-day course (over a weekend) of naproxen sodium (Anaprox DS, 375–500 mg) and hydroxyzine (Vistaril, 50–100 mg) every 6 hours will allow withdrawal of the analgesic medication and provide some relief for the rebound headache, nausea, and vomiting. In situations in which the overuse of medication is more severe and compliance is questionable, the patient may need to be placed in an inpatient setting so medication decreases can be monitored and toxic consequences prevented. In some cases, the patient may have an additional addictive disorder and require a drug rehabilitation program.

Management

The psychiatric management often works best with a multidisciplinary approach, incorporating medication, education, stress management, counseling, and physical therapy. When major psychological difficulties are present, a greater emphasis may need to be placed on stress management and life skills training, psychotherapy, and antidepressant medication.

Stress Reduction

Stress management techniques encompass relaxation training (autogenic phrases, progressive muscle relaxation, deep muscle relaxation, imagery, meditation, hypnosis), biofeedback, and cognitive-behavioral therapy. These techniques may be most useful if combined. For example, biofeedback uses instrumentation to provide feedback about physiological processes and typically is most effective if combined with relaxation strategies.[31] In this manner, maximal increases in hand warmth and lowering of muscle tension can be obtained. Biofeedback not only is beneficial as a tool in reducing stress but also is effective in decreasing excessive muscle tension and improving peripheral blood flow, which can be altered with headaches.[32] In addition, biofeedback may be used as an instrument-aided form of psychotherapy.[31]

Obviously, if an individual learns to reduce stress or decrease muscle tension through biofeedback and relaxation but continues to have faulty stress-related cognitions, improvements will only be temporary.[33] For example, if a patient thinks that each minor headache indicates a severe migraine, the headache may snowball and become associated with nausea and vomiting or a full-blown panic attack. These anxious thought processes may result in a vicious cycle in which the patient increasingly tightens muscles (because of worry about the potential headache) and makes it more likely that he or she will in fact develop a severe headache. The patient should also be taught techniques to enhance generalization of stress reduction skills (e.g., the patient should be able to reduce stress at the office or home and not only in the therapist's recliner).[34] It may be helpful to incorporate some cognitive-behavioral training into a stress reduction program.

Education

Education of patients with chronic headache is one of the most important and overlooked aspects of treatment. In 1979, Packard[35] surveyed 100 patients with headache and 50 primary care physicians regarding what the patient wanted from their physicians. The patients rated an explanation first, whereas physicians thought patients were primarily seeking pain relief. If the physician assumes the patient is coming for pain medication but the patient wants to know what is wrong, treatment efforts may be doomed to failure.

The more educated one is about headache, the more he or she understands how tension, worry, pressure, overactivity, and excessive fatigue relate to headaches and depression and thus he or she is more likely to make changes or comply with treatment regimens designed at managing or reducing stress. In PTH, it is particularly important to inform the patient about post-traumatic symptoms; otherwise, many patients think they are "going crazy." Psychoeducational groups (which may develop into supportive group therapy) are often an ideal way to educate a number of patients about headache and potential triggering factors and to increase social interactions. In addition, simply dealing with patients' fears and questions about medication, side effects, and the importance of taking abortive medications early can be very helpful.

Psychotherapy

Adler and Adler[36] describe psychotherapy with headache patients as existing at three levels. The first level involves that of support, education, and helping the patient rearrange some of the external contingencies in his or her life. Techniques in the first level involve many previously described, such as stress management techniques (relaxation, biofeedback, brief cognitive/behavioral training), education, pacing/coping skills, and supportive group therapy. Primary care physicians are often capable of providing this level of help; in fact, the primary physician may have advantages over the mental health professional in treating certain emotional aspects of headache. These advantages include more accrued knowledge of the patient and the patient's life situation, an established trust, and the patient feeling more comfortable talking to his or her primary physician than to a mental health professional.

Levels two and three involve in-depth psychotherapy, which should be provided only by a mental health professional.

According to Adler and Adler,[36] the major factors differentiating levels two and three are the intensity of the therapy and the therapeutic goals. Level two often involves patients who are having much difficulty coping with the headache; subsequently, they are depressed and anxious. In PTH, issues of anger (e.g., at the other driver, the insurance company, "the system" in a Worker's Compensation case, and so forth) or grief (e.g., at changes in personality or activity level and possible decline in functioning) often need addressing. Level three typically involves character or personality restructuring. These patients almost always have had significant preexisting psychopathology. Therapy in such cases requires numerous sessions and often is psychodynamic.

The type of psychotherapy provided—cognitive/behavioral or psychodynamic—depends primarily on the needs of the patient and training of the provider. Behavior therapy posits that problems are best understood when viewed as long-term effects of learned responses to positive or negative stimuli. There is almost no discussion of unconscious factors. Behavior therapy is most useful in headache patients whose primary problem is self-defeating behavior.[37] A treatment plan is typically devised to help the patient unlearn maladaptive behaviors and acquire appropriate behaviors. At present, behavior therapy is often conducted in conjunction with cognitive therapy. Cognitive therapy involves the delineation and discussion of illogical or self-defeating thoughts that accompany or precipitate the headache. Cognitive/behavioral therapy is concerned with the impact of behaviors and thoughts on headache.

Psychodynamic psychotherapy examines emotional conflicts in the production or exacerbation of somatic symptoms or headache. In many cases, emotional conflicts are believed to have resulted from childhood incidents or interactions. The contribution of unconscious factors is a primary focus in psychodynamic therapy. Unresolved issues in the unconscious must be dealt with and insight gained. To be successful, the patient with headache must learn to relate feelings to life experiences and understand the nature of important relationships, both past and present.[37]

Regardless of the type of therapy provided, some general strategies are often helpful. Adler et al[38] recommend the following strategies for the therapist when dealing with headache patients (regardless of diagnosis): Be warm but formal, establish structure, never challenge the authenticity of the patient's pain, harness positive attributes, reduce high expectations (i.e., for a "cure"), and set realistic goals—for less severe and/or less frequent headache.

Another consideration in conducting psychotherapy is to look at what benefits, or "needs," the headache may be serving. Packard and Andrasik[39] examined what patients meant when they complained of a "really good headache." When patients were asked to clarify what they meant by "good," they stated their terminology was "just a figure of speech." Further exploration, however, revealed that headaches may have indeed been "good" in a relative sense by allowing the patient a forced period of rest in a hectic schedule, resolving a conflict in an acceptable way (becoming sick), or representing a suppressed affect (anger). When a headache is described as "good," something in a patient's life may be worse.

Medications

Antidepressants are often quite effective in managing chronic daily headache or migraine with (or without) psychiatric symptoms. The three major classes of antidepressants are the tricyclics (TCAs), monoamine oxidase inhibitors (MAOIs), and selective serotonin reuptake inhibitors (SSRIs). MAOIs are rarely prescribed except in cases of severe and nonresponsive depression and/or headache because side effects are common and dietary restrictions are necessary. TCAs are frequently prescribed for headache, but they have the annoying side effects of sedation, dry mouth, constipation, and weight gain. SSRIs are advantageous in that they are generally better tolerated and have fewer side effects. We have found the SSRIs to be just as effective in headache treatment as the TCAs. Some patients with refractory depression, migraine, or PTH may benefit from treatment with TCAs in combination with an SSRI. The clinician should be aware that SSRIs usually cause an elevation in TCA levels.

Certain drugs (anticonvulsants, antihistamines, β-blockers, immunosuppressives, and sedatives) may produce depressive reactions in susceptible patients or aggravate an existing depression. Because depression and anxiety often coexist, depressed patients may be mistakenly treated with sedatives. A worsening of the condition suggests that antidepressant therapy may be more appropriate.[14]

Summary

Many practitioners with limited training in psychiatry may feel uneasy about addressing psychiatric issues in headache; however, one does not have to be a mental health professional to be observant and listen well. Some of the most pertinent information can be obtained from clinical observation and knowledge of the patient. In addition, primary care providers often have extremely valuable information and insight into the patient's family, occupational, and social situations. Recognize your limits and know when to refer for psychiatric consultation or treatment.

References

1. Hippocrates. Aphorisms. *In* Lloyd G (ed). Hippocratic Writings. London: Penguin Books, 1983;206–236.
2. Breuer J, Freud S. Case Histories. *In* Strachey J, ed. The Complete Psychological Works of Sigmund Freud: Studies on Hysteria. London, Hogarth Press, 1955.
3. Weiss E, English OS. Psychosomatic Medicine. Philadelphia: WB Saunders; 1943:443–458.
4. Wolff HG. Cranial Pain Sensitive Structures in Headache and Other Head Pain, 2nd ed. New York: Oxford University Press; 1963:59–97.
5. Wolff HG. Personality features and reactions of subjects with migraine. Arch Neurol 1937;37:895–921.
6. Friedman AP. The mechanism and treatment of migraine and tension headache. J Miss State Med 1958;80:141–146.
7. Andrasik F, Blanchard EB, Arena JG, et al. Psychological functioning in headache sufferers. Psychosom Med 1982;44:171–182.
8. Kudrow L, Sutkus BJ. MMPI pattern specificity in primary headache disorders. Headache 1979;19:18–24.
9. Pfaffenrath V, Hummelsberger J, Pollman W, et al. MMPI personality profiles in patients with primary headache syndromes. Cephalalgia 1991;11:263–268.
10. Rappaport NB, McAnulty DP, Waggoner CD, et al. Cluster analysis of MMPI profiles in a chronic headache population. J Behav Med 1987;10:49–60.
11. Robinson ME, Geisser ME, Dieter JN, et al. The relationship between MMPI cluster membership and diagnostic category in headache patients. Headache 1991;31:111–115.
12. Breslau N, Andreski P. Migraine, personality, and psychiatric comorbidity. Headache 1985;35:382–386.
13. Diamond S. Depression and headache: A pharmacological perspective. *In* Adler CS, Adler SM, Packard RC, eds. Psychiatric Aspects of Headache. Baltimore: Williams & Wilkins; 1987.
14. Mebane AH. Antidepressant therapy for chronic pain syndromes. Clin Adv Treat Psychiatr Dis 1990;4:12–16.
15. Blumer D, Heilbronn M. Chronic pain as a variant of depressive disease: The pain prone disorder. J Nerve Ment Dis 1982;170:381–406.
16. Schulman B. Psychiatric management of the headache patient. *In* Diamond S, Dalessio DJ, eds. The Practicing Physician's Approach to Headache, 5th ed. Baltimore: Williams & Wilkins; 1992.
17. Diagnostic and Statistical Manual of Mental Disorders, 4th ed. Washington, DC: American Psychiatric Association; 1994.
18. Diamond S. Depression and headache. Headache 1983;23:122–126.
19. Breslau N, Davis GC, Schultz LR, et al. Migraine and major depression: A longitudinal study. Headache 1994;34:387–393.
20. Breslau N, Merikangas K, Bowden CS. Comorbidity of migraine and major affective disorders. Neurology 1994;44(suppl 7):S17–S22.
21. Stewart S, Breslau N, Keck PE. Comorbidity of migraine and panic disorder. Neurology 1994;44(suppl 7):S23–S27.
22. Packard RC, Ham LP. Posttraumatic headache: Determining chronicity. Headache 1993;33:133–134.
23. Packard RC. Posttraumatic headache: Permanency and relationship to legal settlement. Headache 1992;32:496–500.
24. Packard RC, Ham LP. Posttraumatic headache. J Neuropsychiatry Clin Neurosci 1994;6:229–236.
25. Ham LP, Andrasik F, Packard RC, et al. Psychopathology in individuals with post-traumatic headaches and other pain types. Cephalalgia 1994;14:118–126.
26. Chibnall JT, Duckro PN. Post-traumatic stress disorder in chronic post-traumatic headache patients. Headache 1994;34:357–361.
27. Hickling EJ, Blanchard EB, Schwarz SP, et al. Headaches and motor vehicle accidents: Results of the psychological treatment of post-traumatic headache. Headache Q 1992;3:285–289.
28. Boag TJ. Psychogenic headache. *In* Vinken PJ, Bruyn GW, eds. Handbook of Clinical Neurology. Amsterdam: North Holland Publishing; 1968.
29. Packard RC. Conversion headache. Headache 1980;20:266–268.
30. Elkind AH. Drug abuse and headache. Med Clin North Am 1991;75:717–732.
31. Adler CS, Adler SM, Packard RC. The psychological use of biofeedback and other self-regulatory techniques in headache treatment. *In* Adler CS, Adler SM, Packard RC, eds. Psychiatric Aspects of Headache. Baltimore: Williams & Wilkins; 1987.
32. Andrasik F. Relaxation and biofeedback for chronic headaches. *In* Holzman AD, Turk DC, eds. Pain Management: A Handbook of Psychological Treatment Approaches. New York: Pergamon; 1986.
33. Meichenbaum D. Cognitive-Behavior Modification: An Integrative Approach. New York: Plenum Press; 1977.
34. Stroebel CF, Stroebel NC. The psychophysio-

logical diary for monitoring home practice of self-regulation techniques, generalizing and transferring of state dependent learning, and enhancing mind-body awareness and therapeutic outcome. Annual Meeting of the American Association for Applied Psychophysiology and Biofeedback. 1996.
35. Packard RC. What does the headache patient want? Headache 1979;19:370–374.
36. Adler CS, Adler SM. Psychotherapy and the headache patient. *In* Adler CS, Adler SM, Packard RC, eds. Psychiatric Aspects of Headache. Baltimore: Williams & Wilkins; 1987.
37. Gill JR. An overview of treatment options for the psychologically influenced headache patient. *In* Adler CS, Adler SM, Packard RC, eds. Psychiatric Aspects of Headache. Baltimore: Williams & Wilkins; 1987.
38. Adler CS, Adler SM. From theory to technique: A psychotherapeutic miscellany for headache. *In* Adler CS, Adler SM, Packard RC, eds. Psychiatric Aspects of Headache. Baltimore: Williams & Wilkins; 1987.
39. Packard RC, Andrasik F, Weaver RG. When headaches are good. Headache 1989;29:100–102.

19

Psychological Assessment of the Headache Patient

Paul N. Duckro, Ph.D.

Theresa Tschannen, Ph.D.

Introduction

We present a comprehensive and comprehensible model for the psychological evaluation of patients with headache. This model is based on several premises particular to psychological work with such patients; it is easily generalizable to other chronic medical disorders in which behavioral treatment plays an important role. First, the psychological evaluation is never independent of the medical evaluation. The psychologist and physician may be part of an organized team or may work through cross-referral, but in either case communication and collaboration are vital. Second, headache is at base a medical disorder; however, it is a chronic medical disorder in which frequency, severity, and duration significantly influence and are influenced by psychosocial factors. These psychosocial factors may be psychiatric disorders, emotional distress, or the stress of everyday life. Third, it is the integration of the medical and behavioral perspectives that greatly potentiates evaluation and treatment. Fourth, psychological factors are important in many other aspects of headache management. These other areas include but are not limited to adherence to medication regimens, maintenance of healthy lifestyle, generalization of relaxation training, and management of nonpsychological "triggers" that initiate or exacerbate headache.

The first focus of this chapter is the nature of the psychological interview, which is central to the evaluation process. Next, psychological testing is considered in its role as a component of the psychological assessment. Finally, there is an overview of the psychological report. Each psychologist has a unique way of combining the material of the evaluation, and his or her presentation varies further with each patient. Nevertheless, we outline characteristics of a report that can speak clearly and compellingly to the patient with headache and collaborating physicians. In contrast to the more basic psychological report used in the assessment of patients presenting with psychiatric disorders, such a report reflects the unique application of psychological techniques to the evaluation of the headache patients.

The Psychological Interview

Psychological assessment of the headache patient is not limited to psychological testing. In the hands of an experienced clinician, the testing materials, although valuable, represent only one tool in the assessment. As in most areas of psychological work, the most important tool is the clinician and the careful observations that he or she makes.

The psychologist brings to the assessment a patient-centered focus and a method of critical thinking adapted to dealing with probabilities rather than certainties. This approach is very useful with the headache patient, with whom a singular relationship between any particular factor and headache onset is often hard to identify.

In addition, the psychologist brings a sensitivity to the vicissitudes and nuances of human behavior, including but not limited to diagnosable psychopathology. From the data of the psychological interview, in conjunction with psychological tests, the psychologist is able to develop a specific series of statements detailing the nature of the psychological factors affecting (and affected by) the frequency, duration, and severity of the headache syndrome.

The Psychologist's Perspective

The psychologist's contribution to the assessment of headache occurs in the context of previous medical examination. No matter how significant the psychological factors or diagnosable psychiatric illness, it is simply not possible to claim them definitively as causes of the headache syndrome. The identification of such psychological factors does not rule out medical disease of which the headache may be a symptom, nor (in most cases) can those factors fully account for the headache syndrome.

However, once medical disease has been ruled out as a specific source of the headache, the psychologist participates in the naming of the headache syndrome on the basis of the criteria of the International Headache Society. At this stage, the headache may be seen as a chronic disorder, a syndrome of concurring symptoms initiated or "triggered" by an agglomeration of endogenous or exogenous factors. The focus of assessment shifts from the search for one particular underlying cause to the identification of the various pathways by which headache is initiated, duration is prolonged, severity is exacerbated, and disability is increased.

In the case of chronic, benign headache, the physician reviews the biochemical and physiological pathways that lead to headache and treats them with medications to prevent or abort the headache and with physical therapies. The contribution of the psychologist lies in identification of the various behavioral, emotional, cognitive, and psychophysiological pathways that also affect headache parameters.

In addition to generating specific content for the treatment plan, the psychological assessment affects the patient's perception of treatment. If the evaluation process includes questions about only medical factors, there is the implication to the patient that psychological factors are considered only when medical factors alone do not satisfactorily account for the headache syndrome or medication or other medical procedures do not resolve the syndrome. The patient will develop or maintain a correspondingly dismal view of psychological care for the headache syndrome. When the time comes to refer the patient, he or she will be more likely to view it quite negatively, seeing in this referral the physician's belief that the headache pain is not "real" or the patient is not psychologically competent. The negative perception of referral dramatically reduces the percentage of patients who accept referral, persist in treatment, and do well in psychological care.

Elements of the Psychological Interview

With regard to the clinical history, the psychological assessment overlaps somewhat with the medical examination; however, there are also important differences. In the psychological assessment, there typically is greater emphasis on the subjective experience of the patient. Beyond the historic facts, there is attention to the way in which the patient has reacted to the pain and to the impact of the life events that occurred before, during, and after exacerbations or remissions of headache parameters.

This type of subjective, experiential history essentially invites the patient, in the form of a story, to share the implicit hypotheses he or she has developed regarding the headache and how on the basis of these hypotheses he or she has tried to manage it. If the patient is encouraged to tell the full story of his or her life with headache, without editing out parts they have decided are irrelevant or too personal, the clinician is able to see other potentially important factors that the patient has not recognized or is unconsciously avoiding.

From this base, the clinician will be able to formulate his or her own hypotheses. With the physician, the psychologist can begin to integrate them with the biomedical hypotheses. With the patient, the psychologist can introduce new ideas and discuss the patient's hypotheses with the intention of confirming, discrediting, or subjecting them to mutually designed clinical "experiments."

This detailed experiential history requires more time than a skeletal outline of basic facts, but it is very rich in terms of data. Even so, it is still a retrospective view subject to all the distortions of any memory. Usually, the history will be supplemented by at least several weeks of a headache diary, allowing patient and psychologist a current view of headache activity and related events. This diary will be continued throughout the behavioral treatment. The diary amounts to a type of "concurrent memory" that offers more reliable data from which to describe present headache activity. These data serve to further define the current syndrome, identify factors affecting headache, and record the response to treatment.

The identification of *triggers* (factors initiating headache attacks) and other factors affecting the headache syndrome more indirectly is an important aspect of taking the headache history. The range of potential factors affecting headache is great, and the same factors do not equally affect all patients. In addition, studies of headache triggers suggest that even in a particular individual, most such factors are not so potent as to trigger headache whenever they are present; rather, they seem to operate in a probabilistic fashion, interacting with other triggers and the current condition of the patient.[1] These characteristics of headache triggers make it very difficult to identify them reliably a priori or even on the basis of one or two evaluation interviews. More often, they must be identified and verified over time, with careful observation using a systematic method like the headache diary.

Among the many triggers of chronic, benign headache, psychological factors are perhaps the most common. This does not mean that the headache is actually a psychological problem; in many cases, these psychological factors are not pathological in nature but reflect the stresses of everyday life. Presumably, as the pathophysiology of headache is determined with greater certainty, it will be seen more clearly why psychological factors are so common and potent as triggers. For the present, it is simply important to look for these factors and help the patient (and other involved physicians and psychologists) avoid the mistake of reasoning backward from trigger to cause and treating the headache as a psychological disorder.

On the other hand, it is important to remember that primary psychiatric illness is no less likely to be present among headache patients than in the general population. The increased prevalence of certain affective conditions is discussed in Chapter 20. Personality disorders or relatively fixed personality characteristics may also be present in any particular patient. To identify these conditions, the psychological interview will usually include a modified mental status examination and a history of psychiatric and psychological treatment. When these conditions are found, whether they are secondary to the headache disorder or constitute a coexisting primary disorder, they certainly affect the course of the syndrome and must be addressed in the treatment plan.

Other than the more formal assessment for psychiatric illness, the psychosocial history is reviewed in the same manner as the headache history. Essentially, the client is invited to tell a brief story of his or her life. The way in which this story is told reveals much important information. For example, paucity or shallowness of the material provided may indicate limited psychological-mindedness or guardedness regarding psychological care. The focus of the story may suggest tendencies toward internalization or externalization of blame. These and other "styles" of relating to the self and the world will usually be manifested in the way the patient relates to the treatment team and to the headache itself.

Of course, the specific content of the psychosocial history can be critical. Early trauma such as sexual abuse or parental alcoholism can have long-lasting effects on psychological coping and can affect the way in which the patient copes with the headache. Each family has a unique culture in which the patient's behavior can be understood more clearly. As we noted previously, any events that occurred around the time of significant changes in headache activity may be important in understanding the psychological dimensions of the syndrome.

Assessment of the current life situation is equally important. The concept of secondary gain is overused, and it is often used in a pejorative sense when the patient is not responding or complying. However, it is an important concept. If the family situation is such that attention, even if it is negative attention, is forthcoming only when there is pain, then the patient will experience more pain and express that pain more dramatically. If the work situation is one in which the patient feels wronged or there has been an accident after which the patient feels badly treated, he or she may demonstrate those feelings in pain that does not improve.

On the other hand, there are many dimensions of psychosocial health that are important in themselves but also offer a protective effect from headache activity or associated disability. Social support is one such factor. It is not the quantity of family or friends but rather the quality of those relationships that seems to make the most difference. Friendships in which there is a real sense of mutuality and trust are sources of great support in difficult circumstances. Religious commitment has not been studied specifically with regard to headache management, but it continues to be a positive correlate of health and coping in many studies. Other behaviors of some importance include adequate recreation, exercise, and sleep. Diet is a critical subject given the potential for food triggers of headache, but it is also worthwhile to review the patient's caloric intake, nutritional balance, water intake, and tobacco and alcohol use. Caffeine consumption is an important and problematic area worth extra time. Most patients have not reached the point of "caffeinism," and most have found that a little caffeine helps to reduce headache pain. It is more difficult for them to understand that too much caffeine can increase headache by way of a withdrawal reaction that includes headache. The amount of caffeine that is addictive is not easy to determine in the clinical setting. Milligrams of caffeine in any given beverage will vary. Even in the laboratory, the amount necessary to produce symptoms on withdrawal seems to vary according to the individual. It is usually necessary to ask the patient to conduct his or her own "experiment" by ceasing caffeine use for 1 or 2 days and observing for symptoms of lethargy, headache, and irritability.

An evaluation of psychophysiological arousal is not always part of the psychological assessment. When offered, this assessment is typically conducted with clinical biofeedback equipment. In contrast to its important role in the treatment of headache, clinical electromyography with standard biofeedback equipment has not been sufficiently specific and sensitive as a diagnostic test for significant myofascial involvement.[2] However, for any given individual, it can be a useful guide in planning biofeedback treatment and a useful measure of the learning that has taken place in treatment. In general, simple palpation and range of motion assessment followed by thorough physical therapy evaluation when indicated is likely to be a more fruitful route. Similarly, assessment of autonomic reactivity can be very useful in planning which types of biofeedback to use in treatment, but its value as an assessment procedure in the evaluation of headache appears questionable.

The review of medications is part of the medical examination, yet even here the psychologist plays a role, especially with the patient who presents with refractory headache. The history of prior treatment and the current way in which the patient uses prescribed and over-the-counter medication reveals valuable information regarding his or her understanding of headache and the emotional reaction to headache pain. In our experience, very few headache patients can be diagnosed as having a primary substance abuse disorder; however, many patients with very frequent, severe headache syndromes do overuse medications in their sense of desperation, frustration, and fear that they have no other hope. Similarly, the process of withdrawal from excessive medication use and establishment of a new medication regimen hold many possibilities for psychological intervention. These interventions include education about multidisciplinary care, emotional support, anxiety management, and the development of hope. Material gleaned in the psychological assessment will assist in the estimation of how much anxiety the patient will experience during withdrawal and what type of information and support will be most helpful.

Finally, the patient's overall sense of readiness, especially the readiness for multidisciplinary treatment, must be considered. Excessively pessimistic and excessively optimistic attitudes are equally problematic.[3] If patients come with a history of failed treatment, it is necessary to assess the internalized rationale that they have developed to explain these failures. With the "experienced" patient, a treatment team that combines commitment to the patient with an attitude of cautious optimism is probably more helpful than an attitude of great certainty or one in which the adequacy of prior interventions is offhandedly dismissed. However, each person is different, and the psychological assessment can be the source of useful hypotheses regarding the type of therapeutic relationship and the type of information that will best serve the individual patient.

Psychological Testing

In the course of headache evaluation, psychological testing is most often used to identify psychopathology. Psychological testing complements the clinical interview. A wide range of tests may be used in clinical practice, with each varying widely in length and comprehensiveness. Some are carefully constructed and researched psychometric instruments; others are more casually developed questionnaires that should be considered experimental measures. In the research literature, the Minnesota Multiphasic Personality Inventory[4] (MMPI) may be the most commonly used psychological test. It is available in a revised form, the MMPI-2.[5]

With the MMPI, one type of research strategy that was popular for a time was the effort to differentiate persons with various headache diagnoses from each other and from nonheadache control subjects. Building on earlier work by Kudrow and Sutkus,[6] Andrasik et al[7] compared patients with migraine, tension, mixed, or cluster headache with nonheadache control subjects. They found that only patients with cluster headache did not differ from control subjects and that there were increasing scale elevations along a continuum of patients with cluster, migraine, mixed, and tension headache. This finding was essentially replicated by Blanchard et al.[8] In this study, there was no evidence for a single headache personality. The authors did suggest a relationship between psychological distress and pain; greater distress seemed to be associated with increased frequency and/or duration of headache.

Similarly, Ellertsen and Klove[9] compared a group of patients with chronic musculoskeletal pain with three groups of patients with headache. They found no differences between headache and nonheadache pain subjects. They did find support for the proposed relationship of psychological distress and frequency and/or duration of pain. In general, mean elevations (above 70T) were found on scales 1 (hypochondriasis), 2 (depression), and 3 (hysteria). Dieter and Swerdlow[10] carried out a similar study but added a group of subjects with post-traumatic headache. They found, as did Ellertsen and Klove, mean elevations on scales 1 through 3. They also found a continuum of psychological distress, but the patients with headache were at different points on the continuum than those reported by Andrasik et al[7] and Blanchard et al.[8] Like the Andrasik and Blanchard teams, these authors found that the group with tension headache demonstrated the greatest psychological distress.

Later research has not fully confirmed earlier findings. Invernizzi et al[11] found that a mixed headache group of patients had higher MMPI scores (scales 1, 2, 3, and 7) than did those with migraine or tension headaches. They found no relationship with the length of time the patient had had the headache syndrome and did not test directly for any relationship with the frequency and/or duration of headache attacks. Pfaffenrath et al[12] found no differences among headache diagnostic groups. Mean elevations of scales 1 and 3 were noted in the commonly described "conversion-V" configuration, but the absolute levels did not reach a clinically significant level (70T). They did not attempt an analysis of emotional distress as a function of headache attack frequency and/or duration (the "density" of headache pain).

The MMPI is a very long test containing questions that address the entire range of psychopathological conditions. Furthermore, patients with headache sometimes wonder what relevance the test has for their headache or what it might imply about their physician's opinion of their pain condition. For these reasons, the MMPI is not always used in actual headache clinics. Some authors have reported similarly designed studies with other clinical instruments. Jay et al[13] reported the use of the Millon Clinical Multiaxial Inventory (MCMI).[14] This instrument is similar to the MMPI in focus but much shorter; however, the MCMI must be interpreted cautiously when used clinically with nonpsychiatric populations. Patients with headache have been found to have less overall pathology than patients with chronic pain but more than control subjects. A variety of more focused (and therefore clinically more limited) instruments have been used in research studies and are likely to be found in at least some headache clinics; these include the Beck Depression Inventory,[15] Anger-Expression Scale,[16] State-Trait Anxiety Inventory,[17] Rathus Assertiveness Schedule,[18] and SCL 90 R.[19]

A second line of research with the MMPI attempted to identify psychologically homogeneous subgroups of patients with headache. Rappaport et al[20] found four clusters similar to those identified by a different research team with patients with chronic pain. Two of the groups had no clinically elevated scales. A third was characterized by elevations on scales 1 through 3, whereas a fourth group was characterized by many elevated scales, reflecting more extensive psychological distress. The four clusters could be differentiated on the basis of headache frequency; the trend exhibited the positive relationship between frequency and psychological distress. They could not be differentiated on the basis of headache diagnosis.

Robinson et al[21] replicated the four clusters found in the previous study but included a fifth cluster characterized by an elevation on scale 2. They did not find a relationship of cluster membership to headache parameters. Kinder et al[22, 23] considered men and women separately in their cluster analysis. Both the male and female samples could be clustered into four subgroups generally consistent with the findings of Rappaport et al[20] and Robinson et al.[21] Among male subjects, there was no association between cluster assignment and headache diagnosis. Among female subjects, patients with migraine were more likely to be in a cluster without mean scale elevations, whereas patients with tension headache were more likely to have higher scale elevations.

In summary, the cited literature suggests that a subset of patients with headache demonstrate psychopathology. Depression may be the most common psychological factor found among patients with headache or pain in general, but anxiety also is very important in the experience of and reaction to pain. These findings have been supported by epidemiological and clinical studies of psychiatric diagnoses among patients with headache.[24] Anxiety may be a clinically significant factor among some patients with persistent posttraumatic headache.[25] Other studies have suggested a relationship among suppressed anger, depression, and headache-related disability.[26, 27]

Overall, the relationship between the frequency, duration, and intensity of headache pain (pain density) and psychological distress appears to be more reliable than the relationship between headache diagnostic groups and distress.[28] In many studies, higher levels of psychopathology are associated with greater pain density. It is not possible to infer from this relationship which is the causative factor; nevertheless, many authors have offered the opinion that the psychopathology may be secondary to the pain rather than a cause of more frequent pain. Caution in accepting this interpretation remains necessary. For example, there is other evidence of a bidirectional relationship between migraine and depression.[24] It is also possible that other genetic or learned characteristics predispose selected headache patients to respond with greater distress. Ziegler and Paolo[29] demonstrated that when clinic patients were compared with a control group who had headaches but did not seek treatment, the groups were differentiated only by the intensity of the "most severe headache" and psychological distress as measured with the MMPI-2.

Personality and Headache

The term *personality* is often used in discussion of the results of the studies cited above. None has demonstrated a singular *migraine personality,* a concept that continues to enjoy a place in clinical lore. Unfortunately, the results of these studies cannot be considered conclusive in this regard. All of them have used the MMPI or other instruments that measure psychopathology, a construct that must be differentiated from personality. The MMPI, for example, is designed to detect psychological symptoms, assist differential diagnosis, and identify current level of psychological adjustment.[5, 30] Although the term *personality* may sometimes be used in discussing the results and the test measures certain personality characteristics, the scales of the MMPI do not reflect any coherent theory of personality. There are relatively few instruments that have been developed to measure aspects of a systematic theoretical schema of personality as contrasted with specific or general measures of psychopathology.

A long line of research with many prominent contributors has resulted in an instrument that appears to have promise for the assessment of personality. The instrument, currently named the NEO Personality Inventory-Revised (NEO-PI-R), is based on the five-factor theory of personality.[31, 32] As operationalized in the NEO-PI-R, the five factors are named neuroticism (N), extraversion (E), openness to experience (O), agreeableness (A), and conscientiousness (C). Each factor scale may be further defined in "facet" scales. Costa and McCrae[33] have been active in encouraging application of the five-factor model to both clinical and research problems.

The NEO-PI-R may be contrasted with the MMPI and similar instruments in that it seeks to measure "normal" personality variation rather than psychopathology. Johnson et al[34] and Costa et al[35] compared earlier versions of this instrument with the MMPI. Although they found some overlap between the tests on neuroticism and extraversion, the MMPI does not clearly distinguish the various facets of either construct. The NEO-PI-R also addresses other constructs not found in the MMPI and does so in the context of an overarching theory of personality.

Tschannen[36] used the NEO-PI-R in a cluster analytical study of persons (largely women) with refractory headache. The first of three clusters identified was characterized by high scores on extraversion, openness to experience, and conscientiousness. Persons with this profile might be described as stable, assertive, outgoing, open to new ideas, and goal directed. The second (and largest cluster) had no particularly high or low scores. Persons with this profile might be described as generally calm, balanced in terms of relationships and private time, dependable, moderately well organized, and practical while remaining reasonably open to new ideas. The third cluster was notable for high scores on neuroticism and low scores on the other scales. Persons with this profile are more likely to exhibit signs of psychological distress, behave conservatively, and be more introverted, disorganized, and irritable.

The clusters were further described in post hoc analyses. Tschannen[36] found that the high-neuroticism/low-extraversion cluster was more likely to catastrophize in the face of pain and reported more days with headache pain. Across the sample as a whole, persons scoring higher on neuroticism reported greater disability associated with headache and used less-effective cognitive coping strategies.

Summary

Taken as a whole, the studies of psychological test data for patients with headache lead to several conclusions. First, a significant subset of patients with headache demonstrate measurable psychological distress. Second, psychological distress seems to be most reliably related to the density (frequency/duration/intensity) of pain. This relationship has most commonly been interpreted as one in which the distress is secondary to the pain. Third, a subset of patients with psychological distress have elevations on scales 1 and 3 of the MMPI, scales often associated with somatoform disorders; however, these elevations seem to be partially explained by questions that can reflect actual symptoms of headache syndromes. Therefore, positive answers to those questions by patients with headache might reflect the headache syndrome rather than a psychiatric disorder. Fourth, there is no clear empirical evidence for an association of a particular personality type with migraine or any other headache diagnosis; however, studies with the MMPI or other instruments designed to measure pathology should not be relied on to answer questions about the relationship of personality and headache diagnosis. Fifth, the NEO-PI-R is a relatively new instrument that had not been used with patients with headache before the study by Tschannen.[36] Because it is developed on the basis of a coherent theoretical understanding of personality, it has the potential to answer questions regarding the relationship of personality types and headache parameters.

In the study by Tschannen,[36] there again was no evidence for a single personality type related to headache. The cluster structure indicated three different personality patterns among patients with refractory headache; however, neuroticism was associated with more frequent headache pain, less effective cognitive coping, and greater disability. Neuroticism has been found to be a stable factor with nonclinical populations, although it may increase as depression increases. If neuroticism, as measured by the NEO-PI-R used with patients with headache, can be taken to be a relatively stable factor rather than a transient measure of psychological distress, the data of Tschannen could be interpreted to suggest a causal relationship in which neuroticism predisposes the patient with headache to less-effective coping, greater headache frequency and/or duration, and greater disability.

There are data that indirectly support such a hypothesis.[37] Breslau et al[37] found that neuroticism (as measured with the Eysenck Personality Questionnaire) was associated with increased likelihood of migraine among women. In a comprehensive review of the literature on headache and personality, Silberstein et al[24] reported that the association between migraine and neuroticism was commonly reported among researchers using the Eysenck Personality Questionnaire or similar measures of personality, contrasting migraine patients with healthy control subjects. Other studies indicated that the association of neuroticism and migraine could not be explained completely by coexisting depression or anxiety.[38, 39] Philips and Jahanshahi[40] found that higher levels of complaint behavior among patients with chronic headache were associated with neuroticism and extraversion on the Eysenck Personality Questionnaire, as well as with depression.

Obviously, these findings must be replicated and explored further before definitive conclusions are warranted. A prospective study in which neuroticism, depression, disability, coping, and headache frequency and/or duration are simultaneously measured would shed much greater light on the direction of causality between neuroticism and headache-related impairment and disability.

Conclusion

From the data generated in the clinical interview and psychological testing, a report is generated. Although the format of such reports will vary, most psychological reports will be rich in subjective detail. This detail springs naturally from the personal nature of the clinical interview and provides the background from which a flexible, individualized treatment plan is developed.

A typical report of the evaluation of a patient with headache will include demographic data, current headache activity, headache history, patient hypotheses regarding headache initiators and exacerbators, current treatment, history of treatment, concurrent medical disorders, family headache history, social history, mental status, psychiatric and psychological history, and lifestyle as it relates to physical, psychological, social, and spiritual health and happiness. In the mental status and history of mental health treatment, there is an effort to identify any concurrent psychiatric illness, whether primary or secondary to headache. The symptoms noted in the interview and testing are combined to document or rule out known psychiatric disorders according to the criteria listed in the *Diagnostic and Statistical Manual of Mental Disorders*.[41]

Often, psychiatric disorders are secondary to the headache pain. The reaction to pain is itself an important variable in management of the patient, and anxiety associated with the headache syndrome is a critical affective reaction that will affect the extent to which treatment must be more highly structured. Prolonged pain associated with very frequent headache that is not responding to treatment often leads to depression. Emotions associated with the conditions under which headache started are also important to detail; anger, post-traumatic anxiety, and depression are three of the more common emotions.

The psychological report ends with a plan for treatment. A complete description of behavioral treatment is beyond the scope of this chapter, but models are outlined for professional[42] and patient[43] reading. The management of most patients will start with a basic program of education (including readings), record-keeping (diary), and relaxation training (usually with biofeedback as a teaching tool). These three elements not only provide the patient with useful basic tools but also enhance more accurate and sensitive awareness of physical responses before and during the early phases of headache. (For a more complete description of the construct *accurate somatic awareness*, see Bakal et al.[44])

The behavioral plan must go beyond this basic foundation; specific plans must be constructed and implemented to help the patient use relaxation and other techniques to respond to precursors and early signs of headache. Daily habits relevant to physical health can be modified behaviorally in accordance with the medical plan. It is also possible to develop a more balanced, less stressful way of living, but such changes will not occur without a plan and guidance. One cannot simply change a basic personality style, but compensatory strategies can be developed to modify aspects of the personality not well suited for current social challenges or headache management itself. Finally, any psychological plan is laid out with the full expectation that it will be modified on the basis of ongoing new information. This information comes to the consultation room by way of collaborating professionals, family, the headache diary, and other patient reports.

Clinical experience indicates that when the professional skills of the psychologist are applied as part of a multidisciplinary team and in a manner highly specific to the needs of the headache patient, there is a very powerful contribution to positive outcome and satisfaction. As with any other collaborative effort, careful attention must be paid to areas of overlap in clinical effort among members of the treatment team. With ongoing discussion, issues that might otherwise become contentious are transformed into complementary and even synergistic interventions. The physician and psychologist, with other members of the treatment team, form a powerful and far-reaching clinical collaboration. This is the reality and promise of multidisciplinary treatment of headache.

References

1. Scopp AL. Headache triggers: Theory, research, and clinical applications: Part I. Headache Q 1992;3:32–38.
2. Jensen J, Rasmussen BK. Muscular disorders in tension-type headache. Cephalalgia 1996; 16:97–103.
3. Duckro PN. Biofeedback in the management of headache: Part II. Headache Q 1991;2:17–22.
4. Hathaway SR, McKinley JC. The Minnesota Multiphasic Personality Inventory. Minneapolis: The University of Minnesota; 1943.
5. Graham JR. MMPI-2: Assessing Personality and Psychopathology. New York: Oxford Press; 1990.
6. Kudrow L, Sutkus BJ. MMPI pattern specificity in primary headache disorders. Headache 1979;19:18–24.
7. Andrasik F, Blanchard EB, Arena JG, et al. Psychological functioning in headache sufferers. Psychosomat Med 1982;44:171–182.
8. Blanchard EB, Andrasik F, Arena JG. Personality and chronic headache. Prog Exp Personality Res 1984;13:303–364.
9. Ellertsen B, Klove H. MMPI patterns in chronic muscle pain, tension headache, and migraine. Cephalalgia 1987;7:65–71.
10. Dieter J, Swerdlow B. A replicative investigation of the reliability of the MMPI in the classification of chronic headaches. Headache 1988; 28:212–222.
11. Invernizzi G, Gala C, Buono M, et al. Neurotic traits and disease duration in headache patients. Cephalalgia 1989;9:173–178.
12. Pfaffenrath V, Hummelsberger J, Pollman W, et al. MMPI personality profiles in patients with primary headache syndromes. Cephalalgia 1991;11:263–268.
13. Jay GW, Grove RN, Grove KS. Differentiation of chronic from non-headache pain patients using the Millon Clinical Multiaxial Inventory (MCMI). Headache 1987;27:124–129.
14. Millon T, Green J, Meager R. The Millon Clinical Multiaxial Inventory. Minneapolis: NCS; 1983.
15. Beck AT, Ward CH, Mendelson M, et al. An inventory for measuring depression. Arch Gen Psychiatry 1961;4:561–571.
16. Spielberger CD, Johnson E, Russell S, et al. The experience and expression of anger: Construction and validation of an Anger Expression Scale. *In* Chesney MA, Roseman RH, eds. Anger and Hostility in Cardiovascular and Behavioral Disorders. New York: Hemisphere/McGraw-Hill; 1985:5–30.
17. Spielberger CD, Gorsuch RL, Lushene RE. STAI Manual for the State-Trait Anxiety Inventory. Palo Alto, CA: Consulting Psychologists Press; 1970.
18. Rathus SA. A 30-item schedule for assessing assertive behavior. Beh Ther 1973;4:398–406.
19. Derogatis LR. SCL-90-R Administration, Scoring, and Procedure Manual-I for the R(evised) Version. Baltimore: L.R. Derogatis; 1977.
20. Rappaport NB, McAnulty DP, Waggoner CD, Brantley PJ. Cluster analysis of Minnesota Multiphasic Personality Inventory (MMPI) profiles in a chronic headache population. J Beh Med 1987;10:49–60.
21. Robinson ME, Geisser ME, Dieter JN, Swerdlow B. The relationship between MMPI cluster membership and diagnostic category in headache patients. Headache 1991;31:111–115.
22. Kinder BN, Curtiss G, Kalichman S. Cluster analyses of headache-patient MMPI scores: A cross-validation. Psychol Assess J Consult Clin Psychology 1991;3:226–231.
23. Kinder BN, Curtiss G, Kalichman S. Affective differences among empirically derived subgroups of headache patients. J Personality 1992;58:516–524.
24. Silberstein SD, Lipton RB, Breslau N. Migraine: Association with personality characteristics and psychopathology. Cephalalgia 1995;15: 358–369.
25. Chibnall JT, Duckro PN. Post-traumatic stress disorder in chronic post-traumatic headache patients. Headache 1994;34:357–361.
26. Tschannen T, Duckro P, Margolis R, Tomazic T. The relationship of anger, depression, and perceived disability among headache patients. Headache 1992;32:501–503.
27. Duckro PN, Chibnall JT, Tomazic TJ. Anger, depression, and disability: A path analysis of relationships in a sample of chronic post-traumatic headache patients. Headache 1995; 35:7–9.
28. Scharff L, Turk DC, Marcus DA. Psychosocial and behavioral characteristics in chronic headache patients: Support for a continuum and dual-diagnostic approach. Cephalalgia 1995;15:216–223.
29. Ziegler DK, Paolo AM. Headache symptoms and psychological profile of headache-prone individuals: A comparison of clinic patients and controls. Arch Neurol 1995;52:602–606.
30. Ben-Porath Y, Waller NG. 'Normal' personality inventories in clinical assessment: General requirements and the potential for using the NEO Personality Inventory. Psychol Assess 1992;4:14–19.
31. Costa PT, McCrae RR. Revised NEO Personality Inventory (NEO-PI-R) and NEO Five-Factor Inventory (NEO-FFI) Professional Manual.

Odessa, FL: Psychological Assessment Resources; 1992.
32. Goldberg LR. The structure of phenotypic personality traits. Am Psychol 1993;48:26–34.
33. Costa PT, McCrae RR. Normal personality assessment in clinical practice: The NEO Personality Inventory. Psychol Assess 1992;4:5–13.
34. Johnson JH, Butcher JN, Null C, Johnson KN. Replicated item level factor analysis of the full MMPI. J Personality Social Psychol 1984; 47:105–114.
35. Costa PT, Busch CM, Zonderman AB, McCrae RR. Correlations of MMPI factor scales with measures of the five factor model of personality. J Personality Assess 1986;50:640–650.
36. Tschannen T. Chronic Headache and Personality. Thesis. St. Louis: St. Louis University; 1995.
37. Breslau N, Chilcoat HD, Andreski P. Further evidence on the link between migraine and neuroticism. Headache 1996;36:263. Abstract.
38. Breslau N, Andreski P. Migraine, personality, and psychiatric comorbidity. Headache 1995; 35:382–386.
39. Breslau N, Davis GC, Shultz LR, Peterson EL. Migraine and major depression: A longitudinal study. Headache 1994;34:387–393.
40. Philips HC, Jahanshahi M. The effects of persistent pain: The chronic headache sufferer. Pain 1985;21:163–176.
41. Diagnostic and Statistical Manual of Mental Disorders, 4th ed. Washington, DC: American Psychiatric Association; 1994.
42. Duckro PN. Biofeedback in the management of headache: Part I. Headache Q 1990;1:290–298.
43. Duckro PN, Richardson WD, Marshall JE, et al. Taking Control of Your Headaches. New York: The Guilford Press; 1995.
44. Bakal D, Demjen S, Duckro P. Chronic daily headache and the elusive nature of somatic awareness. *In* Grzesiak RC, Ciccone DS, eds. Psychological Vulnerability to Chronic Pain. New York: Springer; 1994:116–136.

20

Biofeedback, Relaxation Training, and Other Psychological Treatments for Chronic Benign Headache

Edward B. Blanchard, Ph.D.

John G. Arena, Ph.D.

Introduction

The psychological procedures biofeedback, relaxation training, mental imagery techniques, and cognitive stress coping therapy were first described as treatments for chronic benign headache disorders in the late 1960s to early 1970s. These procedures should be part of the total treatment armamentarium in a clinic or center specializing in headache.

Despite their availability in headache specialty centers, psychologists, clinicians, and researchers would not expect the the practicing physician to apply these treatments. In a moderate-to-large primary care group, there probably is good justification for having these treatments available from a staff psychologist or nurse who is trained as a biofeedback therapist. Otherwise, the physician should make an informed referral for these treatments.*

From this perspective, we believe the practicing physician should be aware of the history and research evidence supporting the use of these procedures with patients with headache and have a general understanding of what is involved in the procedures. We conclude with recommendations concerning the patients for which these procedures are most appropriate.

*If the physician does not know a practitioner in the area or community who provides these kinds of treatment, two national organizations can provide names of appropriate referrals in the area: Association for Applied Psychophysiology and Biofeedback, Wheat Ridge, CO (800) 477–8892, or Association for Advancement of Behavior Therapy, New York, NY (212) 647–1890.

What Are Biofeedback, Relaxation Therapy, and Cognitive-Behavioral Therapy?

Biofeedback, as it is generally used, is a procedure in which the therapist monitors the patient's bodily responses (e.g., muscle tension, surface skin temperature, or heart rate) through the use of a machine and then feeds this information back to the patient. Feedback is usually presented to the patient through an auditory modality (e.g., a tone that is higher or lower as muscle tension increases or decreases) and/or a visual modality (e.g., a computer screen on which surface skin temperature is presented in a graph format on a second-by-second basis during each minute). Through this physiological feedback, it is expected a patient will learn how to control his or her bodily responses. A more formal definition of biofeedback is "a process in which a person learns to reliably influence psychophysiological responses of two kinds: either responses which are not ordinarily under voluntary control or ordinarily are easily regulated but for which regulation has broken down due to trauma or disease."[1, p. 2]

Relaxation therapy is a systematic approach to teaching people to gain awareness of their physiological responses and achieve both a cognitive and physiological sense of tranquillity without the use of the machinery used in biofeedback. There are various forms of relaxation therapy.[2, 3] The major forms, however, are progressive muscle relaxation therapy,[4] meditation,[2] autogenic training,[5] and guided imagery.[6] By far, the most widely used relaxation procedures in headache therapy are variants of jacobsonian progressive muscle relaxation therapy and guided imagery; we emphasize those procedures in this chapter.

Because relaxation therapy and biofeedback are believed to directly influence both an individual's physiology and psyche, they are commonly referred to as *psychophysiological interventions,* and we refer to them as such throughout this chapter.

Cognitive-behavioral therapies for headache are based on the assumption that an individual's thoughts, emotions, and behaviors influence his or her physiology. Therefore, cognitive-behavioral treatments generally involve the identification of thoughts, emotions, and behaviors that routinely precede or exacerbate headache activity, with the therapist subsequently teaching patients in a systematic manner to modify these thoughts, feelings, and behaviors. Because cognitive-behavioral therapies are usually combined with relaxation or biofeedback procedures, we emphasize these procedures much less than the two psychophysiological techniques.

Historical Overview

Reports on the scientific (rather than anecdotal) evaluation of the systematic application of psychological procedures to chronic headache first appeared in the late 1960s and early 1970s. Since then, more than 100 reports of uncontrolled and controlled evaluations, along with prospective follow-ups of 5 or more years, have appeared. A comprehensive scientific review of this literature was presented by Blanchard and Andrasik in 1982,[7] with an update by Blanchard in 1992.[8]

Biofeedback. The initial report on the use of frontal electromyographic (EMG) biofeedback (described later) with tension-type headache appeared in 1970.[9] It was followed with the report on a small-scale, controlled clinical trial in 1973.[10]

The initial report on the use of thermal biofeedback (described later) with migraine headache appeared in 1972.[11] Controlled clinical trials confirming its efficacy were reported by Blanchard et al[12] in 1978 and Sargent et al in 1986.[13]

Diamond and colleagues[14] reported the results of a large, uncontrolled trial with a large series (556 patients) of patients with headache; in this trial, biofeedback was used in a tertiary headache center in 1979 and later in a larger series.[15] Sovak et al[16] showed thermal biofeedback to be equivalent to propranolol in a controlled trial.

Relaxation Training. Although progressive muscle relaxation (PMR) training, as developed by Edmund Jacobson,[4] had been used with some patients with headache, the first systematic report of its use with tension-type headache was by Tasto and Hinkle in 1973.[17] One of the first controlled clinical trials of the use of relaxation with tension-type headache was reported by Chesney and Shelton in 1976.[18] Blanchard et al[12] evaluated abbreviated PMR in a controlled trial involving migraineurs and found it to be effective and equivalent to thermal biofeedback.

An alternative form of relaxation, known as *autogenic training,* was described by Schultz and Luthe.[19] It involves a more passive, self-instructive form of relaxation that emphasizes autonomic function. It is frequently used as an adjunct to thermal biofeedback for migraine. In a controlled evaluation of it as a primary therapy for migraine, it was found to apparently not be as effective as thermal biofeedback.[13]

Cognitive Stress Coping Therapy. Kenneth Holroyd popularized the adaptation of elements of cognitive therapy to the treatment of chronic headache. Beginning in 1977, Holroyd and colleagues[20, 21] showed in controlled trials that cognitive therapy was effective with tension-type headache. Blanchard et al[22] showed that it added appreciably to relaxation training with this group of headache patients. Its role in the treatment of migraine headache is less well supported.

Detailed Descriptions of Psychological Treatments

EMG Biofeedback

Arena and Blanchard[23] provide a more detailed, "how-to" description of both the EMG

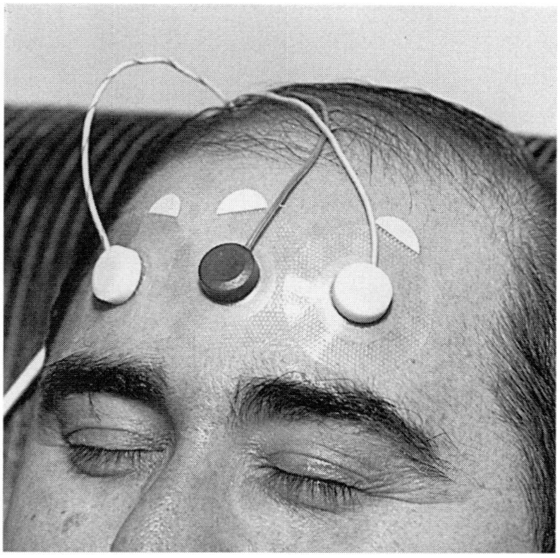

Figure 20–1 Placement of forehead sensors for biofeedback training.

and thermal biofeedback procedures. When Arena and Blanchard refer to EMG, surface EMG is meant, which involves the use of noninvasive (surface) electrodes, is painless, and involves the pattern of many motor action potentials. EMG as a diagnostic procedure in neurology involves the use of invasive needle electrodes, considers a single motor action potential, and often is quite painful.

EMG (or muscle-tension) biofeedback is essentially used with patients with tension-type headache. It is based on the assumption that tension headache is caused or exacerbated by elevated levels of muscle tension in the forehead, neck, and shoulder regions, situationally stressful events, or both. There is much controversy in the literature concerning the role of muscle tension in the etiology or maintenance of tension headache.[24] There is less controversy about the role of situational stress in exacerbating tension headache, although there is a surprising paucity of empirical research in this area. In a study by Arena and colleagues,[25] 74 subjects with tension headache self-monitored and recorded for 28 to 35 days their daily headache activity and stress levels four times a day; results indicated that 76% of subjects with tension headache have some significant stress-pain relationship. Regardless of which of the two assumptions is correct, teaching individuals to reduce muscle tension in areas implicated in headache through the use of EMG biofeedback leads to a decrease in subjective stress levels as well as a decrease in tension headache activity (see efficacy rates).

The actual hook-up process of EMG biofeedback is quite simple: for forehead feedback, the trainer swabs the forehead with an alcohol prep, instructs the patient to look straight ahead, and place the two active sensors on the forehead over each eye, approximately in line with the pupil of the respective eye (Fig. 20–1). The nonactive (ground) sensor is placed between the two active sensors. For upper trapezius (neck and shoulder) placement, patients simply shrug their shoulders, and the active leads are placed over the belly of the trapezius muscle between the spine and the shoulder joint, approximately 1.5 inches apart; again, the ground sensor is placed between the two active sensors (Fig. 20–2). There are some data to suggest that feedback from the trapezius muscle may be more efficacious than feedback from the forehead.[26]

As with any treatment, the rationale that the trainer gives the patient is very important. Typically, the therapist describes to the patient both the elevated levels of muscle-tension theory and the stress theory. Patients easily understand that stress plays a role in their headache by leading to higher levels of muscle tension; they also readily grasp that their headaches and stress are interconnected. The trainer usually emphasizes that biofeedback is a self-regulation technique that will allow the patient to prevent the occurrence of a headache. Patients are informed that they

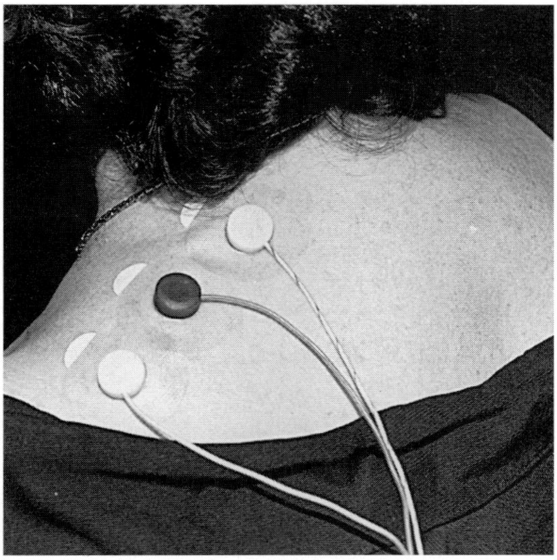

Figure 20–2 Placement of shoulder sensors for biofeedback training for headaches.

need to incorporate these skills into their daily activities as a lifestyle change. Explanations of the physiological bases of muscle tension and the role of self-regulation allow the patient to gain an understanding of control of bodily responses and increase self-efficacy.

Patients are then given a number of possible strategies to help them in their goal of obtaining the biofeedback response:

Relaxing Imagery. In this technique, the patient imagines a pleasant scene, such as walking through the woods on an autumn evening listening to the leaves crunch with each step they take or on a beach listening to the waves as they roll in and roll back out again.

Relaxing (Autogenic) Phrases. Statements such as, "I feel very relaxed," "My arms and hands feel heavy and warm," and, "I feel an inward quietness" are repeated over and over mentally. Table 20–1 presents selected examples of such relaxing (autogenic) phrases.

Deep Breathing Procedures. During these procedures, the patient, with eyes closed, concentrates on diaphragmatic breathing (breathing by expanding the lungs fully while keeping the muscles of the shoulders and chest relaxed, allowing the abdomen to expand) and repeats a relaxing word such as "relax," "calm," or peaceful" when exhaling. (See detailed description of a diaphragmatic breathing procedure.)

Table 20–1 Relaxing (Autogenic) Phrases

I feel quite quiet . . .
I am beginning to feel quite relaxed . . .
My ankles, my knees, and my hips feel heavy, relaxed, and comfortable . . .
My chest, my stomach, and my whole body feel relaxed and quiet . . .
My breathing is deep, slow and relaxed . . .
My hands, my arms, and my shoulders feel heavy, relaxed, and comfortable . . .
I can feel my neck and shoulders unwind, loosen up, smooth out, and relax more and more . . .
My neck, my jaws, and my forehead feel relaxed . . .
They feel comfortable and smooth . . .
My eyes feel heavy and relaxed . . .
My whole body feels quite quiet, heavy, comfortable, and relaxed . . .
I feel quite quiet . . .
My arms and hands are heavy and warm . . .
I feel quite relaxed . . .
My whole body is relaxed and my hands are warm, relaxed, and warm . . .
My hands are warm . . .
Warmth is following into my hands, they are warm, warm . . .
My mind is quiet . . .
My mind is calm, relaxed, and quiet . . .
I feel an inward quietness . . .
My mind is quiet, and my whole body is relaxed and comfortable.

Awareness of Sensations. Some individuals are able to lower their muscle tension levels by simply concentrating on and *becoming aware of the sensations of tightness and tension* in their forehead, neck, and shoulders and, by focusing on what it is like when those muscles relax, loosen up, and unwind.

Nothingness. Some patients report that if they can make their mind blank and think of nothing—actually stop thinking, then they can relax and lower their muscle tension.

Mental Games. Some patients find that focusing on a color ("warm" colors, such as yellow, green, or brown seem to work best) helps to relax them and decrease their muscle tension levels. Others actually play a game in their mind, such as tic-tac-toe, bowling, chess, cards, or basketball.

Concentrating on the Auditory Feedback. Some individuals just ignore all of the above strategies and simply concentrate on the feedback tone. They even report imagining the tone going down when they practice in their everyday environment without a portable biofeedback device attached to them.

At the first session, patients are instructed to pick only one strategy and stick with it throughout the entire session. Most therapists limit the initial session to about 10 to 15 minutes of biofeedback and increase the length of the biofeedback to a maximum of 25 minutes in later sessions. It is essential for the trainer to emphasize that this is a difficult response to learn, it will take some time before the patient can lower their muscle tension reliably, and patients should not get discouraged if they cannot immediately control their EMG levels.

At the end of each session, patients are usually asked which strategy they found to be the most effective and to rate on a 1-to-10 scale how relaxed they are and what they would rate their level of overall body tension now compared with at the beginning of the session. Recent stressful events and headache pain levels are often explored at both the beginning and end of each session, and the ability to decrease their muscle tension levels during a session is often related to both stress and pain levels.

Home practice has traditionally been considered an essential element of all psychophysiological interventions for chronic headache.[27] Most therapists begin biofeedback home practice once the patient has demonstrated he or she can reliably produce the desired biofeedback response in the office setting. Home practice can be conducted by instructing the patient to practice the office strategy that seemed to work the best at home and in other real world locations such as on the job, at a gas station, and so forth. Sometimes, patients are told to use a small pocket mirror during home practice as a biofeedback aid ("Try to smooth out your forehead as much as you can"). Small portable biofeedback devices are available for $300 to $700, and many therapists routinely lend these to their patients during the course of treatment.

Generalization of the biofeedback response to the *real world* involves preparing the patient to or determining whether the patient can carry the learning that may have occurred during the biofeedback session into the real world. There are many ways to test or prepare for generalization. Homework may be construed as a generalization procedure. Other common methods are a *self-control* condition (e.g., "Please try to lower your forehead muscle tension without any feedback") that is interspersed between a baseline and a feedback condition. If the patient can control the response, the clinician may infer that between-session learning (i.e., generalization) has occurred. Another way of preparing the patient to generalize the biofeedback response is to attempt to make the office biofeedback training simulate real world situations. For example, initially training patients on a recliner and progressing to a comfortable office chair (with arms), an uncomfortable office chair (without arms), and, last, the standing position.

It usually takes 8 to 16 sessions of EMG biofeedback (average of 12) for maximal results to be obtained. Patients are usually seen once or twice a week for 45 to 60 minutes each time.

Thermal Biofeedback

Temperature or thermal biofeedback is used primarily with migraine and mixed migraine-tension headache sufferers. Its use in vascular headache is based on two theories, both of which emphasize that biofeedback is a prophylactic rather than abortive procedure. The two-stage theory of migraine postulates that there are two stages that occur in migraine headache: (1) vasoconstriction of the temporal arteries and arterioles, which causes the prodrome, and (2) the massive vasodilation of the temporal arteries and arterioles, which causes the pain. When a patient who has been successful in thermal biofeedback training warms his or her hands after noticing they are beginning to turn cold, the patient is not only increasing peripheral blood flow to the extremities but also increasing blood flow to the temporal arteries and arterioles, thus preventing the first stage of the migraine. The second theory underlying the use of thermal biofeedback for migraine headache postulates that situational stress either causes or exacerbates the headache and that when patients warm their hands, they are also decreasing sympathetic nervous system arousal (and perhaps increasing parasympathetic arousal) and therefore reducing general stress levels. There is considerable controversy regarding a number of assumptions with the first theory of why thermal biofeedback is efficacious for migraine headache and some controversy regarding the second, although surprisingly there have been a number of studies in which a daily headache diary was used that demonstrated the role of stress in migraine headache,[28, 29] whereas empirical studies are for tension headache.

Regardless of which of the two theories regarding the effective mechanism of change in thermal biofeedback training is correct, as with EMG biofeedback training for tension headache, teaching individuals through the use of thermal biofeedback to increase their hand temperature leads to a decrease in migraine headache activity (see below for efficacy rates).

There is a great deal of overlap between EMG and thermal biofeedback procedures; we present only the differences between the two techniques.

The initial session typically begins with the therapist telling the patient that he or she is going to learn to warm the hands with the assistance of the biofeedback training and is followed by acknowledgment that the connection between hand warming and migraine relief is not obvious. The trainer points out that to warm one's hands, the tiny blood vessels in the periphery must dilate; that this vasodilation is under the control of the autonomic nervous system; and that the sympathetic nervous system is the part of the autonomic nervous system, which controls the "fight or flight" response and peripheral vasoconstriction and vasodilation. It is explained that when there is sympathetic nervous system activity, or *sympathetic outflow*, the blood vessels constrict. Patients are told the biofeedback therapist is attempting to reduce sympathetic nervous system activity (outflow), which is monitored through measurement of hand temperature, and to increase parasympathetic arousal.

The therapist also stresses that this treatment is designed to bring about a tonic charge, or generalized reduction in sympathetic activity; thus, regular daily practice is important. Patients are told that the treatment is not especially designed to be a phasic or short-term, coping strategy. The overall goal is to reduce the frequency and intensity of headache—a prophylactic or preventative self-regulatory strategy, not to abort headaches or reduce their discomfort once they have begun.

The thermometer or "thermistor" placement is somewhat arbitrary (Fig. 20–3); we have routinely used the ventral pad of the last digit on the index finger of the nondominant hand. We know of no empirical research that demonstrates an advantage of one placement over another. The thermistor should be held in close contact with the skin with a Velcro band or paper tape. Care should be taken when using tape not to fully encircle the finger and create a tourniquet. The room should be kept reasonably warm, at least 72°F and preferably 75° to 78°F. It is very hard for a patient to warm her or his hands in a cool or cold room; in a cold room, the patient is fighting a very strong reflex (heat conservation by peripheral vasoconstriction).

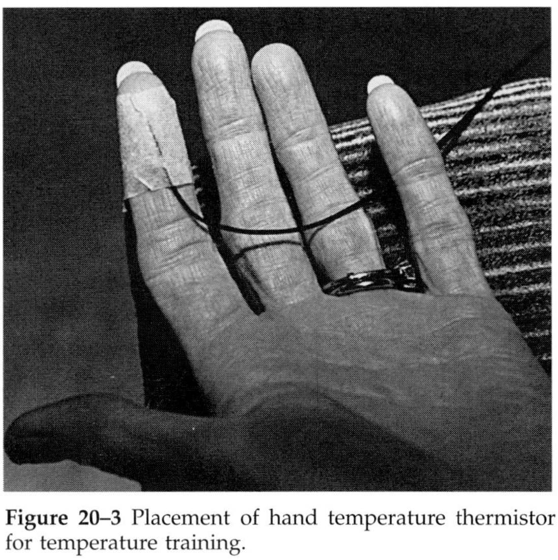

Figure 20–3 Placement of hand temperature thermistor for temperature training.

With temperature biofeedback, patients usually prefer a visual display (a computer monitor that graphs their hand temperature every second over a 60 second interval, or a series of lights that range from bright green to yellow to bright red, with green indicating cooling the hands and red indicating warming the hands) (Fig. 20–4). Unlike with EMG biofeedback, patients in thermal biofeedback training tend to have more success with imagery strategies that focus on warmth (e.g., a beach scene, being in a sauna), autogenic relaxation phrases,[24, 28] and feelings of warmth or blood pulsations in the fingertips.

There is some evidence that patients with vascular headache who achieve a criterion of 95° or 96°F or higher at any point during training have a significantly higher likelihood of experiencing a clinically meaningful reduction in headache activity (at least 50%) than those who reach lower maximum levels.[30–32]

It usually takes 12 to 16 sessions of thermal biofeedback (average of 12) for maximal results to be obtained. Patients are usually seen once or twice a week for 45 to 60 minutes each time. Although there are no empirical data to support their clinical impression, we feel strongly that twice-a-week sessions are best, especially during the first 2 weeks, to maximize learning.

Relaxation Procedures

This section describes a nine-session relaxation therapy regimen that has been successfully used with patients with tension headache.[7, 33, 34] Although this relaxation regimen is based on an abbreviated form of jacobsonian progressive muscle relaxation therapy (i.e., tension-release exercises), it also routinely incorporates other forms of relaxation into the training, such as relaxing imagery, relaxation by recall, and cue-controlled relaxation techniques. Moreover, because two forms of relaxation—relaxing (guided) imagery and diaphragmatic breathing—are so important, more-detailed descriptions of these techniques are given.

As with biofeedback, it is important to emphasize to patients the rationale for the

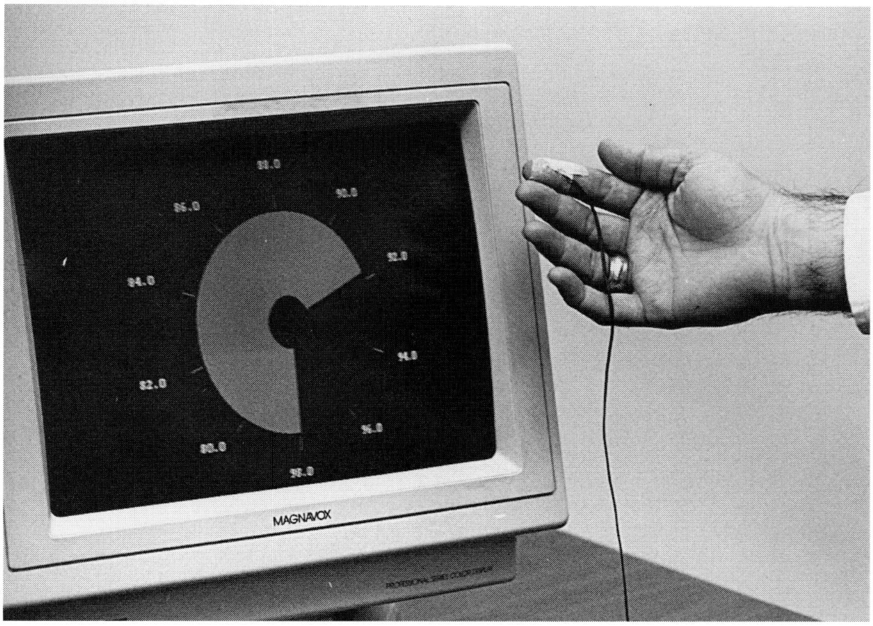

Figure 20–4 Hand temperature thermistor with computer feedback screen.

use of relaxation therapy with chronic headache. The trainer points out that relaxation therapy involves learning how to achieve a mental and physical state of tranquillity in a very brief period of time, as well as how to apply these relaxation skills to daily living. It is highlighted that *relaxation* means a systematic set of procedures and that the technique is a learned response. The relationship between muscle tension and headache is described, as is the relationship between stress and headache. For migraineurs, the relationship between decreased sympathetic nervous system arousal and relaxation therapy is especially emphasized.

The first session of relaxation therapy generally involves the tensing and then relaxing of 14 to 16 muscle groups throughout the body, with special attention paid to the muscles of the neck, shoulders, and face. Patients are informed that in essence, when they tense their muscles and relax them, they are forcing those muscles to relax, and this is important because most headache sufferers have been tense for so long that they have forgotten what it feels like to be relaxed. Patients are instructed to pay special attention to the contrast between a tense and a relaxed state. Between each muscle group, the therapist typically includes 20 seconds or so of *relaxation patter*—statements such as, "Just let yourself become more and more relaxed," "The relaxation is flowing into all the areas of your body," and "Notice the pleasant feelings of warmth and heaviness that are coming into your body as your muscles relax completely." After the tensing of the last muscle group, the trainer usually includes a *deepening procedure,* in which he or she counts from 1 to 5, informing the patient that they will become more relaxed as the counting continues. Then, the therapist introduces an *attention to breathing procedure,* in which the patient is made aware of his or her breathing; told to take deep, slow, relaxing breaths; and instructed to mentally pair the word *relax* with each exhalation. Finally, an *alerting procedure* is performed, in which the trainer counts back from 5 to 1, telling the patient that as he or she does so the patient will become more alert. A relaxation tape, tailored to the patient's individual needs by the therapist, is usually recorded during each session to assist in home practice. A sample of a relaxation therapy session is given in Table 20–2.

The second session of relaxation is similar to the first, with the addition of a guided relaxation imagery scene at the end, just before the alerting procedure (see the section on guided imagery).

The third session of relaxation is essentially same as the second, with the addition of a muscle discrimination procedure performed on the neck and eyes. In muscle discrimination training, patients are taught to distinguish between the different levels of muscle

Table 20–2 Sample Relaxation Therapy Session

1. Now I want you to tense the muscles of your *lower arms and hands* by holding both arms out over your lap and making a fist with each hand. Study the tensions located in your lower arms and hands. Study those tensions. (Wait 5 to 10 seconds.) Now relax the muscles of your lower arms and hands and study the difference between the tension and the relaxation.
   Just let yourself become more and more relaxed.
2. Now I want you to tense the muscles of your *upper arms* by bringing both arms to your shoulders and applying pressure at each elbow as if you were making muscles. Study the tensions located in your upper arms. Study those tensions. (Wait 5 to 10 seconds.) Now relax the muscles of your upper arms and study the difference between the tension and the relaxation.
   Just let the relaxation flow into all the areas of your body.
3. Now I want you to tense the muscles of your *calves* by pointing your toes toward your knees. Study the tensions located in your calves. Study those tensions. (Wait 5 to 10 seconds.) Now relax the muscles of your calves and study the difference between the tension and the relaxation.
   Notice the pleasant feelings of warmth and heaviness that are coming into your body as your muscles relax completely. You will always be clearly aware of what you are doing and what I am saying as you become more deeply relaxed.
4. Now I want you to tense the muscles of your *lower legs* by pointing your toes away from your knees. Study the tensions located in your lower legs. Study those tensions. (Wait 5 to 10 seconds.) Now relax the muscles of your lower legs and study the difference between the tension and the relaxation.
   (Pause 20 seconds.)
5. Now I want you to tense the muscles of your *thighs* by pressing your thighs together tightly. Study the tensions located in your thighs. Study those tensions. (Wait 5 to 10 seconds.) Now relax the muscles of your thighs and study the difference between the tension and the relaxation.
   Just let yourself become more and more relaxed, deeper and deeper. Just give yourself up completely to the very pleasant, relaxed, quiet, comfortable feelings.
6. Now I want you to tense the muscles of your *stomach* by drawing your stomach in tightly, while breathing normally. Study the tensions located in your stomach. Study those tensions. (Wait 5 to 10 seconds.) Now relax the muscles of your stomach and study the difference between the tension and the relaxation.
   (Pause 20 seconds.)
7. Now I want you to tense the muscles of your *chest* by taking a deep breath and holding it in. Study the tensions located in your chest. Study those tensions. (Wait 5 to 10 seconds.) Now relax the muscles of your chest and study the difference between the tension and the relaxation.
   Just let yourself become more and more relaxed. If you feel like you're floating, that will be fine, too. As you become more relaxed, you may feel yourself settling deep into the chair. All your muscles are becoming more and more deeply relaxed. Loose . . . heavy . . . and relaxed.
8. Now I want you to tense the muscles of your *shoulders* by drawing your shoulders up towards your ears. Study the tensions located in your shoulders. Study those tensions. (Wait 5 to 10 seconds.) Now relax the muscles of your shoulders and study the difference between the tension and the relaxation.
   Just let yourself become more and more relaxed, letting the relaxation flow into all the areas of our body, deeper and deeper.
9. Now I want you to tense the muscles of your *neck* by pressing your head tightly backwards against the chair (pillow). Study the tensions located in your neck. Study those tensions. (Wait 5 to 10 seconds.) Now relax the muscles of your neck and study the difference between the tension and the relaxation.
   The relaxation is growing deeper and still deeper. You are relaxed—calm, tranquil, and relaxed. With each breath you take in, your relaxation increases, and each time your breathe out, you spread the relaxation throughout your entire body.
10. Now I want you to tense the muscles of your *lips* by pressing your lips together tightly without biting down on your teeth or clamping down with your jaw. Study the tensions located in your lips. Study those tensions. (Wait 5 to 10 seconds.) Now relax the muscles of your lips and study the difference between the tension and the relaxation.
    (Pause 20 seconds.)
11. Now I want you to tense the muscles of your *eyes* by closing your eyes somewhat tightly. Study the tensions located in your eyes. Study those tensions. (Wait 5 to 10 seconds.) Now relax the muscles of your eyes and study the difference between the tension and the relaxation.
    Now the very deep state of relaxation is moving into all the areas of your body. You are becoming more and more deeply relaxed . . . completely relaxed. You can feel the comfortable sensations of relaxation as you go into a deeper and still deeper state of relaxation.
12. Now I want you to tense the muscles of your *jaw* by opening your mouth as wide as possible. Study the tensions located in your jaw. Study those tensions. (Wait 5 to 10 seconds.) Now relax the muscles of your jaw and study the difference between the tension and the relaxation.
    Just let yourself become more and more relaxed.
13. Now I want you to tense the muscles of your *lower forehead* by frowning and trying to lower your eyebrows. Study the tensions located in your lower forehead. Study those tensions. (Wait 5 to 10 seconds.) Now relax the muscles of your lower forehead and study the difference between the tension and the relaxation.
    (Pause 20 seconds.)

Table 20–2 Sample Relaxation Therapy Session *(Continued)*

14. Now I want you to tense the muscles of your *upper forehead* by wrinkling your forehead and trying to raise your eyebrows. Study the tensions located in your upper forehead. Study those tensions. (Wait 5 to 10 seconds.) Now relax the muscles of your upper forehead and study the difference between the tension and the relaxation.

Now I want you to relax all the muscles of your body. Just let them become more and more relaxed. I'm going to help you to achieve a deeper state of relaxation by counting from one to five. As I count, you will feel yourself becoming more and more deeply relaxed, going further and further down into a deep, restful state of deep relaxation.

One—you are going to become more deeply relaxed.
Two—down, down into very relaxed state.
Three—deeper and deeper.
Four—more and more relaxed.
Five—completely relaxed, a deep restful state of deep relaxation.
(Pause 45 to 60 seconds.)

Now I want you to remain in your very relaxed state. I want you to begin to concentrate only on your breathing. Breathe through your nose. Notice the cool air as you breath in (pair with inhalation) . . . and the warm, moist air as you breathe out (pair with exhalation). (Pause 20 seconds.) Just concentrate on your breathing, taking deep, slow, relaxing breaths. (Pause 30 seconds.) Now, each time you breathe out mentally repeat the word "relax." Breathe in (pair with inhalation) . . . Breathe out (pair with exhalation). Relax. (Pause 30 to 60 seconds.) Just continue to concentrate on your breathing, taking deep, slow, relaxing breaths, and mentally repeating the word relax each time you breathe out.

(Pause 45 to 60 seconds.)

Now I am going to help you to return to your normal state of alertness. In a little while, I am going to begin counting backwards from five to one. You will gradually become more alert. When I reach two, I want you to open your eyes. When I get to one you will be entirely roused up in your normal state of alertness, feeling quite refreshed. OK now. Five. Four. You are becoming more and more alert, you feel very refreshed. Three. Two. Now your eyes are open and you begin to feel very alert, returning completely to your normal state. One. (Wait 10 seconds.) When you feel like it, you may sit up and stretch.

Please Note: Sometimes patients state that they are unable to feel any tension when they tense a particular muscle group. If this occurs, we give them an alternative way of tensing the muscle in question. Please see Arena and Blanchard (1996) for alternative muscle tensing strategies for each of the 14 muscle groups detailed above. The two muscle groups which individuals have the most trouble tensing are the shoulders and neck. Alternative tensing strategies for the shoulders are: (a) Please press your shoulders firmly back into the hair (couch). (b) Holding both arms out in front of you, please roll your shoulders. (c) Holding your arms at your side, please pull your shoulders down. An alternative tensing strategy for the neck is: Please try to touch your chest with your chin, going as close as you possibly can, but never actually doing so.

tension in their bodies. First, they tense their muscles to full strength; then, 50%; and finally, 25% tension. This procedure is useful for two types of headache patients: those who cannot discriminate between the various levels of muscle tension and characterize any muscle tension as intense tension and those who refuse to characterize any state of muscle tension as tension unless it is tension near a cramping level. Both types of patients must be able to accurately label their physiological levels. For those who have trouble discriminating between the different levels of muscle tension, they are instructed to practice these exercises at home until they can reliably differentiate between the various levels of muscle tension.

The fourth session of relaxation therapy has only one goal—to reduce the number of muscle groups to eight or even six. The patient is informed that to make the relaxation a portable coping skill, one thing that must happen is for the relaxation to be shorter. This is usually accomplished by combining single muscle groups into one (e.g., combining arm and leg muscle groups).

The fifth session of relaxation simply continues the goal of session 4 and reduces the number of muscle groups to four.

Most therapists probably would characterize the sixth session of relaxation therapy as the most important of all the sessions; patients are introduced to the concept of portability through a technique known as *relaxation by recall*, and the trainer begin to stress the importance of daily practice in the everyday world.

Relaxation by recall is based on the tension-release exercises, with the difference being that patients are taught to become relaxed without actually tensing their muscles. After going through the previous five sessions, patients with headache have learned what it feels like for their muscles to be tense and what it feels like for their muscles to be relaxed. During the sixth session, they are instructed to focus their attention on the six to eight muscle groups in their body used in session 4 and to determine whether their muscles are relaxed or there is some residual tightness or tension present. If they notice that a particular muscle group is tense, they just "let go" of the muscle tension that is present and recall what it feels like for that muscle group to relax. In other words, to relax their muscles by recall, a patient simply remembers what the muscles felt like when they were relaxed and "lets go" of remaining tension in the muscle.

Most patients are able to learn fairly quickly how to relax their muscles by recall. They easily grasp that it is a very important skill; most patients do not want to go around all day actually tensing their muscles to relax them. Patients are told that relaxation by recall is the main step toward making the relaxation therapy a coping skill because it is now "portable" and they can easily use it in daily living. A relaxation tape is usually made of the session, and patients are informed that as with the tension release exercises, they should try to practice the relaxation by recall exercises at least twice a day.

The second major component of the sixth session is to stress the importance of practice in the everyday world. Patients are told that by practicing in the "real world," they will gain awareness of increased muscle tension and will be able to relax muscles before they develop increased muscle tension or cramping, which can lead to headaches. It is pointed out that this is the ultimate goal of the relaxation therapy.

Patients are urged to think about their muscle state throughout the day. To help them to do so, they are told to (1) set and reset a wristwatch alarm every 45 minutes or so and check their muscle tension when it goes off; (2) buy "smiling face" or other stick-ons, place the stick-ons in strategic places, and check their tension whenever they see one; and/or (3) check their muscle tension every time they open and close a door, see themselves in a mirror, or answer a telephone.

The seventh session of relaxation therapy involves using relaxation by recall on the four muscle groups used in the fifth session with the introduction of a strategy called *cue-controlled relaxation.* This procedure involves (1) taking a deep breath, (2) holding it for 1 or 2 seconds, (3) consciously breathing out, (4) mentally repeating the word *relax* on exhales, and (5) doing a quick body scan and using the relaxation by recall procedures to find and eliminate any remaining muscle tension in the body.

Patients are also given additional strategies to become more relaxed in their daily living, such as tensing briefly some of the muscle groups that they may be having difficulty in relaxing by using the recall procedure, using the "deepening exercise" that is part of the relaxation procedure by itself, or saying repeatedly to themselves the relaxing (autogenic) phrases that are outlined (see Table 20–1). Two major additional strategies—diaphragmatic breathing and relaxing imagery—are described in detail later.

The eighth session of relaxation is essentially the same as the seventh, except that even greater emphasis is placed on performing the relaxation techniques in the everyday world. It is strongly advocated that patients stop using the relaxation tapes except on an infrequent basis (i.e., once or twice a week) and begin to practice the relaxation strategies in situations that one would not normally think of as being conducive to relaxation, such as while standing up, sitting in a hardback chair, or driving a car; during meetings; and so forth.

The ninth and last session of relaxation is usually spent reviewing what the patient has learned in the previous eight sessions and emphasizing to the patient that he or she needs to be constantly practicing the relaxation procedures. The final session is typically very brief. Sometimes, if deemed by the therapist to be useful, it includes a 5-minute cue-controlled relaxation procedure or a 15-minute relaxation session consisting of autogenic relaxation phrases (see Table 20–1). Patients are instructed to contact the trainer immediately if their headaches increase or return, and a 6- or 12-month "booster session" is scheduled.

Although two other relaxation techniques usually are not used by themselves, they are so intertwined with the various relaxation techniques that they deserve special attention. These techniques are *relaxing imagery* and *diaphragmatic breathing.*

Relaxing Imagery

With the exception of prayer, relaxing, or guided, imagery may be the oldest of all relaxation techniques. It has been used in the various forms of Yoga and Zen meditation to supplement other approaches to relaxation. Feuerstein[35] points out that 2000 years ago, pleasant nature scenes were common relaxing strategies in Tantra Yoga. Interestingly, Lichstein[2] notes that pleasant nature scenes remain the most commonly used subjects for adults in guided imagery.

The earliest example of imagery being applied in modern times is that of Chappell and Stevenson.[36] Patients with peptic ulcer were taught in a group format to use relaxing imagery scenes to counteract anxiety that was assumed to exacerbate their ulcers. At a 3-year follow up, 26 of 28 subjects remained markedly improved, whereas subjects in an untreated control group continued to have ulcers. Imagery is now nearly always combined with other relaxation strategies.

The theoretical logic behind relaxing or guided imagery in the treatment of chronic headache is straightforward: Through imaging of a relaxing scene, one will be able to achieve a state of both mental and physical relaxation that is similar to what would be felt if actually experiencing the relaxing event, which would consequently lead to reduction in headache pain. If one is imagining an image that has been previously experienced, then relaxing imagery is quite similar to relaxation by recall procedures (i.e., one is recalling what it was like when the mind and body were calm and relaxed).

It is essential to obtain a relaxing scene from the patient rather than just using a standard relaxing scene; some common scenes are beach scenes, waterfalls, mountains streams, fishing, and walking through the woods on an autumn evening. Relaxing imagery has one obvious pitfall; some individuals are simply poor imaginers and may get very discouraged because they are unable to imagine the pleasant scene at all, even after repeated practice. If this happens, the therapist will discontinue the guided imagery and switch to another relaxation technique.

Keeping in mind the above caveat regarding tailoring the guided imagery to each patient, the following dialogue concerns a sample relaxing scene:

> Now, I want you to imagine that it's a very, very cold winter evening, and you're sitting in front of a fireplace, in a cabin, in the mountains of North Carolina. You can feel the warmth of the fire on your face and hands, and you can smell the pleasant odor of burning firewood. The fire is crackling and you seem mesmerized by the color of the flames—sometimes red, sometimes yellow, sometimes blue, sometimes gold. And now you can feel the warmth of the fireplace pouring down onto every muscle of your body. Off to the side is a window, where you can see that it's just begun to snow. You get up, walk to the window, and press your nose against the windowpane. And the coldness of the windowpane contrasts delightfully with the warmth of the fire. You wipe your breath off the window and look outside at the newly fallen snow. There's nothing more beautiful than newly fallen snow. It's like a blanket of white covering everything—your car, the woodpile, the branches of the trees, the trail to the door of the cabin. And it's so quiet . . . so peaceful . . . so still. . . . And there's nothing for you to do but concentrate on the great feelings of warmth and relaxation flowing into every muscle of your body as you relax there, in that cabin, in the woods, in the winter, when it's just begun to snow and the fire in the fireplace is on.

Diaphragmatic Breathing

Many relaxation techniques place special emphasis on breathing. Therapists often tell patients that learning to breath correctly is the most important relaxation technique that they can master and that if they become proficient in proper breathing techniques, they have half the relaxation challenge won. Most adults do not breath diaphragmatically; to do so, one needs to take deep, slow, relaxing breaths and push the air down into the chest, expanding the belly, not the thoracic cavity and shoulders. Headache sufferers are informed that with each deep breath they take, they will feel more relaxed. Breathing in this way will trigger the relaxation response at other times during the day when they do not have time to do the entire procedure.

It is pointed out to the headache patient that it is difficult to become very anxious if one is breathing correctly. Frequently, the therapist asks whether the patient has ever had a panic attack or ever seen someone become very nervous. (Nearly everyone has had one of these experiences.) It is pointed out that one of the first things that occurs during a panic attack is that breathing becomes very rapid and shallow (i.e., one begins to hyperventilate). Patients are told that they can prevent high levels of anxiety by breathing diaphragmatically.

The following is a diaphragmatic breathing exercise:

"Diaphragmatic breathing is a technique you can use to control tension in your body. First, place one hand on your chest and one on your abdomen. Take a breath in, and notice which hand moves the most. If you see the chest move out more, you are breathing in a tense manner. The chest is constructed such that the lungs are in the upper chest and a muscle (the diaphragm) separates the stomach from them. This muscle is used in gaining more volume of air as you breathe in. If you have ever played a wind instrument, sung in a choir, or swam under water, you probably have learned this technique. Also this is the way you breathe immediately before going to sleep as you become deeply relaxed. If you have a child you can watch them because they have not learned to breathe in a tense manner. Again, take a long deep breath in and try to push your stomach out so that it pushes against your belt. If you do this slowly you will feel the air expand in your lungs, and your stomach will naturally extend outward. This is not a fashion statement but until you learn to breathe in this way it is helpful. Another thing you can do is lie down and place a large book on your abdomen and a small paperback on your chest. As you breathe in, allow the big book to rise and keep the small book still. Try this for 20 breaths.

"Close your eyes and take a deep breath. Feel the coolness of the air as it passes into your nose and expands into your lungs. Feel your stomach expand as you breathe in as the chest becomes full and tight. Breathe out very slowly and easily. Take a second deep breath. Slowly breathe out. With each breath you can feel yourself becoming more relaxed. Concentrate on your breathing. . . . Allow your breathing to become smooth and rhythmic. Practice this breathing exercise 5 to 10 times a day."[23, p. 195–196]

Cognitive-Behavior Therapy for Chronic Headache

The majority of studies that have used cognitive therapy for the treatment of headache have done so in combination with psychophysiological intervention. This section is a relatively brief overview of the procedures. As noted previously, cognitive-behavioral therapies for headache are based on the assumption that an individual's thoughts, emotions, and behaviors influence their physiology. Therefore, cognitive-behavioral treatments generally involve identifying thoughts, emotions, and behaviors that routinely precede or exacerbate headache activity, with the therapist subsequently teaching patients in a systematic manner to modify these thoughts, feelings, and behaviors.

The most important tool of the cognitive-behavior therapist is the headache diary. Although a headache diary is ubiquitously used in psychological headache research, it is frequently used only as an outcome measure with the psychophysiological interventions (i.e., patients monitor only their headache activity on, for example, a 0-to-5 scale four times a day). In cognitive-behavioral procedures, however, the headache diary is used to monitor more than pain levels; the therapist frequently has the patient monitor cognitive activity such as thoughts or self-statements that occur before a severe headache or an emotional event such as anxiety or depression. Patients are then informed that what they think about a situation determines the stressfulness of the situation and that they can learn to control their headaches by learning mental strategies for control of stress. The job of the therapist is to assist the patient in identifying unreasonable expectations or beliefs that may explain their bodily responses to a variety of stressful situations. For example, the patient may believe that he or she must be loved by everyone. When experiencing a situation that is interpreted as not supporting this core belief, the patient becomes depressed, which can lead to a headache. The therapist aids the patient in examining the logical validity and behavioral and emotional consequences of continuing to hold these maladaptive expectancies and beliefs. Patients are taught to identify these maladaptive cognitions or beliefs in the real world as soon as possible to interrupt the chain of maladaptive thoughts. They are given coping strategies to implement that can counteract the maladaptive thoughts. Typically, these strategies involve reappraisal of the actual risks and consequences of the situation, self-instructions designed to counteract the specific maladaptive beliefs or thoughts (e.g., "I don't have to be loved by everyone to be a good person"), or relaxing imagery (see above) designed to counteract generalized worries and anxiety when there are no immediate or specific performance demands.[23, 28]

Expected Efficacy of Psychological Treatments

The following is adapted from Blanchard[37] and summarizes the average range of good clinical response (at least a 50% reduction in headache activity as documented by daily headache diary) for the psychological treatments under consideration in this chapter.

A review of Table 20–3 provides the practicing physician with information regarding the efficacy of each psychological treatment for a given type of headache patient. The physician can then make appropriate recommendations to his or her patient regarding which treatment will be most effective.

Appropriate and Inappropriate Headache Patients for Psychological Treatments

Appropriate Candidates

Tension-Type Headache. Patients with tension-type headaches, either episodic or chronic, are good candidates for EMG biofeedback, relaxation training, and/or cognitive stress coping therapy. In fact, there is some evidence[38] that the combination of these techniques is superior to amitriptyline. In a meta-analytic review of tension headache literature, Bogaards and ter Kuile[39] found that pharmacological therapy was comparable to the use of placebo in studies in which a headache diary was used and that psychophysiological treatments were clearly superior to pharmacological interventions. Along these lines, in a large, double-blind multisite study, Pfaffenrath and colleagues,[40] examined the efficacy of amitriptyline, amitriptylinoxide, and placebo for chronic tension headache and found no differences among the three conditions. Regardless of whether medication is more efficacious than placebo for tension headache, the findings of the majority of studies indicate that there are a substantial proportion of tension headache sufferers (55% to 70%) who are not being helped by pharmacological interventions. The practicing physician should be familiar with treatments such as biofeedback and relaxation therapy to make appropriate recommendations for treatment of their patients. We suggest that patients who prove refractory to a trial of one or two pharmacological agents be referred for these treatments.

Patients with tension-type headache can create a problem by gradually consuming increasing amounts of analgesic medication until they begin to experience analgesic-rebound headache,[41] or what Michultka et al[42] termed *high medication consumption headache* (see Chapter 21). Although these patients are relatively refractory to psychological treatment,[43] in another study, Blanchard and colleagues[43] have shown that relaxation training, plus intensive psychological support, can be used to wean a majority of these patients from their dependence on analgesics and other headache medications. After this discontinuation process, the psychological treatments are very effective. Reduced headaches and reduced medication consumption were well maintained in the study by Blanchard et al[43] at 1-year follow-up.

Migraine Headache. Patients with migraine headaches respond well to thermal biofeed-

Table 20–3 Percentage of Patients Who Respond with Noticeable Headache Relief

Headache Type	Therapy Type: *Relaxation*	*EMG Biofeedback*	*Thermal Biofeedback*	*Cognitive Therapy*
Tension-type	40–55%	50–60%	NA	60–80%
Migraine	30–50%	NA	40–55%	50%
Mixed tension-type and migraine	20–25%	NA	30–45%	NA
COMBINATION THERAPY				
Tension-type	Adding EMG biofeedback to relaxation increases success from 50% to 75%. Adding cognitive therapy to relaxation increases success from 40% to 65%.			
Migraine	Adding thermal biofeedback to relaxation increases success from 30% to 55% Adding relaxation to thermal biofeedback increases success from 40% to 55%.			
Mixed Tension-type and migraine	Adding thermal biofeedback to relaxation increases success from 20% to 55%. Adding relaxation to thermal biofeedback increases success from 25% to 55%. (We recommend the combination therapy for mixed headache.)			

Adding cognitive therapy to relaxation and thermal biofeedback does *not* improve success with migraine or mixed headache.

back, with or without adjunctive relaxation training. Evidence is mixed as to whether thermal biofeedback is equivalent in headache prophylaxis to propranolol[16] or inferior to it.[44]

There is a continuing controversy in the literature about the efficacy of thermal biofeedback for migraine headaches associated with a woman's menstrual cycle. In a reanalysis of their data, Solbach et al[45] found that thermal biofeedback is not effective in patients with menstrual cycle migraine. Later studies[46, 47] found that biofeedback is equally effective for menstrual and nonmenstrual migraine.

Pediatric Migraine. Migraine headache in children and adolescents, ages 8 to 16 or 17, responds very well to thermal biofeedback. A review[48] showed this treatment to be superior to all other psychological treatments and possibly to propranolol. Significant improvement was reported in 65% to 80% of pediatric headache patients treated with thermal biofeedback. We recommend thermal biofeedback as the treatment of choice for pediatric migraine.

Other Appropriate Candidates

Clearly, the patient who is reluctant to take prophylactic medication for his or her headaches is a good candidate for psychological treatments; this may represent a growing proportion of younger patients.

Other appropriate candidates include patients for whom standard drug therapy has failed, patients who are noncompliant with their drug regimen, and patients who have developed analgesic-rebound headache.

Finally, the female patient who is pregnant is a good candidate. Hickling and colleagues[49] have shown in a small uncontrolled trial that pregnant patients with severe migraine headache respond readily to psychological therapies.

Post-traumatic Headache. There is very little published research on the use of psychological treatments with post-traumatic headache. The uncontrolled series that have been described report generally good results. For example, Hickling et al[50] reported 67% of subjects with post-traumatic headache were improved based on daily headache diary data. Interestingly, 8 of the 12 subjects were found to also have *post-traumatic stress disorder* (PTSD). These latter patients required almost twice as many treatment sessions (26 versus 11) before a good response was obtained. It appears that PTSD must be dealt with before good headache relief can be obtained. The clinician should be careful to assess for possible PTSD in the patient with post-traumatic headache.

Inappropriate Candidates

Cluster Headache. Although there are case reports of successful treatment of secondary cluster headache with psychological treatments,[51] the largest series (11 participants) of cluster headache patients treated with a combination of relaxation training and thermal biofeedback (22 sessions)[52] reported only 2 of the 11 were slightly improved over a 30-month follow-up. *We do not recommend these treatments for cluster headache.*

Psychological Disturbance. There is minimal literature[35] on the prediction of good versus poor outcome with psychological therapies. Patients with tension-type headache who are depressed and migraineurs who are high in somatization and hysterical traits have consistently been found to respond less well to relaxation and/or EMG biofeedback. Headache patients in whom these characteristics are pronounced may well be good candidates for psychotherapy or behavior therapy.

Conclusion

It was our intention to introduce the practicing physician to various forms of psychological treatments for chronic benign headache. Chronic headache is the most frequent pain complaint in the clinical setting. An understanding of appropriate psychological procedures, the expected efficacy of these procedures, and the appropriate application of these procedures to different headache populations may provide physicians with additional methods to use in the constant challenge to alleviate the suffering of patients.

References

1. Blanchard EB, Epstein LH. A Biofeedback Primer. Reading, MA: Addison-Wesley; 1978:2.

2. Lichstein KL. Clinical Relaxation Strategies. New York: John Wiley & Sons; 1988.
3. Smith JC. Cognitive-Behavioral Relaxation Training: A New System of Strategies for Treatment and Assessment. New York: Springer; 1990.
4. Jacobson E. Progressive Relaxation. Chicago: University of Chicago Press; 1929.
5. Luthe W, ed. Autogenic Therapy. New York: Grune & Stratton; 1969–1973.
6. Bellack A. Reciprocal inhibition of a laboratory conditioned fear. Behav Res Ther 1973;11:11–18.
7. Blanchard EB, Andrasik F. Psychological assessment and treatment of headache: Recent developments and emerging issues. J Consult Clin Psychol 1982;50:859–879.
8. Blanchard EB. Psychological treatment of benign headache disorders. J Consult Clin Psychol 1992;60:537–551.
9. Budzynski T, Stoyva J, Adler C. Feedback induced muscle relaxation: Application to tension headache. J Behav Ther Exp Psychiatry 1970;1:205–211.
10. Budzynski TH, Stoyva JM, Adler CS, et al. EMG biofeedback and tension headache: A controlled outcome study. Psychosom Med 1973;6:509–514.
11. Sargent JD, Green EE, Walters ED. The use of autogenic feedback training in a pilot study of migraine and tension headaches. Headache 1972;12:120–124.
12. Blanchard EB, Theobald DE, Williamson DA, et al. Temperature biofeedback in the treatment of migraine headaches. Arch Gen Psychiatry 1978;35:581–588.
13. Sargent J, Solbach P, Coyne L, et al. Results of a controlled, experimental, outcome study of non-drug treatments with a control of migraine headaches. J Behav Med 1986;9:291–323.
14. Diamond S, Medina J, Diamond-Falk J, et al. The value of biofeedback in the treatment of chronic headache: A five-year retrospective study. Headache 1979;19:90–96.
15. Diamond S, Montrose D. The value of biofeedback in the treatment of chronic headache: A four-year retrospective study. Headache 1984;24:5–18.
16. Sovak M, Kunzel M, Sternbach RA, et al. Mechanism of the biofeedback therapy of migraine: Volitional manipulation of the psychophysiological background. Headache 1981; 21:89–92.
17. Tasto DL, Hinkle JE. Muscle relaxation treatment for tension headaches. Behav Res Ther 1973;11:347–349.
18. Chesney MA, Shelton JL. A comparison of muscle relaxation and electromyogram biofeedback treatments for muscle contraction headache. J Behav Ther Exp Psychiatry 1976; 7:221–225.
19. Schultz JH, Luthe U. Autogenic Training, Vol I. New York: Grune & Stratton; 1969.
20. Holroyd KA, Andrasik F, Westbrook T. Cognitive control of tension headache. Cognit Ther Res 1977;1:121–133.
21. Holroyd KA, Andrasik F. Coping and the self-control of chronic tension headache. J Consult Clin Psychol 1978;5:1036–1045.
22. Blanchard EB, Appelbaum KA, Radnitz CL, et al. A placebo-controlled evaluation of abbreviated progressive muscle relaxation and relaxation combined with cognitive therapy in the treatment of tension headache. J Consult Clin Psychol 1990;58:210–215.
23. Arena JG, Blanchard EB. Psychophysiological intervention in the treatment of chronic pain syndromes. *In* Gatchel RJ, Turk DC, eds. Chronic Pain: Psychological Perspectives on Treatment. New York: Guilford Publications; 1996:179–230.
24. Arena JG, Hannah SL, Bruno GM, et al. Effect of movement and position on muscle activity in tension headache sufferers during and between headaches. J Psychosom Res 1991; 35:187–195.
25. Arena JG, Bruno GM, Hannah SL, et al. The relationship between self-reported stress and headache activity in tension headache sufferers: Results of 28 to 35 day pain logs. In press.
26. Arena JG, Bruno GM, Hannah SL, et al. A comparison of frontal electromyographic biofeedback training, trapezius electromyographic biofeedback training and progressive muscle relaxation therapy in the treatment of tension headache. Headache 1995;35:411–419.
27. Blanchard EB, Andrasik F. Management of Chronic Headache: A Psychological Approach. New York: Pergamon Press; 1985.
28. Levor RM, Cohen MJ, Naliboff BD, et al. Psychosocial precursors and correlates of migraine headache. J Consult Clin Psychol 1986;54:347–353.
29. Kohler T, Haimerl C. Daily stress as a trigger of migraine attacks: Results of thirteen single-subject studies. J Consult Clin Psychol 1990; 58:870–872.
30. Blanchard EB, Andrasik F, Neff DF, et al. Biofeedback and relaxation training with three kinds of headache: Treatment effects and their prediction. J Consult Psychol 1983;50:562–575.
31. Libo LM, Arnold GE. Does training to criterion influence improvement? A follow-up study of EMG and thermal biofeedback. J Behav Med 1983;6:397–404.
32. Morrill B, Blanchard EB. Two studies of the potential mechanisms of action in the thermal biofeedback treatment of vascular headache. Headache 1989;29:169–176.
33. Arena JG, Hightower NE, Chang GC. Relaxation therapy for tension headache in the elderly: A prospective study. Psychol Aging 1988;3:96–98.
34. Blanchard EB, Andrasik F, Evans DD, et al. Behavioral treatment of 250 chronic headache

patients: A clinical replication series. Behav Ther 1985;16:308–327.
35. Feuerstein G. Textbook of Yoga. London: Rider; 1975.
36. Chappell MN, Stevenson TI. Group psychological training in some organic conditions. Mental Hygiene 1936;20:588–597.
37. Blanchard EB. Behavioral therapies in the treatment of headache. Headache Q 1992;3:53–56.
38. Holroyd KA, Nash JM, Pingel JD, et al. A comparison of pharmacological (amitriptyline HCl) and nonpharmacological (cognitive-behavioral) therapies for chronic tension headaches. J Consult Clin Psychol 1991;59:387–393.
39. Bogaards MC, ter Kuile MM. Treatment of recurrent tension headache: A meta-analytic review. Clin J Pain 1994;10:174–190.
40. Pfaffenrath V, Diener H-C, Isler H, et al. Efficacy and tolerability of amitriptylinoxide in the treatment of chronic tension-type headache: A multi-centre controlled study. Cephalalgia 1994;14:149–155.
41. Kudrow L. Paradoxical effects of frequent analgesic use. *In* Critchley M, Friedman AP, Gorini S, et al, eds. Advances in Neurology: Headache: Physiopathological and Clinical Concepts, Vol 33. New York: Raven Press; 1982: 335–361.
42. Michultka DM, Blanchard EB, Appelbaum KA, et al. The refractory headache patient. II. High medication consumption (analgesic rebound) headache. Behav Res Ther 1989;27:411–420.
43. Blanchard EB, Taylor AE, Dentinger MP. Preliminary results from the self-regulatory treatment of high medication consumption headache. Biofeedback Self-Regul 1992;17:179–202.
44. Mathew NT. Prophylaxis of migraine and mixed headache: A randomized controlled study. Headache 1981;21:105–109.
45. Solbach P, Sargent J, Coyne L. Menstrual migraine headache: Results of a controlled, experimental outcome study of non-drug treatments. Headache 1984;24:75–78.
46. Gauthier JG, Fournier A, Roberge C. The differential effects of biofeedback in the treatment of menstrual and non-menstrual migraine. Headache 1991;31:82–90.
47. Kim M, Blanchard EB. Two studies of the nonpharmacological treatment of menstrually-related migraine headache. Headache 1992; 32:197–202.
48. Hermann C, Kim M, Blanchard EB. Behavioral and prophylactic pharmacological intervention studies of pediatric migraine: An exploratory meta-analysis. Pain 1995;60:239–256.
49. Hickling EJ, Silverman DJ, Loos WR. A nonpharmacological treatment of vascular headache during pregnancy. Headache 1990;30:407–410.
50. Hickling EJ, Blanchard EB, Schwarz SP, et al. Headaches and motor vehicle accidents: Results of the psychological treatment of post-traumatic headache. Headache Q 1992;3:285–289.
51. King AC, Arena JG. Behavioral treatment of chronic cluster headache in geriatric patients. Biofeedback Self-Regulat 1984;9:201–208.
52. Blanchard EB, Andrasik F, Jurish SE, et al. The treatment of cluster headache with relaxation and thermal biofeedback. Biofeedback Self-Regulat 1982;7:185–191.

21

Medication Overuse and Dependency in the Headache Patient

R. Michael Gallagher, D.O.

Introduction

For as long as there have been headache sufferers, there has been a quest to find relief from pain. The ancients offered remedies to appease or counter supernatural forces; the Greeks and Romans offered bleeding, purging, roots, and herbs. As humans observed and learned, these primitive treatments evolved into modern-day medications and nonmedicinal modalities. The clinician can choose from a broad array of analgesics that can provide safe and effective symptomatic therapy.

Despite advances in the pharmacological armamentarium, patients with headache continue to present a difficult and challenging problem for the clinician. Head pain is extremely complex and not adequately understood. The very nature of head pain can leave patients unable to think, interact, or function. The location of head pain—in close proximity to the center of sensory control and contact with the world—can leave patients with severe anxiety. In addition, individual neurobiological and psychosociological differences, as well as underlying psychological difficulties, can influence the effect of treatment.

The ideal headache pain medication is easy to take, relieves pain, causes no adverse effects, and is nonaddictive; unfortunately, this ideal medication has yet to be developed. Many new analgesics are introduced and sometimes hailed as being the ideal or at least close to it, but as the use of these new medications increases and there is opportunity for study, this proves not to be the case. For this reason, the clinician must be knowledgeable and exercise caution.

When taken properly, analgesics usually provide relief from headache pain without complications. When they are misused or inappropriately prescribed, analgesics may aggravate the headache problem; therefore, it is critical that patients use these medications correctly. Consideration should be given to effectiveness, rapidity of action, safety, and potential for addiction. Clinicians must be cognizant of analgesic limitations and protect their patients, especially those who experience severe and/or frequent headaches.

Analgesic Misuse

Analgesic medications can be considered "life-saving" when a sufferer is confronted with severe pain. *Relief* from the pain can have different meanings to different people. To some, it may mean "getting by" or being able to sleep, whereas to others it may mean complete freedom of pain. Regardless, it is important that clinicians discuss this issue with their patients. It is extremely helpful for patients to have reasonable and realistic expectations.

Patients who take symptomatic pain medication too frequently or in excessive amounts may habituate to their therapeutic action and begin a cycle of increased consumption, resulting in addiction. *Habituation* is the psychological and emotional dependence on a drug to maintain a state of well-being. *Addiction* refers to an uncontrollable dependence on a drug that, when discontinued, causes emotional, mental, and physiological reactions. As a result, the analgesic fails to provide pain relief and actually seems to perpetuate and intensify the headache. This seemingly paradoxical effect is termed *analgesic-rebound headache.*[1] The term *rebound* refers to the worsening of or recurrence of headache as the analgesic effect wears off. There is an apparent withdrawal phenomenon in which the patient experiences an escalation of pain when the medication is withheld. Similar effects can occur with caffeine and ergotamine overuse.[2,3]

In addition to the analgesic-rebound phenomenon, patients who use analgesics on a daily basis may not respond to appropriate prophylactic therapy until the analgesics are withdrawn.[4] Such patients often mistakenly believe that "nothing" will help their problem and experience repeated treatment failures. These patients may respond to medications previously deemed to be ineffective; the significant difference between failure and effectiveness is the withdrawal of frequent or daily analgesics.

In the treatment of patients with headache, there is an important difference between the frequency and quantity of analgesic use. The frequency with which medications are used seems to be more problematic than the amount taken. In general, it is probably worse for a patient to take a small number of analgesic tablets (one or two) on a continuing daily basis than to take a larger number of tablets (six or eight) in 1 day intermittently or for a limited number of days.

Numerous factors, which vary according to the type of headache, may promote excessive analgesic use. For patients with migraine, these factors include the fear of worsening pain, gastric stasis that slows absorption of oral medications, prolonged migraine physiology (especially with menstrual migraine), status migrainosis, and the consumption of too much caffeine.[5,6]

Factors that influence the misuse of analgesics in individuals with tension-type (muscle contraction) headache include the presence of anxiety and depression, a frenetic lifestyle, use of medications that are inappropriate for the degree of pain, and excessive ingestion of caffeine and over-the-counter drugs.

Patients with cluster headache often mistakenly believe that taking an analgesic early in the cluster attack will lessen its duration. As a result, the frequency of cluster attacks, when not controlled prophylactically, can lead to the misuse of medication if the individual takes analgesics for each episode. Other factors that influence the overuse of analgesics in patients with cluster headache are the consumption of alcohol and the failure to implement prophylactic treatment.

Factors that result in the overuse of analgesics in individuals with mixed headache include anxiety and depression, fear of the headache becoming worse, inability to determine the type of headache being experienced, and, again, consumption of large amounts of caffeine and over-the-counter drugs.

The improper use of analgesics is also likely to occur when patients are unable to find a therapeutic regimen that provides satisfactory results. Most physicians have had new patients with headache who complain that they have tried everything and nothing works for them. A major reason for headache therapy failure is that the treatment plan is based on an inaccurate diagnosis of the type of headache. It is not uncommon for patients with headache to be misdiagnosed and treated with inappropriate analgesics that provide little relief. An accurate diagnosis, although difficult and time consuming, is essential for the effective management of headache. In other cases, headache therapy fails because the clinician does not recognize that the patient requires prophylactic rather than symptomatic treatment alone. A preventative regimen is appropriate in patients who need to use analgesics more than 2 or 3 days each week or whose headaches do not respond to appropriate abortive and/or symptomatic treatment. Prophylactic therapy should also be considered in patients who require an excessive amount of analgesics to treat an headache (four to six pills per dose) or have a history of habituation. Some clinicians may base the necessity of prophylactic treatment on analgesic use (Table 21–1).

Indications for Analgesics

All patients who experience headache pain deserve an analgesic for symptomatic treat-

Table 21–1 Indication for Prophylactic Headache Treatment Based on Analgesic Use

Analgesics needed more than 3 days each week
Excessive amount of analgesics needed
Unresponsiveness to analgesics
History of habituation

From Gallagher RM. Proper use of analgesics in the treatment of headache. Headache Q 1992;3 (suppl 1):22–27.

Table 21–2 Analgesic-Prescribing Guidelines

Select appropriate medication for degree of pain.
Ensure patient can tolerate medication.
Prescribe in limited quantities.
Educate patient regarding limitations on frequency and quantity of use.
Require regular follow-up visits.

ment alone or headaches that do not respond to abortive treatment. In most cases, analgesics can be taken concomitantly with abortive or reversal medication when the pain is sufficiently severe. It is helpful to inform patients who take prophylactic medications to continue their regularly scheduled doses during severe headache attacks.

Analgesic Guidelines

The following guidelines are provided to assist the clinician in the appropriate use of analgesics[7] (Table 21–2).

1. Select a medication that is appropriate for the degree of pain experienced and the frequency of attacks. In general, a 650-mg dose of aspirin or 200-mg dose of ibuprofen will be ineffective in resolving an incapacitating migraine headache, no matter how early the medication is taken. On the other hand, an opioid or opioid-like medication is not appropriate for a mild tension-type headache that would probably respond to 650 mg aspirin or 200 mg ibuprofen. Avoid the use of habit-forming medications whenever possible. In the early stages of headache, the less potentially habit-forming analgesics often are effective. During the later stages of headache or when pain is more severe, it may be necessary to prescribe opioids or other potentially habit-forming medications.

2. Ensure that the patient can tolerate the medication prescribed. A patient's age, medical status, and psychological health must be considered. Caution should be used in patients who have never previously taken a potent or sedating analgesic. These medications may sedate excessively or cause dizziness or lightheadedness.

3. Prescribe analgesics in limited quantities with few or no refills. When patients are given larger amounts of analgesics, they often are tempted to take medication prematurely or unnecessarily. Many patients with headache are extremely aware and fearful of any sensation in their heads. Consequently, they begin to medicate at the slightest sign of impending headache or even in anticipation of a headache. In addition, when some patients want to feel well on a given day and reach a certain level of activity, they may take medication on awakening in the morning even when there is no indication of headache. If a clinician has treated a patient for several years and established that the patient is responsible and compliant, he or she may want to prescribe a limited quantity of medication with one or two refills. However, many patients with chronic headache do not fit into this category.

4. Educate the patient about the medication that is being prescribed; this involves not only explaining potential side effects but also clearly delineating how and when the medication is to be used. The best approach is to treat the headache before the pain intensifies. Once the pain has escalated, it may become difficult to treat successfully regardless of its source. Instead of simply telling the patient to not take too much of the drug or to not take it too often, specific limitations and guidelines should be explained. For example, patients can be told to limit analgesic use to no more than 2 days per week. They should be instructed to call the clinician if they feel they need larger quantities or more frequent doses to control their headaches. Appropriate adjustment of dosage or the selection of a different medication can then be recommended.

Potentially habit-forming medications should not be prescribed for patients who are overusing analgesics or have a history of abuse. The potential for addiction with these medications can vary significantly with the type of headache (Table 21–3).

Patients with migraine in general have a low risk of addiction when their headaches are episodic, occur fairly infrequently, and are controlled with a therapeutic regimen. Pa-

Table 21–3 Potential for Analgesic Addiction by Headache Type

Migraine headache	Low
Cluster headache	Low to moderate
Tension-type headache*	Moderate to high
Mixed headache	Highest

*Frequent or chronic.

From Gallagher RM. Proper use of analgesics in the treatment of headache. Headache Q 1992;3 (suppl 1):22–27.

tients with cluster headache have a low-to-moderate potential for becoming addicted to analgesics. Often, these patients, who do use excessive medications during headache periods, stop their use once the cluster bout is over. Individuals with tension-type headaches and facial neuralgia have a high risk for addiction when their symptoms are frequent or prolonged. Mixed headache is associated with the highest potential for addiction because of the continuous, unpredictable, and often severe pain.

It is useless to instruct patients to "not become addicted" or "to cut down on their intake of medication" on their own once they have become habituated or addicted. Patients have little control over their use of analgesics because they are responding to real or perceived pain and have a fear of the pain. It is the clinician's responsibility to prescribe the appropriate analgesic in small quantities without refills and monitor the patient's use.

Regular follow-up visits without long lapses between visits are essential. Lack of continuity of care undermines the best of treatment plans. To effectively monitor the use of analgesics, the clinician must see patients on a regular basis, especially new patients and those taking potentially habit-forming medications. If patients are unwilling to schedule follow-up visits, the clinician can refuse to treat them. Conversely, if the clinician is too busy to regularly see patients with headache, it is best to refer them to another clinician who has or is willing to spend the necessary time.

Appropriate Analgesic Use

The armamentarium of medications that can be used for the symptomatic treatment of headache is large. A reasonable starting approach for the clinician is to prescribe a medicament that is deemed to be sufficiently strong to provide adequate relief. If not effective, a methodical progression through the various levels of therapy in the order of increasing potency, with close attention paid to the circumstances of attacks and response to treatment, can then be used until an effective regimen is established.

Simple Analgesics and Nonsteroidal Anti-inflammatory Drugs

Numerous simple analgesics and nonsteroidal anti-inflammatory drugs (NSAIDs) are available for the treatment of headache. Traditionally, only medications such as acetaminophen and aspirin have been available on an over-the-counter or off-the-shelf basis, but in recent years, NSAIDs such as ibuprofen, naproxen sodium, and ketoprofen have become available without prescription. In the past, many of these medications were the prescription drugs of first choice for numerous clinicians. With the availability of these agents without prescription, clinicians should be sure to continue to consider them in a headache sufferer's total treatment plan. In addition, when some of these medications do not help a particular patient, they may actually be effective when the same patient is taking prophylactic medications.

The addition of caffeine as an adjuvant to simple analgesics or NSAIDs can enhance analgesic activity.[8] Various nonprescription and prescription medications of long-standing popularity contain caffeine. In fact, some specialists recommend that abortive and analgesic medications that do not contain caffeine be taken with a caffeinated beverage. In general, caffeine-containing compounds are more effective in patients who consume minimal amounts of caffeine, but it should be noted that not all headache authorities agree with this concept.[9]

Although over-the-counter medications can be effective and adequate for many sufferers, their frequent use can present a problem for patients. The potential is present for significant adverse reactions, such as gastric irritation, ulcer, or major organ complications. In addition, *analgesic rebound* can occur, especially in medications containing caffeine.[1] For this reason, patient education and monitoring are extremely important.

Muscle Relaxant Medications

The central-acting muscle relaxants are a group of prescription medications that are frequently overlooked as therapeutic options. These medications induce muscle relaxation through depression of the central nerve pathways and through their effect on higher centers in the brain. Because of this effect on the higher brain centers, they are sometimes used as analgesics or axiolytics.[10]

The muscle relaxants can be effective in tension-type headaches and may help in the early stages of migraine. Medications such as carisoprodol, chlorzoxazone, metaxalone, orphenadrine, and methocarbamol frequently provide relief with relative safety when used judiciously. Although habituation is not common with most of these medications, it should be noted that carisoprodol is related to meprobamate and, when overused, could become a problem for certain patients.[11] The agent chlorzoxazone can be associated with unpredictable hepatic toxicity, and some authorities recommend its avoidance.[12] Some of the muscle relaxants are compounded with caffeine, aspirin, acetaminophen, or codeine to enhance their therapeutic effect. Appropriate caution regarding rebound, gastric irritation, organ toxicity, and habituation should be exercised when prescribing these medications.

Combination, Opioid, and Opioid-like Analgesics

Most patients experience a similar pain cycle regardless of the exact biochemical nature of their headache. When an individual experiences pain, he or she usually becomes anxious, causing the scalp, head, and neck muscles to tighten. The muscle spasm causes additional pain, and the cycle repeats. Consequently, medications that are often most effective for headache pain are those that interrupt more than one part of the pain cycle (e.g., reducing pain and anxiety or reducing muscle spasm and pain).

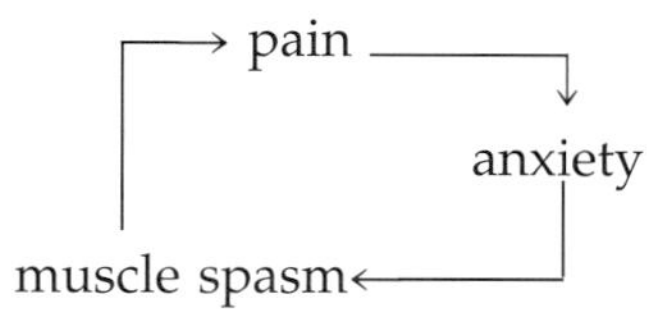

The combination analgesics are considered by some to be more effective for severe headache pain than the component agents alone. The combination of more than one analgesic or the addition of an anxiolytic agent, such as a barbiturate or benzodiazepine, can interrupt the vicious cycle of pain and anxiety. In general, these medications are relatively safe and effective for episodic headache pain and most patients; however, because these medicaments usually contain potentially habit-forming agents, their judicious use is imperative. Daily or near-daily use can result in habituation or addiction and analgesic-rebound headaches. This group of analgesics is quite extensive and includes many drugs in various combinations.

The daily or near-daily use of potentially addicting medications is not warranted in headache patients; however, there may be a very small subset of individuals who can tolerate opioid or opioid-like analgesics without demonstrating addictive behavior.[13] Very few sufferers fall into this category, and some specialists are skeptical of the existence of such a group in chronic headache sufferers. Although it is tempting to consider any difficult patient a candidate for daily use, great caution must be exercised because a prior history of substance abuse excludes this possibility (Table 21–4).

Dealing with the Drug-Seeking Patient

Most clinicians who see headache sufferers will find it necessary on occasion to manage the drug-seeking patient. Drug-seeking patients can be divided into two general categories: the fraudulent sufferer and the iatrogenically addicted sufferer.

The *fraudulent drug-seeking patient* is an individual who feigns headache disorders to obtain analgesics for inappropriate use. This person is often a night-time or weekend caller who is very familiar with the various headache disorders. They usually indicate how ineffective most therapies and physicians have been in the past and identify exactly which medication will help their pain. It is also very common for their history to be accompanied by an extreme story of unfortunate circumstances and an uncanny ability to elicit sympathy from the clinician and staff.

To effectively deal with fraudulent sufferers who are seeking analgesics, the clinician must begin with a high degree of suspicion

Table 21–4 General Criteria for Daily Opioid and Opioid-like Analgesics

All reasonable and appropriate treatment has failed.
There is no prior history of substance abuse.
The patient is knowledgeable and fully informed of the deviation from general analgesic standards of care.
Appropriate consultations and evaluations have been made.
There is a positive therapeutic response.
The patient is restored to functionability.
There is no escalation in use.
There is one physician managing all analgesics and medications.

of any new patient with a story that warrants a prescription for an analgesic. This suspicion should be communicated directly to the patient, and an effort should be made to immediately corroborate any story of previous medical encounters or misfortunes (e.g., a call to their previous pharmacy or physician in the presence of the patient). If the hour is late or the pharmacy or previous physician's office is closed, call and leave a message describing your situation and ask for a return call. Schedule a revisit within 24 to 48 hours, emphasizing to the patient the need for follow-up and further information. If it is thought that the patient might be truthful and truly in need of immediate pain medication, a limited prescription (four to six tablets or capsules) can be given. In most cases, fraudulent sufferers subsequently abandon further efforts and move to another clinician target. Suspicion and close scrutiny of newer patients usually represent the best safeguard.

Iatrogenically addicted sufferers are a completely different group; they are in need of empathy and help from the clinician. These patients are excessive users of analgesics, often take multiple medications, often use excessive caffeine, and often use various over-the-counter medications. They frequently are depressed and skeptical of the entire medical system because of previous treatment failures. A history elicited from such patients is often filled with omissions and "storytelling" to convince the clinician to prescribe the analgesic to which they are addicted. These patients can be desperate, and a knowledgeable and caring clinician can help them a great deal.

Ideally, these iatrogenically addicted patients can be treated in a dedicated inpatient headache unit. Such units have knowledgeable and empathetic staff who can manage detoxification safely and institute an appropriate comprehensive therapeutic regimen. Unfortunately, these units are small in number, and distance and various insurance limitations make them inaccessible to many (see Chapter 23).

It is possible to deal with the addicted patient on an outpatient basis, but it takes much effort and time on the part of the staff and clinician. Such patients invariably will undergo a limited withdrawal period of which headache is the predominant symptom. The first step after identification of the problem is to involve another family member or a person who is in a position to render support and guidance to the patient. A comprehensive treatment plan, including appropriate prophylaxis and realistic goals regarding headaches, should be developed by the clinician, patient, and family member. A rapid withdrawal of the offending analgesic or agent should be instituted while simultaneously initiating appropriate prophylactic treatment. No potentially addicting analgesics should be administered. If sedation is needed, consideration can be given to antihistamines such as hydroxyzine or a phenothiazine.[14] Seizure precautions, such as the temporary administration of an anticonvulsant such as phenobarbital, should be taken. Non–habit-forming or non–caffeine-containing analgesics, muscle relaxants, or antihistamines can be given for pain; in the early stages of withdrawal, these medications will be of minimal help. Frequent contact with the office and frequent follow-up visits should be planned. The success of such a program will depend on the firm resolve of the clinician with the cooperation of the patient's family or support person.

Conclusion

Head pain is a very disturbing and fearsome symptom that has plagued humans throughout recorded history. Humans are differentiated from lower animals by their ability to rationalize and talk. The centers for these activities are located in the head; when pain occurs in this area, it often makes it that much more disturbing. Head pain can interfere with the normal functions of the brain and incapacitate or alter lifestyle. For this reason, it is important that clinicians recognize and provide realistic and adequate treatment to suffering patients. This treatment should include the judicious and limited use of analgesics when appropriate.

References

1. Rapoport AM. Analgesic rebound headache. Headache 1988;28:662–665.
2. Griffiths RR, Woodson PP. Caffeine physical dependence: a review of human and laboratory animal studies. Psychopharmacology 1988;94:437–451.
3. Gallagher RM. Ergotamine withdrawal causing 'rebound headache.' JAOA 1983;82:677.

4. Kudrow L. Paradoxical effects of frequent analgesic use. Adv Neurol 1982;33:335–341.
5. Volans GN. Research review: Migraine and drug absorption. Clin Pharmacokinet 1978; 3:313–318.
6. Boyle R, Behan PO, Sutton JA. A correlation between severity of migraine and delayed emptying measured by an epigastric impedance method. Br J Clin Pharmacol 1990;30:405–409.
7. Gallagher RM. Proper use of analgesics in the treatment of headache. Headache Q 1992;3 (suppl 1):22–27.
8. Laska EM, Sunshine A, Mueller F, et al. Caffeine as an analgesic adjuvant. JAMA 1984; 251:1711–1718.
9. Migliardi JR, Armellino JJ, Friedman M, et al. Caffeine as an analgesic adjuvant in tension headache. Clin Pharmacol Ther 1994;56:576–586.
10. Gallagher RM. Muscle relaxant medications. *In* Tollison CD, Satterthwaite JR, eds. Painful Cervical Trauma. Baltimore: Williams & Wilkins; 1992:184–191.
11. Physicians Gen. ℞. Smithtown, NY: Data Pharmaceutica, Inc.; 1994.
12. Chlorzoxazone hepatoxicity. Med Lett 1996; 38:43–46.
13. Portenoy RD. Drug treatment of pain syndromes. Semin Neurol 1987;7:139–149.
14. Gallagher RM, Mueller L, Ciervo CA. Hydroxyzine as an analgesic for headache (abstract). Clin Pharmacol Ther 1994;55:130.

22

Emergency Treatment of Headache

Merle L. Diamond, M.D.

Introduction

Headache is a frequent presenting complaint in the emergency department (ED). The occurrence of headache as the chief complaint on admission is between 0.36% and 2.5% of patients.[1] In a survey of 16,755 patients presenting at a walk-in ED, 323 (1.9%) had migraine complaints.[2] Fifty-four of the migraine patients included in the study made more than one visit to the ED. Migraineurs appear to use the ED and other health care services two to five times as often as nonmigraineurs.[3]

The incidence of headache with significant morbid or fatal outcome is not frequent.[4] Determining the differential diagnosis of the patient presenting with headache is essential to rule out organic disease. Appropriate treatment regimens can be instituted once the diagnosis has been established. In the ED, relief of acute pain usually must be addressed. Referring the patient for follow-up care and preventing repeat ED visits and possible narcotic habituation are recurrent problems for the emergency physician.

To adequately treat the patient presenting to the ED with headache as the chief complaint, the emergency physician must be familiar with the various categories of headaches. Several headache classifications have been established and are discussed in Chapter 2. For simplicity, the division of headaches into three categories—organic, vascular, and tension-type headaches—is very useful for the ED setting.

Multiple disease processes are included in the category of organic headaches (Table 22–1). In evaluating the headache patient, the emergency physician must be aggressive in diagnosing the patient to rule out life-threatening illness. The emergency physician can be reassured that organic causes of headache occur rarely.

Between 4.5% and 20% of patients with headache who visit the ED will have vascular headaches.[5] Referral for follow-up is essential to prevent frequent repeat visits to the ED and dependence on habituating analgesics. At the ED, tension-type headache is the most prevalent diagnosis among these headache patients. Narcotic analgesics must be totally avoided in these patients.

Patient Evaluation

History and Physical Examination

All patients presenting to the ED with the complaint of headache should be interviewed carefully regarding their headache history. This history is an essential tool in establishing the diagnosis. Patients presenting with recent onset headache or a change in the character of their headache should be thoroughly evaluated for possible organic disease. If the pa-

Table 22–1 Organic Causes of Headache

Stroke	Embolic Thrombotic Hemorrhagic
Infection	Meningitis Encephalitis Sinusitis Brain abscess
Inflammation	Vasculitis Temporal arteritis Cervical arthritis
Tumor	Primary Metastatic
Hypertension	

tient complains of the "worst headache of my life" with associated stiff neck, possible nausea and vomiting, and focal neurological symptoms, subarachnoid hemorrhage (SAH) should be ruled out. The patient with an extensive history of headaches who presents at the ED with a recurrent acute headache that has been triggered by dietary indiscretion or is associated with menses and is accompanied with nausea, vomiting, and photophobia probably can be diagnosed with migraine.

During the history, certain factors should be identified. Completion of the interview in a timely, organized manner will aid in establishing the diagnosis. The time of onset of this particular headache, character of the pain, severity, duration, and any associated symptoms with this particular headache should be outlined. The interviewer should determine whether the patient has a prior history of headache and should obtain information about the original onset of the headache, as well as any previous tests and treatment. The patient should also be questioned about a family history of headache, any exertional aspects to the acute attacks, and current therapeutic regimens.

The patient presenting at the ED with the complaint of headache should receive a physical and neurological examination. If the patient relates a recent onset of headaches or a change in character of the headaches, the emergency physician should be alert to possible organic pathology. The extent of the examination is dependent on the patient's current status. During the evaluation, the fundus, neck, throat, and nose should be examined.

Diagnostic Evaluation

Diagnostic testing will not usually establish the diagnosis in the majority of patients presenting to the ED with headache.[6] The physical examination and the headache history will facilitate the choice of diagnostic tests to be performed. In ordering diagnostic studies, the emergency physician should consider the possibility that the patient will seek follow-up care.

A complete blood count should be performed if there is any suspicion of an infection or a marked anemia, which could cause an hypoxia-related vascular headache. Evaluation of renal function and electrolytes should be obtained in patients who appear to be dehydrated due to status migraine with associated vomiting. Blood chemistries should also be performed on patients consuming excessive amounts of prescribed or over-the-counter analgesics.

As discussed in Chapter 5, neuroimaging is particularly useful in patients with headache. The criteria for ordering neuroimaging are listed in Table 22–2. These more stringent guidelines are a valuable tool for the emergency physician confronted with a patient presenting with acute headache. If elevated intracranial pressure due to focal lesions is suspected, the need for obtaining a computed tomography (CT) scan and a careful ophthalmic disk examination before performing a lumbar puncture is essential to prevent a possible cerebellar herniation.

A CT scan should also be obtained on any hypertensive patient presenting to the ED with a change in sensorium and focal neurological symptoms to rule out increased intracranial pressure and intracerebral bleeding. In 75% to 90% of patients with SAH, the CT scan will demonstrate the abnormality, depending on the resolution of the scanner as well as time of onset of symptoms. Sensitivity of CT decreases as time from onset of symptoms increases. The CT scan also may differentiate between brain abscesses and some tumors.

A lumbar puncture is an important diagnostic tool in the ED. If the emergency physician suspects SAH, meningitis, or both, a lumbar puncture should be performed. In the presence of an SAH, xanthochromic or red blood cells will be demonstrated in the spinal fluid expressed during the lumbar puncture. The fluid also will reveal white blood cells, as well as bacteria, in the patient with bacterial

Table 22–2 Criteria for Ordering CT Scan

1. Clinical suspicion of cerebellar hemorrhage or infarct
2. Stroke in evolution or completed stroke with emergency use of anticoagulants
3. History and examination suggestive of intracerebral hemorrhage or mass lesion
4. Acute signs of increased intracranial pressure
5. Patients at risk for cerebral abscess but requiring lumbar puncture
6. Blunt head trauma with findings of increased intracranial pressure
7. Depressed skull fracture
8. Open skull fracture
9. Penetrating head injury
10. Head injury and Glasgow Coma Scale score of less than 9

meningitis. As stated, the suspected presence of a focal lesion will contraindicate the performance of a lumbar puncture; therefore, a CT scan must be obtained before a lumbar puncture on all patients with suspected increased intracranial pressure or patients at risk for focal lesions.

To rule out temporal arteritis, a sedimentation rate according to the Westergen method should be obtained on all patients older than 50 who present to the ED with recent onset headache or a change in the character of the headache. If the sedimentation rate is elevated, a temporal artery biopsy should be scheduled as soon as possible, and treatment with corticosteroids should be started promptly to prevent irreversible blindness.

Subarachnoid Hemorrhage

At the ED, the most dramatic headache presentation probably is that of the patient with SAH. These patients typically present with a history absent of previous headache complaints.[7] The patient with a previous history of headaches will usually not report any unusual features of the headache or describe difficulties with his or her therapeutic regimen. The emergency physician should be cognizant that thunderclap headache may occur in patients with migraine or with an SAH.[8] Approximately 10% of all cerebrovascular accidents are related to the presence of an SAH, and an approximately 50% mortality rate has been reported.[9] It should be noted that 50% of patients who survive the initial bleed but do not receive treatment will die within the next 2 weeks.

The clinical picture of the patient with SAH is a terrible headache, usually described as "the worst ever," with a typically acute onset. The headache goes from nothing to severe in a very brief interval. Associated symptoms related to increased intracranial pressure, including nausea, vomiting, meningismus, and focal neurological signs, often are reported. A transient loss of consciousness associated with the onset of bleeding also may be noted. Vital signs should be monitored because an elevated blood pressure may occur due to sympathetic hypersensitivity.[9] SAH is discussed in greater detail in Chapter 10.

Meningitis

The life-threatening diagnosis of meningitis will more likely be confronted by the emergency physician than by the office-based clinician. This serious problem may occur in any population and is not limited to any particular season. Meningitis should be suspected in any patient presenting with headache, fever, and stiff neck. The age of the patient can aid in determining which causative agent is responsible.[5] *Haemophilus influenzae* is the most prevalent cause of meningitis in children aged 2 through 5. Older children and adolescents with meningitis are more frequently infected with *Neisseria meningitidis*. In older patients, the cause of their meningitis is usually Streptococcal pneumonia. Patients receiving immunosuppressive treatment and those who are immunosuppressed for other reasons are particularly susceptible to these as well as to other organisms.

Temporal Arteritis

In treating patients with temporal arteritis, early diagnosis and management are essential, and the emergency physician should be conversant with the clinical picture of this disorder. Headache is the most common presenting complaint, and the typical patient has been previously asymptomatic and is older than 50, and the headache is of recent onset. The female-to-male ratio is 2:1. Associated systemic symptoms include weight loss, night sweats, low-grade fever, aching of joints, and jaw claudication.[10] *Polymyalgia rheumatica* is the term used to describe this cluster of symptoms.

During the interview, the patient will complain of head pains or headache usually localized to the affected scalp vessels. Another characteristic symptom is pain in the jaw muscle on chewing. On examination, the physician will observe that the area around the temporal artery is usually tender to touch, and the skin may appear red.[11] The involved arteries will dictate which physical signs will be present.

The absolute necessity for early diagnosis and treatment should not be diminished. Vision is lost in one or both eyes in 50% of untreated cases. Early treatment is critical because the resultant blindness is irreversible. As stated previously, this condition can be easily ruled out through the use of the sedimentation rate according to the Westergen method. A sedimentation rate of more than 40 mm/hr indicates the need for a temporal artery biopsy. Corticosteroid treatment can be initiated during the interim while awaiting the temporal artery biopsy if temporal arteritis is suspected. The corticosteroid therapy may need to be continued for several years, with follow-up sedimentation rates performed at regular intervals.

Tumors and Brain Abscesses

Inflammation, traction, and displacement or distention of the pain-sensitive structures of the cranium will cause the headache due to intracranial sources. The term *traction headache* describes the typical source of the displacement. A rapidly expanding lesion, which produces traction on the pain-sensitive areas of the head, will produce a headache that is a cardinal sign of a brain tumor (see Chapter 10). Headache is a frequent manifestation of increased intracranial pressure. In one retrospective chart review of 101 patients with primary brain tumors diagnosed in the ED, 56 presented with the complaint of headache.[12] If the tumor is slow growing, the headache usually is mild and transient. This headache is easily relieved with over-the-counter analgesics, and the patient will rarely visit an ED.

The morbid outcome of these traction headaches should alert the emergency physician to the generalizations regarding headache due to brain tumor, which are outlined in Chapter 10. The patient with headache due to brain tumor will often describe the pain as deep, aching, steady, dull, and rarely throbbing. This headache can, at times, be severe, but it is not typically as intense as migraine. Over-the-counter analgesics and ice packs often relieve the pain. Eventually, the headache may become progressive due to enlargement of the mass and resultant surrounding cerebral edema. Increases in intracranial pressure, due to Valsalva, exertion, or other maneuvers, may exacerbate the pain. Focal signs may occur in patients with a mass lesion, depending on which area of the brain is involved. Signs of increased elevation in blood pressure may also be demonstrated. CT scanning, and possibly magnetic resonance imaging, is indicated in patients presenting with exertional aspects to their headaches. Other neurological signs, such as headache accompanied by fainting, should alert the emergency physician to the need for further testing and referral to the appropriate specialist.

Disease of the adjacent nasal and aural structures will usually be the cause of the headache due to brain abscess. This pain will typically start at those sites before the involvement of the cerebral parenchyma. The development of papilledema and other signs of localized traction and generalized displacement of the brain will usually herald a brain abscess. These patients will also present with associated symptoms such as fever, leukocytosis, and pleocytosis. Ear infections will usually produce abscesses above or below the tentorium. Hiccoughing, vomiting, and occipital headache are typical signs of abscesses below the tentorium. Pain in the frontal region adjacent to the diseased frontal, ethmoid, and sphenoid sinus usually results from an epidural abscess due to a sinus infection.

At the ED, the patient should be questioned about recent or concomitant ear infections or sinusitis. The presence of fever and purulent nasal drainage is indicative of the need for CT scanning and possibly sinus radiography. The possibility of a brain abscess should be suspected in a patient presenting with recent-onset headache and with no other clinical signs except for an elevated white blood cell count. Referral to the appropriate specialist is indicated, and immediate antibiotic therapy should be instituted.

Hypertensive Headache

A frequently occurring presentation at the ED is the patient with hypertensive headache.[5] Characteristically, the headache is worse on awakening and gradually improves throughout the day.[10] The diagnosis can be confirmed only with a diastolic blood pressure of 110 mm Hg or higher. The degree of elevation in blood pressure may or may not affect the severity of the headache. Typically, the hypertensive headache is bilateral; it usually occurs at the occiput. It also can involve the entire head. Patients will describe the pain as throbbing or "bursting" in nature and very severe. Tremors or palpitations and other symptoms of catecholamine release may occur.

Essential hypertension does not usually cause headache; however, headache due to increased blood pressure may be a manifestation of another disorder. A sudden increase in blood pressure due to acute nephritis or acute pressor reactions may produce a similar headache. Some of these patients may require imaging to rule out associated intracerebral bleeding.

Migraine

Between 4.5% and 20% of patients presenting to the ED with headache will have migraine.[5] The key to diagnosing the patient with migraine is the careful history, which is reviewed in Chapter 3. Distinguishing migraine from an acute life-threatening medical emergency is simplified with an accurate history and physical examination. The patient with migraine will consistently report a prior history of this type of headache. Usually, patients with an acute migraine will consult the emergency physician because of the severity of the headache as well as the associated gastrointestinal and neurological symptoms.

The neurological examination of these migraine patients is typically negative. However, the blood pressure may be elevated during an acute attack. The patient presenting with status migraine may appear dehydrated due to prolonged vomiting. Laboratory evaluation of serum electrolytes is indicated. Hospitalization may be indicated to stabilize the patient, initiate intravenous fluid replacement, and provide analgesia.

Complicated Migraine

The patient with complicated migraine may present at the ED because of the severity of the associated neurological symptoms. These symptoms are typified by hemiplegic migraine, manifested by hemiparesis, and ophthalmoplegic migraine, with defects of the third and, occasionally, fifth cranial nerve. Because of the severe nature of these symptoms, the patient consults the emergency physician. These symptoms often persist after the resolution of the headache attack. Owing to the difficulty in differential diagnosis of these conditions, the emergency physician should obtain a history of previous headaches before attempting to establish this diagnosis. CT scanning may be indicated, and a lumbar puncture may be considered if these symptoms persist.

Basilar Artery Migraine

Many patients with a specific form of complicated migraine, basilar artery migraine, are misdiagnosed in the ED. Basilar artery migraine is manifested by several neurological deficits that render diagnosis very difficult. The headache is characteristically severe and paroxysmal[13] and occurs predominantly in females during adolescence and the third decade. The diagnosis can be established by the presence of any three of the following symptoms: (1) bioccipital headache, (2) impairment or loss in the temporal and nasal fields of both eyes, (3) disturbed oculomotor function, such as diplopia or nystagmus, (4) dysarthria, (5) vertigo, (6) tinnitus or impaired hearing, (7) ataxia of gait, (8) bilateral paresis, (9) bilateral paresthesia, or (10) altered consciousness, such as amnesia, confusion, somnolence, stupor, or syncope.

Owing to this variety of symptoms, the patient with basilar artery migraine may be misdiagnosed with a mental disorder, brain tumor, or drug abuse. Differential diagnosis includes tumors of the posterior fossa, thrombosis of the basal artery or cerebral veins, cerebellar hemorrhage or infarction, drug intoxication, or metabolic disorders. It is essential that the emergency physician obtain a history of similar headaches in the patient or in the patient's family. Once the diagnosis is established, treatment with standard migraine prophylactic agents is recommended, and the patient should be referred for follow-up care.

Cluster Headache

Cluster headache is a form of vascular headache that is not as common as migraine. This type of headache is usually easy to differentiate from other headache conditions because of its characteristic presentation of severe, unilateral headache, typically localized around one eye. The emergency physician should be cognizant that cluster headaches are predominant among males and that the initial onset usually occurs between the third and fifth decades.

Cluster headache is personified by its episodic pattern, occurring in series usually lasting from 3 weeks to 3 months. During the series, the acute headache occurs several times per day and often awakens the patient in the first few hours after falling asleep. Characteristically, the acute cluster headache has a very limited duration. The headache may have been abated before the patient could arrive at the ED. However, the pain of cluster headache is extremely excruciating, and this patient may present at the ED in severe distress. The emergency physician should be aware that many patients with cluster headache have contemplated suicide during a cluster series because of the severity and regularity of the pain.

The emergency physician may note an increase in the number of patients with cluster headache visiting the ED during spring and fall. Cluster headaches have been described in detail in Chapter 7. A previous history of cluster headaches will help the physician establish the diagnosis. The associated symptoms of nasal congestion, rhinorrhea, ptosis, and conjunctival injection may confuse the examining physician, and acute sinusitis must be ruled out.

Tension-Type Headache

The patient with episodic tension-type (muscle contraction) headaches will usually obtain relief with over-the-counter analgesics and simple relaxation methods. Most patients with this type of headache experience the pain on an episodic basis; however, some patients report a daily, chronic headache. Because of the chronicity of these headaches, habituating analgesics must be avoided, particularly in the ED. The diagnosis and treatment of these headaches are detailed in Chapter 11. Many patients with chronic tension-type headaches have an underlying depression, as demonstrated by the presence of a sleep disturbance.[14] Narcotic analgesics, sedatives, and tranquilizers should be strictly avoided in all settings and particularly in the ED. At the ED, patients with chronic tension-type headaches require an appropriate referral to a physician or clinic familiar with the treatment of headache.

Emergency Treatment of Headache

Two steps are involved in the emergency treatment of headache: *initial stabilization* and *treatment*, which may be started immediately. Basic resuscitative measures should be undertaken with intravenous access and antibiotics if bacterial meningitis is suspected. The use of monitoring and oxygen therapy may be indicated. Pain relief is the goal of most patients who present with the chief complaint of headache. Establishing the diagnosis is essential before initiating treatment (Table 22–3).

For patients with an organic basis for their discomfort, appropriate referral is vital. In patients presenting with symptoms of SAH, admission to a neurosurgical intensive care unit is required, at which appropriate sedation, prophylaxis of seizures, and further evaluation can be provided. If meningitis is suspected, aggressive antibiotic treatment should be initiated as soon as possible. Although the results of cultures obtained via lumbar puncture may take several hours, treatment should be started without delay.

Admission is also indicated in patients with a suspected focal lesion to facilitate further evaluation of the etiology of the lesion. Neurosurgical consultation will probably be required. In the ED, the staff will attempt to decrease elevated intracranial pressure with measures that include hyperventilation, dexamethasone, diuretics, or a combination.

For patients presenting with hypertensive headaches without intracerebral pathology, treatment with either oral or intravenous agents may be used. At the ED, monitoring and establishment of intravenous access should be undertaken. Effective therapies include sublingual nifedipine, clonidine loading, and diuresis. The neurological status of the patient and other end-organ damage will affect the selection of the route of administration (parenteral, oral, or sublingual), as well as the need for rapid decrease in blood pressure. Most patients with hypertensive emergencies (i.e., end-organ damage) require admission.

Early diagnosis and prompt treatment with high doses of corticosteroids are essential in the patient with suspected temporal arteritis. Awaiting results of temporal artery biopsy should not preclude initiation of therapy. The urgency of treatment is due to the possibility of irreversible blindness associated with untreated temporal arteritis.

Narcotic and ergotamine abuse is frequent in patients with coexisting migraine and tension-type headaches. Because these patients experience recurrent migraine attacks, as well as a daily headache pattern, they require frequent analgesia and may become habitual visitors to the ED. Attempts must be made to provide appropriate, nonhabituating therapy to the headache patient and to refer the patient for adequate follow-up

Table 22–3 Differential Diagnosis of Headache

	SAH	Meningitis	TA	HTN	Migraine	Cluster	TT
Onset	Acute	Acute or chronic	Acute or chronic	Acute or chronic	Acute	Acute	Chronic
Location	Global	Global	Localized	Occipital frontal	Unilateral	Unilateral	Global unilateral
Associated symptoms	N, V, LOC, meningismus, focal neuro/SX	N, V, fever, photophobia, meningismus, focal SX, seizures	Weight loss, PMR, fever, decreased vision, jaw claudication	N, V, focal neuro SX	N, V, photophobia phonophobia	Rhinorrhea, lacrimation of ipsilateral side	Multisomatic C/O
Pain characteristics	Worst ever	Severe throbbing	Severe throbbing over area affected	Throbbing	Throbbing	Sharp, stabbing	Ache
Duration	Brief	Brief	Prolonged	Brief	Prolonged	30 min–2 hr	Daily
Prior history	(−)	(−)	(−)	(+)	(+)	(+)	(+)
Diagnostic test	CT 80–90%	LP(+)I CBC	WSR(+)	CT scan to R/O bleeding	–	–	–
PE	(+) Focal signs, + decreased LOC, + meningismus	Meningismus, decreased LOC, irritability, rash	Tender temporal arteries, myalgias, fever	Papilledema, decreased venous pulsations, decreased LOC, CV changes	Nausea, vomiting, photophobia, phonophobia	Unilateral rhinorrhea, lacrimation, partial Horner's syndrome	(−)

PE = Physical examination; N = nausea; V = vomiting; LOC = loss of consciousness; SX = symptoms; LP = lumbar puncture; PMR = polymyalgia rheumatica; WSR = Westergren sedimentation rate; CV = cerebrovascular; C/O = complaints; R/O = rule out; TA = temporal arteritis; HTN = hypertension; TT = tension-type headaches.

care to prevent recidivism and habituation problems.

There are many options for administering migraine abortive therapy in the ED[15] (Table 22–4). The introduction of the serotonin (5-HT) agonists has broadened the choices for this type of therapy.[16] For more than seven decades, ergotamine was used in migraine abortive therapy. Ergotamine can be administered in several forms: oral and rectal (combined with caffeine) and sublingual. Parenteral therapy can be accomplished with an ergotamine derivative, dihydroergotamine (DHE), which is also available in a nasal spray.

Sumatriptan also is available for parenteral, oral, and nasal administration. It should be determined before the administration of sumatriptan or other triptans if the patient has used an ergot or DHE before presenting at the ED. None of these agents should ever be used diagnostically. Unlike the ergotamine preparations, sumatriptan can be used at any time during an attack; of course, the introduction of the oral and nasal preparations of sumatriptan and the availability of other triptans (naratriptan, rizatriptan, and zolmitriptan) as oral preparations may preclude an ED visit.

At the ED, selection of the route of administration is especially influenced by the need for rapid analgesia. The emergency physician also should be cognizant that the effectiveness of the agent is dependent on the stage of the attack at which it is taken. Ideally, the abortive medication should be taken as early as possible in the attack. Ergotamine may not provide any relief if it is taken several hours into an acute headache; however, the triptans have demonstrated efficacy if used in the later stages of an acute migraine attack. Also, the emergency physician should be familiar with the use and restrictions of this therapy. A 4-day hiatus between days of use of ergotamine and DHE must be maintained to prevent the rebound phenomenon. At the ED, the migraine patient must be questioned about which agents and which doses have been used to relieve this particular migraine attack.

The phenothiazines have been used successfully in the ED for migraine abortive therapy, probably because of their dopaminergic and adrenergic actions. Due to the associated gastrointestinal symptoms, which are relieved by the phenothiazines such as chlorpromazine and prochlorperazine, these agents are often used in the ED. In a 1990 study, DHE was compared with two other agents, chlorpromazine and lidocaine, for treatment at the ED of migraine attacks.[17] Rectal prochlorperazine has also been suggested for acute migraine treatment in the ED, providing relief within 2 hours.[18] Metoclopramide has also demonstrated efficacy as a single-agent therapy for migraine in an ED because it relieved both the headache and the associated gastrointestinal symptoms. Metoclopramide and prochlorperazine, given intramuscularly, have been compared, but neither drug was recommended for single-agent therapy.[19] One investigation suggested the use of intravenous haloperidol for treatment of migraine in the ED.[20]

Table 22–4 Migraine Abortive Therapy in the Emergency Department

Agent	Dose	Route of Administration	Contraindications	Side Effects
Sumatriptan	6 mg	Subcutaneous	1. Coronary artery disease 2. ↑ Blood pressure 3. Concomitant use of ergotamine or other triptan	Flushing
Dihydroergotamine with antiemetic (metoclopramide) →	1 mg/mL 10 mg	Intravenous, subcutaneous, or intramuscular	1. Coronary artery disease 2. ↑ Blood pressure 3. Concomitant use of ergotamine or other triptan	1. Flushing 2. Diarrhea
Prochlorperazine	10 mg IM	Intramuscular	Dystonic	↓ Blood pressure
Chlorpromazine	1 mg/kg	Intramuscular	Dystonic	↓ Blood pressure
Ketorolac	30 mg	Intravenous	1. Peptic ulcer disease 2. Renal disease 3. Liver disease	Gastrointestinal complaints

It is important to remember that, on occasion, abortive treatments are contraindicated and/or have been maximized. Patients who have had these treatments will need appropriate rescue medications. For those patients requiring pain relief, a parenteral nonsteroidal anti-inflammatory drug, ketorolac, may provide benefit.[21] In a survey, narcotics were the most common therapy for migraine patients visiting an ED.[22] Butorphanol, which is available for transnasal administration, may be preferred to parenteral narcotic analgesics. Butorphanol is a synthetic mixed agonist-antagonist opioid analgesic. Because of its lipophilic nature, this agent has been used successfully in the transnasal preparation. The nasal mucosa are highly vascular, producing rapid intake and absorption of this agent.

Some migraine patients will experience a migraine attack that continues for longer than 24 hours. The treatment of choice for prolonged migraine attack is corticosteroid therapy. The protracted duration of these attacks is believed to be due to a sterile inflammation. The use of an agent such as long-acting dexamethasone (16 mg IM) or methylprednisolone (80 mg IM) may be effective.

Patients with unrelenting migraine that is refractory to therapy are diagnosed with status migraine. In addition to the severe pain of migraine, the associated symptoms may also be debilitating. After a prolonged attack lasting several days, the patient may become dehydrated and will need to be evaluated for fluid loss. Hospitalization may be indicated to initiate intravenous fluid replacement and monitor the serum electrolytes. In 1984, Raskin and Raskin[23] reported on their study of 55 patients with intractable migraine. Dihydroergotamine (0.5 mg IV) was administered with 10 mg of metoclopramide, in repetitive doses, every 8 hours for 2 days. Forty-nine patients were headache free after 48 hours. By using this type of therapy, the use of habituating analgesics, such as narcotics, will be avoided, and the sustained recovery of these patients may be achieved.

As stated previously, the use of narcotic analgesics should be avoided, if possible. The parenteral administration of these agents may be considered in the ED for migraine patients in severe pain. In addition to maintaining caution with these habituating agents, the ED staff must be aware of possible infection at the injection site.

Owing to the characteristic brief duration of cluster headache, patients with this problem are rare visitors to the ED. By the time the patient arrives at the ED, the acute headache has probably subsided. Occasionally, a cluster headache patient will seek treatment at the ED. The emergency physician should be cognizant that there is an approximate 75% success rate for these patients through the use of oxygen therapy, administered by mask at 8 to 10 L, for 10 to 15 minutes. Dihydroergotamine IV or other ergot preparations may also be used in treating acute cluster headaches. Kittrelle and co-workers[24] reported on the effective use of 4% lidocaine solution applied to the sphenopalatine fossa via nasal drops. Barre[25] reported on the successful use of cocaine hydrochloride, in a saline solution, administered in a similar method. Because of the severity of these headaches, narcotic analgesics may be administered in the ED setting. The self-limiting nature of episodic cluster headaches will minimize the risk of habituation.

As discussed, the patient with chronic tension-type headaches or coexisting migraine and tension-type headaches may be a frequent visitor to the ED. The chronicity of the headache as well as the apparent recidivism to conventional therapy may frustrate an ED staff and inhibit the patient from receiving appropriate therapy and referral for follow-up care. For patients being treated with antidepressants, the emergency physician should be cognizant of the drug interactions between the traditional tricyclics and the monoamine oxidase inhibitors. In a recent report, the serotonin syndrome was discussed for patients transitioning from phenelzine to venlafaxine.[26] The serotonin syndrome consists of a group of symptoms that are due to increased serotonin activity in the brain and include neuromuscular abnormalities, cognitive behavioral alterations, and autonomic nervous system instability. The patient may present as restless, agitated, with poor coordination, tremor, myoclonus, diarrhea, shivering, diaphoresis, fever, confusion, seizures, hypertension, arrhythmias, and coma. To prevent these symptoms from occurring, a 2-week drug hiatus is imperative before initiating the new antidepressant.

Chronic pain problems are impossible to manage in the ED setting and escalate the burdens of a crowded ED. Unfortunately, without adequate treatment, these patients are in danger of becoming part of a system that reinforces their habituation, and they will continue to be recurrent visitors to various practitioners and EDs.

Postpuncture Headache

In the ED, the physician may have the occasion to examine a patient who complains of headache following lumbar puncture. The probable cause of postdural puncture headache has been identified as continued leakage of cerebrospinal fluid (CSF) from the subarachnoid space following the procedure, resulting in traction on the intracranial vessels. These headaches can occur immediately after the lumbar puncture, but usually they appear from 24 to 48 hours after the procedure. Patients describe the headache as postural, with severe pain experienced when the patient assumes an upright position. Lying flat resolves the acute pain. Typically, the pain is located over the occipital area and may radiate to the neck, forehead, or behind the eyes. Headaches are often accompanied by nausea, blurred vision, and neck pain or stiffness.

The treatment of postdural puncture headaches has been a subject of much debate. Prevention is the major key to this form of headache, a factor that should be considered in the ED when performing a lumbar puncture. Some physicians have recommended bedrest for up to 24 hours following the procedure, but this is probably not helpful. The spinal needle diameter and its design have been considered major elements in the prevention of postpuncture headaches (e.g., the newer "atraumatic" needles).[27]

In the majority of postpuncture headache patients, the symptoms resolve spontaneously within 3 to 7 days with conservative treatment measures such as bedrest and oral analgesics and/or an abdominal binder as well as aggressive oral hydration. Antiemetics are indicated if the headache is associated with nausea. If the headache is moderate to severe, IV hydration may be required as well as analgesics and methylxanthines, such as caffeine or theophylline.[28] The definitive treatment for these headaches is an epidural blood patch, usually performed by the consultant anesthesiologist, in which 10 to 20 mL of autologous blood is injected into the epidural space to "patch" the dural tear.

References

1. Fodden DI, Peatfield RC, Milsom PL. Beware the patients with a headache in the accident and emergency department. Arch Emerg Med 1989;6:7–12.
2. Kaa KA, Carlson JA, Osterhaus JT. Emergency department resource use by patients with migraine and asthma in a health maintenance organization. Ann Pharmacother 1995;29:251–256.
3. Stang PE, Osterhaus JT, Celentano DD. Migraine: Patterns of healthcare use. Neurology 1994;44(suppl 4):S47–S55.
4. Leicht MJ. Non-traumatic headache in the emergency department. Ann Emerg Med 1980;9:404–409.
5. Dhopesh V, Anwar R, Herring C. A retrospective assessment of emergency department patients with complaint of headache. Headache 1979;19:37–42.
6. Johnson CE, Zimmerman RD. Decisions in the evaluation of headache. MRI Decisions 1989;2:16.
7. Fontanarosa PB. Recognition of subarachnoid hemorrhage. Ann Emerg Med 1988;18:1199–1205.
8. Wijdicks EF, Kerlhoff H, Van Gyn J. Long-term follow-up of 71 patients with thunderclap headache minimizing subarachnoid hemorrhage. Lancet 1988;2:68–70.
9. Little N. Acute head pain. Emerg Med Clin North Am 1987;4:687–698.
10. Lance JW. Mechanism and Management of Headache, 5th ed. Oxford: Butterworth-Heinemann; 1993.
11. Paulley JW, Hughes JP. Giant-cell arteritis, or arteritis of the aged. Br Med J 1960;2:1562.
12. Snyder H, Robinson K, Shah D, Brennan R, Handrigan M. Signs and symptoms of patients with brain tumors presenting to the emergency department. J Emerg Med 1993;11:253–258.
13. Bickerstaff ER. Basilar artery migraine. Lancet 1961;1:15–17.
14. Diamond S. Tension-type headaches. *In* Dalessio DJ, Silberstein S, eds. Wolff's Headache and Other Head Pain, 6th ed. New York: Oxford University Press; 1993:235–261.
15. Thomas SH, Stone CK. Emergency department treatment of migraine, tension, and mixed-type headache. J Emerg Med 1994;12:657–664.
16. Akpunonu BE, Mutgi AB, Federman DJ, et al. Subcutaneous sumatriptan for treatment of acute migraine in patients admitted to the emergency department: A multicenter study. Ann Emerg Med 1995;25:464–469.
17. Bell R, Montoya D, Shuaib A, Lee MA. A comparative trial of three agents in the treatment of acute migraine headache. Ann Emerg Med 1990;19:1079–1082.
18. Jones EB, Gonzalez ER, Boggs JG, Grillo JA,

Elswick RK Jr. Safety and efficacy of rectal prochlorperazine for the treatment of migraine in the emergency department. Ann Emerg Med 1994;24:237–241.
19. Jones J, Pack S, Chun E. Intramuscular prochlorperazine versus metoclopramide as single-agent therapy for the treatment of acute migraine headache. Am J Emerg Med 1996;14:262–265.
20. Fisher H. A new approach to emergency department therapy of migraine headache with intravenous haloperidol: A case series. J Emerg Med 1995;13:119–122.
21. Davis CP, Torre PR, Schafer NC, Dave B, Bass B Jr. Ketorolac as a rapid and effective treatment of migraine headache: Evaluations by patients. Am J Emerg Med 1993;11:573–575.
22. Barton CW. Evaluation and treatment of headache patients in the emergency department: A survey. Headache 1994;33:91–94.
23. Raskin NH, Raskin KE. Repetitive intravenous dihydroergotamine for the treatment of intractable migraine. Neurology 1984;34:245.
24. Kittrelle JP, Grouse DS, Seybold ME. Cluster headache, local anesthetic abortive agents. Arch Neurol 1985;42:496–498.
25. Barre F. Cocaine as an abortive agent in cluster headache. Headache 1982;22:69–73.
26. Diamond S, Pepper BJ, Diamond ML, et al. Serotonin syndrome induced by transitioning from phenelzine to venlafaxine: Four patient reports. Neurology 1998;51:274–276.
27. McConaha C, Bastiani AM, Kaye WH. Significant reduction of post-lumbar puncture headaches by the use of a 29-gauge spinal needle. Biol Psychiatry 1996;39:1058–1060.
28. Leibord RA, Yealy DM, Coppola M, Cantees KK. Post-dural-puncture headache: Characteristics, management, and prevention. Ann Emerg Med 1993;22:1863–1870.

23

Headache Clinics and Inpatient Treatment Units for Headache

Frederick G. Freitag, D.O.

Historical Perspective

In 1945, the first hospital-affiliated headache clinic in the United States was established at Montefiore Hospital.[1] Approximately 20 years later, Seymour Diamond established the Diamond Headache Clinic as the first private headache clinic in the United States. The development of this clinic was fostered by Diamond's recognition of the prevalence of individuals from within his practice who experienced problems with their headaches and required specialized treatments to provide relief. The establishment and growth of this clinic fostered the interest in the development of a large number of practices throughout the United States at which patients could receive specialized care.

This growth of specialized headache treatment programs paralleled the growth and development of other pain treatment programs, at which headaches were treated in addition to a wide variety of other chronic pain states. In some cases, the chronic pain programs focused on specific, isolated modalities such as behavioral approaches or local anesthetic management with nerve blocks and eschewed the role of medical therapies. Many of these pain programs were also developed with a focused plan of inpatient management.

By the 1980s, it was apparent that select headache patients required more treatment than could be offered on an outpatient basis, even within the confines of a specialized headache practice. For these selected patients, programs evolved that combined the medical expertise of the outpatient headache programs and advanced to the levels of more aggressive medical intervention. These programs also involved other modalities, such as the behavioral approach. In 1983, the largest comprehensive inpatient headache treatment program was opened in conjunction with the Diamond Headache Clinic at Weiss Memorial Hospital, an affiliate of the University of Chicago Hospitals. The 35-bed inpatient facility was moved in October 1993 to Columbus Hospital, a member of Catholic Health Partners. During the remainder of the decade, these inpatient programs expanded to other areas of the country.

The growth of managed care programs will certainly continue to have an impact on the medical care of the patient with headache. In a study conducted at a managed care organization, patients with migraine generated nearly twice as many medical claims as other group patients, and their pharmacy claims were almost 2.5 times those of other groups.[2] Compared with other patients, the migraineurs used more emergency medical services. Many headache centers are exploring alternative approaches to the management of the patient with headache problems; the goal is to provide not only appropriate care for the patient but also a reduction in patient utilization of health care facilities and medications in addition to cost-effective provision of comprehensive services.

Reasons for Referral to a Headache Clinic

The reasons for referral to a headache clinic are varied, and the perspective differs for the referring physician, patient, and headache specialist. Blau and MacGregor[3] found marked differences among these three groups (Table 23–1). According to their study, the

Table 23–1 Three Perspectives on the Role of Referral to the Headache Specialist

Primary Care Physician	Patient	Headache Specialist
Failure to respond	Increased headache frequency	Headache in addition to migraine
Patient request	Knowledge deficit	Reassurance
Diagnostic question	Disability	

referring physician usually requests the consultation for one of three reasons: (1) the patient's failure to respond to treatment, (2) a request by the patient, and (3) uncertainty on the physician's part of the diagnosis.

The patient's perspective differs significantly. Their reasons for consultation are (1) increasing frequency of headaches, (2) attainment of greater understanding of his or her headache disorder, and (3) increasing disability related to the headache and absences from work or school. The headache specialist's outlook overlaps those of the referring physician and the patient. The specialist believes that the occurrences of headaches and the need to provide reassurance of underlying patient fears are the two primary reasons for consultation.

Patients with the complaint of headache consult a variety of specialists. The primary care specialties of family medicine, internal medicine, pediatrics, and gynecology are among the foremost in providing care for patients with headache; however, specialized areas of practice are also commonly used by patients seeking relief from their headaches. Neurologists constitute the majority of the specialists who are consulted for headache management. Patients also seek care from ophthalmologists, otorhinolaryngologists, allergists, and psychiatrists. Some patients confer with those in alternative branches of health care, including chiropractic, behavioral medicine, and homeopathy.

The primary physician is usually able to adequately address the complaint and provide a mutually satisfactory outcome of the condition. However, substantial numbers of patients are not helped by physicians who are not experienced with complicated headache problems. Table 23–2 provides reasons patients are referred to a specialized headache facility.

The use of the various classifications for headaches as well as the patient's history and examination facilitates establishment of the diagnosis and appropriate selection of a treatment program. At times, however, the patient's description of the headache does not coincide with typical patterns and impedes determination of the diagnosis. Other patients, such as those with coexisting migraine and tension-type headaches, may focus on one component of their headaches and not consider other relevant aspects. The severity of migraine headaches and associated symptoms may cause the patient to ignore or minimize the occurrence of the daily or almost daily tension-type headaches. It is possible that the tension-type headaches do not interfere with the patient's daily activities and the acute headaches may respond to over-the-counter analgesics. Some patients with cluster headaches complain of significant nasal congestion and rhinorrhea; these symptoms may confuse a physician who is not experienced with the presentation of cluster headache. This scenario may be further distorted by the seasonal aspects of cluster headache and responses to sympathomimetic agents.

Despite an accurate diagnosis, some patients fail on therapies considered the "drug of choice" for a specific condition. This failure may result from insufficient doses, inadequate therapeutic trials on the drug, managed care formulary-mandated decisions, and patient refractoriness to therapy.

Referral to a specialized headache center may be related to the patient's perspective. Some patients who have responded to the drugs of choice demonstrate an increasing tolerance to standard agents. This situation prompts the use of increasingly higher doses to maintain the response and may occur with

Table 23–2 Reasons for Referral to a Headache Clinic

The history and physical examination do not establish a working diagnosis (e.g., mixed-headache syndromes, cluster headaches).
Patient is refractory to conventional treatment.
Patient has an increasing tolerance to treatment.
Concomitant medical conditions necessitate special care (e.g., headaches combined as well as hypertension, asthma, coronary artery disease, diabetes).
The patient has dependencies on 5-hydroxytryptamine agonists, narcotics, barbiturates, or tranquilizers for relief of pain.
Pyschological and psychiatric problems necessitate a comprehensive approach.
Headaches have an economic impact.

both prophylactic regimens and abortive agents for acute headaches. In some patients, the increasing tolerance may occur independent of dependency issues or from *rebound headache.* The patient who has previously responded to therapeutic agents at the low end of the therapeutic range may now require doses at the high end.

Some patients with headache problems present with concomitant medical conditions that affect the selection of appropriate therapeutic agents. The frequency of this situation is quite substantial, as demonstrated in a 1995 study.[4] In this study of 846 patients with migraine and matched control subjects, comorbid medical disease was substantially more prevalent among migraine patients than among the controls. Slightly more than one half of the control group had one or more comorbid medical diseases, and nearly three fourths of the migraine patients reported one or more comorbid medical diseases. In an earlier study at a managed care organization,[2] comorbid conditions were the cause of significant costs within the migraine patients. This high prevalence of comorbidity raises significant issues related to the establishment of therapeutic regimens that consider these concomitant and sometimes therapeutically conflicting situations. Medical regimens for the treatment of chronic respiratory and cardiovascular disorders not only may include agents with the potential to exacerbate the headache problem but also may preclude the use of more standard headache agents. In certain disorders of the gastrointestinal and renal systems, the treatment of headaches may induce or exacerbate disorders of these systems, such as peptic ulcer disease or renal insufficiency.

A major referral aspect involves dependency on medications used for acute headache pain and rebound headache phenomen. Often the patient's headache frequency escalates from the repetitive use of acute headache agents until the patient has a daily headache that characteristically responds only to the overused medication. The occurrence of rebound headaches has been linked to abortive migraine therapy with the 5-hydroxytryptamine agonists, from ergotamine through sumatriptan. Rebound headaches have also been observed with the use of prescription analgesics containing opiates and barbiturates. Caffeine, in both prescription and over-the-counter analgesics, is particularly noted for rebound headaches if the combined dietary and medication amounts of this substance exceed 200 to 300 mg/day. Dependence on prescription analgesics containing narcotics, barbiturates, or minor tranquilizers is another major referral factor. In addition to the occurrence of rebound headaches, other signs and symptoms of physical addiction may be demonstrated. The physician may become entrapped in a vicious cycle with the habituated patient; Dalessio[5] cited a number of "headache games" that may play contributory roles in this process. These analgesic-related problems may occur within specialized headache centers[6]; Oates et al found that, despite patient and staff education and adequate treatment provided in a specialized center, 17% of the patients continued to use analgesics prescribed by other physicians and 22% continued to use over-the-counter analgesics beyond their prescribed medications. Unfortunately, for many patients, the initiation of prophylactic treatment without termination of the offending agent is unsuccessful.

The presence of psychological problems and psychiatric conditions in a patient with headache may prompt referral to a headache clinic, facilitating a comprehensive medical approach with psychotherapeutic evaluation and treatment. Patients refractory to therapy often present with the headache as the predominating focus of their life. It may also serve as an integral component of their family situation. The preoccupation with pain (headache) frequently leads to a complex emotional situation with the patient being angry and resentful of family, friends, and coworkers because of the headache and the failure of others to be able to comprehend and accept the headaches. The patient's family and friends may be resentful because of the impact the headache has on daily activities, as well as social and business commitments. Increasing isolation of the headache patient and an escalation of the emotional response may result. Depression is a frequent component of the emotional situation that inhibits the appropriate responsiveness of the patient.

Finally, the financial burden of headaches on worker productivity may prompt referral to a headache clinic. In a survey,[7] the impact of migraine on productivity was substantial. Among men, an estimated 2.7 million annual workdays were worked at less than full productivity because of migraine headaches. The number significantly increased to 18.8 million days of decreased productivity within 1 year among women in the work force. In homemakers, 38.5 million days were lost owing to decreased productivity from migraine. The impact on the economy from lost workdays and decreased productivity alone accounted for nearly $115.6 million per month.

Treatment received at a specialized headache center has been demonstrated to have a positive impact on these economic factors[8]; in this report, the investigators demonstrated that workdays missed among the studied patients declined by 75% from a mean of 5.24 days per month, and the number of workdays with decreased productivity fell 51% to 5.89 days per month.

Organization of a Headache Clinic

Outpatient programs dedicated to the treatment of headaches have characteristics that distinguish them from other types of clinical practices. The patient with headache presents with different needs and expectations than those presenting in a general medical practice and, in some cases, those with other chronic pain conditions. The patient with chronic pain requires a multidisciplinary approach to treatment. The medical, physical, social, and psychological aspects of his or her pain problem must be addressed on a continuing basis. The complexity of this approach is time consuming and intensive on its demands on the staff. Typically, general medical practices are not structured for these rigorous services. In one study,[9] it was demonstrated that the office environment and personnel must be predisposed to dealing with these types of patients and their treatment needs. Patient satisfaction with the sophistication and depth of evaluation correlated with outcome measures of headache frequency, duration, and severity. Patients who were satisfied with their evaluation demonstrated statistically significant decreases in severity and duration of their headaches at 1 year after the evaluation. It was found that a variety of factors influence the likelihood of follow-up care at a headache treatment program[10] (Table 23–3). Approximately 40% of patients failed to return or continue follow-up treatment after an initial visit. Factors that played a role in failure of patient return for follow-up at a specialized headache center included professional fees that were excessive and not covered by managed care, excessive waiting time, relationship with the assigned physician, and inability to achieve a positive response after the first visit.

Table 23–3 Factors Influencing Follow-up Care

Managed care coverage of professional fees
Waiting time
Patient-physician relationship
Degree of improvement after a single visit

In a specialized headache center, physician availability and scheduling flexibility are increasingly necessary. Patients may have schedules that prevent them from missing time from work to address their ongoing medical needs. Patient access to the physician and adjunctive health care staff is essential to address concerns and questions regarding interim treatment. Managed care contracts are placing limitations on the number of patient follow-up visits, thus requiring alternative approaches of communication between the patient and staff to ensure continuity of care. The complexity of the health care insurance field has lead to increasing demands on clerical personnel to monitor and assist the patient and physician in the financial aspects of treatment; this is observed particularly in referral patterns within the management care environment.

Nurse practitioners trained specifically to deal with patients with headache are of significant benefit in the successful outcome of treatment for both the physician and patient. Their skill and expertise in obtaining headache histories and their knowledge of the various treatment approaches and problems can provide a more relaxed atmosphere for the patient. The nurse's firm understanding of patient expectations and potential problems as well as provision of patient education can have an enormous impact on the treatment outcome. The nurse's perspective may also help identify additional factors that will assist the physician in selecting and implementing the optimal treatment for individual patients.

Evaluation of the Patient

Patients presenting to a headache clinic usually report previous care by other health care practitioners. The failure to obtain adequate relief for their headaches has, in the least, caused the patient to feel frustrated and hopeless. An understanding and caring approach to these patients will be beneficial. At times, a period of successful therapy may be needed to provide the patient with some hope of success and underscores the importance of the evaluation and treatment of the patient with headache as an ongoing process. Too often, previous treatment has consisted of a primary care physician with one-time consultations with various specialists. This process may be successful in the patient with a simple headache problem, although it is not the case with the typical patient presenting to a specialized headache clinic. Ongoing management of the headache problem by a physician at the headache clinic is needed for an optimal outcome.

The first step in the evaluation process of the headache patient is a comprehensive history[11, 12] and examination. The headache history, with the medical and surgical history, must be considered particularly owing to the high level of comorbid disease in patients with headaches, as previously noted. Assessment of headache triggers should be included. Previous diagnostic studies should be itemized, including personal review of the radiographs, computed tomography (CT) scans, and magnetic resonance imaging (MRI) films with a neuroradiologist. Factors concerning the patient's work, recreational habits, and diet should also be determined. Typical aspects of the patient's social history should be sought to identify factors that may have an impact on the headache and treatment, although these issues may be considered unimportant by the patient.

Additional diagnostic studies may be needed as part of the patient's evaluation. Medical disorders such as endocrinopathies, including hyperprolactinemic states and thyroid disease, are regularly discovered as contributing factors in patients with intractable headache. Abnormal MRI findings are often demonstrated in patients with migraine[13]; an MRI may be indicated in these patients, despite a recently performed CT scan. The MRI should be performed both with and without gadolinium enhancement and should include careful views of the posterior fossa, especially in patients with symptoms indicative of vertebrobasilar systems or a history of significant head and neck trauma.

The maintenance of ongoing headache calendars can provide valuable insights into the nature of the patient's headache complaint, especially in patients with coexisting migraine and tension-type headaches. Two patterns are typically demonstrated in these calendars: (1) the presence of daily tension-type headaches in patients who revealed only migraine at their first evaluation and (2) the differentiation between migraine and tension-type headache when the patient experiences daily headaches. In some cases, the patterns of triggering events are evident, thus providing the patient with ongoing guidance for prevention of his or her headaches. Changes in the headache pattern and response to acute therapies can be monitored in a more objective fashion with these calendars. In patients with coexisting migraine and tension-type headache, the calendar may reveal improvements in the response to acute therapies with decreasing headache duration before a reduction in the frequency of the headaches has been observed.

As part of the evaluation process, it may be necessary to determine whether treatment will be initiated on an outpatient basis or as an inpatient treatment program. The factors that are assessed in making this evaluation include the patient's pain and responsiveness to analgesics or acute abortive therapies. The patient who is dependent on analgesics or having rebound headaches due to overuse of abortive therapies may require an inpatient treatment setting. A review of the patient's history of treatment should include an assessment of the patient's responsiveness to attempts to control the headaches. If limited trials for both acute and prophylactic agents have been undertaken, the patient may be successful only with outpatient treatment. Accordingly, the assessment of previous therapies should include the appropriateness of the medications used, dosages, duration of the specific treatment, and the patient's ability to tolerate the therapy in consideration of adverse effects. For the patient with a difficult headache situation, certain factors, including social and psychological issues, can predispose the patient to failure if treatment is initiated in an outpatient setting.

Beyond the social and psychological issues that must be considered in this evaluation, comorbid medical and psychiatric diseases are commonly demonstrated in patients with headache. The multiplicity of disorders often requires close management by a variety of physician specialities to optimize the overall state of health of the patient. In patients who have previously been refractory to acute and possibly prophylactic agents, consideration should be given to dependency issues and the role of drug-induced rebound headaches. If this unresponsiveness has played a role in the patient's headache situation, it may be necessary to evaluate the level of toxicity the patient is experiencing from these therapies. The patient's ability to cope with the headache during the transition period should also be assessed when limited acute treatment success may occur on an outpatient basis.

Treatment in the Outpatient Setting

In the outpatient setting, the patient with the difficult headache problem may require a complex therapeutic regimen. The majority of patients will receive an individualized program of specific pharmacological agents for both prophylactic and abortive therapy, as well as pain relief measures. The agents used in the pharmacological treatment of the various headache disorders have been described in previous chapters. In addition to obtaining patient data, assessing treatment response, and documenting ongoing care, the nursing staff may provide significant help in educating the headache patient. Working in conjunction with the physician, the nurses may obtain a more detailed review of potential side effects of medications and can reinforce compliance with the scheduled medications, thus minimizing adverse reactions and medication abuse.

The identification of lifestyle factors that may contribute to headaches must also be addressed. Diet, sleep habits, and life stressors can be reviewed at the initial consultation as well as at follow-up visits. Patient education is essential in the recognition of these headache triggers. Biofeedback training may also be considered for many patients (see Chapter 20).

The importance of interdisciplinary care in the outpatient venue has been demonstrated by Sharff and Marcus[14]; they reported that 71% of patients participating in a multidisciplinary treatment program had a positive outcome. In comparison, only 26% of those electing to pursue a more limited scope of treatment reported improvement.

In many cases, appropriate multidisciplinary measures can minimize the need for inpatient hospitalization. With adequate facilities for the acute and comfortable care of the patient, certain outpatient centers are developing techniques for expanded levels of outpatient acute care that will preclude admission to an inpatient environment.

Treatment in an Inpatient Setting

Although headache therapy often can be instituted on an outpatient basis, approximately one third of all patients referred to the Diamond Headache Clinic are refractory to attempts to establish treatment in an outpatient milieu. The complexities of some treatment regimens and complicating concomitant medical problems often are contraindications to initiation of treatment in an outpatient setting.

Seven major factors have been identified in determining the indication for treatment in an outpatient versus an inpatient setting (Table 23–4). These factors include the degree and intractability of the patient's pain. Previous response to therapies, usually effective in headaches, must be evaluated according to the patient's experience. As noted, the high incidence of comorbid medical conditions often prompts admission to the inpatient setting to initiate therapy and provide supportive medical therapy. Acute therapies for headaches may produce dependency problems and toxicity, and careful monitoring is facilitated in the inpatient setting. Psychological issues also play a role in the initiation of therapy, and inpatient admission can expedite evaluation of the patient's psychological health and coping strategies.

The use of an inpatient setting for the treatment of chronic headache disorders is a relatively new concept. In Seattle, Fordyce et al[15, 16] pioneered the concept of an inpatient pain unit. A variety of health care professionals and practitioners from other disciplines have further refined this concept.

Table 23–4 Factors Involving Outpatient Versus Inpatient Treatment

Degree and intractability of pain
Refractoriness to established regimens
Need for supportive medical measures
Degree of toxicity and drug dependence
Coping ability
Psychological health considerations
Comorbid medical disease considerations

Table 23–5 Treatment Methods

Detoxification
Pharmacological therapy
Biofeedback
Group psychotherapy
Nursing intervention
Stress management
Physical therapy
Exercise programs
Dietary management and education
Interactions between patients
Lifestyle management
Discharge planning

The use of an inpatient pain specialty assessment and treatment unit may result in improved long-term results compared with alternative treatment programs. Williams et al[17] demonstrated in a controlled clinical trial that patients who were initially treated on an inpatient basis had greater improvement in their pain, were able to maintain control of the pain more effectively over 1 year, and used overall health care services less than patients matched for type, severity, and duration of pain who were treated on an outpatient basis.

With the trend of escalating health care costs, increasing emphasis has been placed on outpatient treatment for a variety of medical problems, including headaches. Inpatient care, compared with outpatient treatment, is more costly for the patient, employer, and insurance industry; nevertheless, hospitalization is indicated for those patients who have failed to respond to outpatient therapy. These patients may demonstrate greater success with inpatient therapy followed by careful outpatient follow-up.[18] Table 23–5 itemizes the types of therapeutic modalities used at the inpatient unit.

Patient selection for admission to the headache unit must adhere to strict criteria (Table 23–6). Certain requirements have been established, and one or more must be met before a patient is admitted to the unit. Some patients complain of intractable pain, despite having received medication at their initial visit with the physician. In most of these cases, pain relief is of short duration or incomplete. These patients may benefit from a change in analgesics or the initiation of prophylactic medications on a routine basis to reduce the frequency or severity of their headaches. The patient who has been using large quantities of over-the-counter analgesics containing caffeine and other sympathomimetic drugs on a daily basis may require hospitalization. According to a survey of 473 physicians who treat patients with headache,[19] between 30% and 60% of patients required inpatient treatment for withdrawal of medication.

A large number of medical conditions may complicate the treatment of headaches. As noted previously, migraine sufferers are more likely than the general population to experience one or several concomitant medical problems. Concomitant psychological and psychiatric conditions may occur up to 25 times more frequently in migraine patients than in the general population.[20] A thorough history and careful physical evaluation may indicate the need for inpatient treatment to achieve the required balance in treating the headache and concomitant medical problems. If the headache unit has been established in a large hospital, consultations with other spe-

Table 23–6 Criteria for Admission to Inpatient Headache Unit

Prolonged, unrelenting headache with associated symptoms, such as nausea and vomiting that, if allowed to continue, would pose a further threat to the patient's welfare
Status migraine
Dependence on analgesics, caffeine, narcotics, barbiturates, and/or tranquilizers
Habituation to ergots; if taken on a daily basis, ergots cause a rebound headache when stopped.
Pain that is accompanied by serious adverse reactions or complications from therapy; continued use of such therapy aggravates or induces further illness
Pain that occurs in the presence of significant medical disease; appropriate treatment of headache symptoms aggravates or induces further disease
Chronic cluster headache that is unresponsive to treatment
Treatment requiring copharmacy with drugs that may cause a drug interaction and necessitating careful observation within a hospital environment (monoamine oxidase inhibitors and β-blockers)
Patients with probable organic cause of their headache requiring appropriate consultations and perhaps neurosurgical interventions
Severe intractable pain in the presence of dehydration, electrolyte loss, or prostration
Severe pain in association with severe psychiatric disease
Pain necessitating frequent parenteral medications

cialists, if warranted, is facilitated. Neurosurgical consultations of organic lesions can be achieved easily. A cooperative effort among staff members ensures optimal and continuous care of the hospitalized patient.

The majority of patients requiring admission to the inpatient unit are consuming excessive quantities of analgesics or ergot preparations. The issues involved in withdrawing patients from these medications are described below.

Detoxification

The primary goal of the inpatient headache treatment program is to control the patient's pain. As with every aspect of the program, a multidisciplinary approach to pain control is undertaken, with the first step being detoxification. Medication withdrawal generally begins during the first week of treatment while the previous analgesic medications are discontinued, including narcotics, barbiturates, caffeine, and benzodiazepines. Careful observation of the patient is required during detoxification to identify withdrawal symptoms with potentially serious consequences.

The method of discontinuation of the habituating drug is selected after consideration of the agent dosage, signs of tolerance, and setting in which withdrawal will occur. For patients on high doses of narcotics, barbiturates, or benzodiazepines or those who show signs of tolerance, the only safe method of drug discontinuation may be a gradual withdrawal. However, for the average patient who has been using moderate amounts of these agents, abrupt cessation of the offending agent may be safely accomplished at the inpatient unit, where adequate precautions for the management of withdrawal symptoms are established.

The most typical signs and symptoms of withdrawal from opiates include sweating, yawning, tearing, rhinorrhea, tremor, muscle twitching, aching, muscle pain, irritability, mydriasis, and increased respiratory rate. These symptoms occur during the first 24 hours and are followed during the next 2 days by tachycardia, hypertension, nausea, vomiting, insomnia, and abdominal cramps. As the process associated with detoxification subsides over 5 to 10 days, only symptomatic treatment will be required. However, specific treatment may be indicated depending on the symptoms and severity. Withdrawal symptoms also occur with termination of narcotics, such as codeine and pentazocine, that are generally considered safe with minimal habituation tendencies.

Barbiturate habituation frequently occurs in headache patients who use one of several prescription analgesics that contain short-acting barbiturates. Withdrawal from these medications is frequently prolonged, and observation of the patient during the course of several weeks may be necessary. The typical signs and symptoms of barbiturate withdrawal include anxiety, insomnia, hyperpyrexia, diaphoresis, nausea, vomiting, tachycardia, tachypnea, and fever. Severe withdrawal symptoms from high doses of barbiturates may induce delirium and convulsive states, including grand mal seizures. Excessive amounts of caffeine, a common additive in both over-the-counter and prescription analgesics, produce withdrawal symptoms such as rebound vascular headaches, grogginess, malaise, rhinorrhea, nausea, and depression.

In evaluation of the patient presenting for inpatient treatment, the current headache must be assessed to determine whether it is only related to analgesic or ergotamine dependency or a prolonged migraine attack is the cause. If the patient is experiencing a protracted migraine attack, the use of therapies aimed at controlling the acute migraine attacks must be reviewed, and therapy for managing the rebound attacks must be instituted. However, if the patient's history reveals overuse of ergotamine, dihydroergotamine (DHE), or sumatriptan, standard interventions such as intravenous DHE may be precluded. The continued use of a serotonin agonist, such as DHE, may only relieve the headache as it is related to the rebound phenomenon. Once DHE is discontinued, the rebound process starts anew and results in prolongation of the process of withdrawal and recovery. In the patient with a protracted migraine that has been complicated by the overuse of serotonin agonists, we find that the administration of parenteral corticosteroids, such as 16 mg of long-acting dexamethasone either alone or with repository corticotropin (ACTH), may be advantageous in terminating the prolonged migraine component, thus allowing the rebound headache to be managed. In rare cases, additional oral or parenteral corticosteroids may be used.

If the patient is not dependent on serotonin agonists and status migraine is evident at admission, the use of intravenous DHE according to the Raskin protocol[21] may be helpful in initiating rapid control of the headaches. Use of this technique for more than 1 or 2 days is not considered safe for outpatient use.[22] This mechanism appears to be related to the control of the acute migraine process, although the majority of severe headaches result from withdrawal. Although this process may not fully eliminate the withdrawal headache, it may provide sufficient reduction in the headache to minimize the need for adjunctive analgesics and phenothiazines.

At our unit, we have modified the Raskin protocol for the use of intravenous DHE according to the individual patient's needs (Table 23–7); variations include the administration of DHE in an intravenous solution over a brief period of time, usually ranging from 30 to 60 minutes. This adaptation may reduce the adverse effect profile of DHE, which includes pain at the infusion site, chest discomfort, and blood pressure changes. In addition, we rarely find it necessary to concomitantly administer intravenous metoclopramide; the vast majority of patients require only trimethobenzamide HCl (intramuscularly or orally). However, some patients may need more potent agents, such as metoclopramide or promethazine HCl.

In managing patients during withdrawal from a variety of analgesics, it has been our experience that the use of a phenothiazine, especially promethazine, is most advantageous. The phenothiazines act, in part, by blocking the 5-hydroxytryptamine$_3$ receptors and provide analgesia by blocking pain transmission. Promethazine has a fairly comparable sedation profile and may also induce hypotension as well as orthostatic changes in the patient. The major advantage to the use of promethazine is the decreased potential for akathisia or other movement disorders. Promethazine, unlike other phenothiazines, has the ability to control vomiting. Most adults can tolerate 100 mg promethazine intramuscularly every 6 hours. Some patients require dosage adjustment for efficacy or improved tolerance. In patients unresponsive to a phenothiazine or patients in whom phenothiazines are contraindicated, the use of a benzodiazepine with a short half-life may be beneficial.

Routine dosing of the analgesic-dependent patient with a nonhabituating agent, such as ketorolac given on a timed basis, may be helpful during the withdrawal process. The use of a fixed schedule for administration rather than an as-needed basis appears to provide better analgesia results according to a variety of studies that examined the management of chronic pain.

In rare cases, a patient may be consuming large quantities of narcotics to control the headache pain. For some patients, clonidine has been used successfully in opiate withdrawal, and it can be used in adjunct with other techniques. Although clonidine has on occasion been reported to be helpful for migraine prophylaxis, it is not beneficial for refractory patients who have become dependent on pain medications.

During withdrawal, some patients who have taken large quantities of narcotics or barbiturates may require the use of adjunctive narcotics or long-acting barbiturates. A thorough, daily assessment of the patient is essential to determine the need for adjunctive opiates and barbiturates. Although there is no reliable method of determining the specific

Table 23–7 Diamond Headache Inpatient Treatment Unit Protocol for Intravenous DHE-45

Establish intravenous access.
Premedicate the patient with choice of:
- Trimethobenzamide (200 mg IM)
- Trimethobenzamide (250 mg PO)
- Metoclopramide (10 mg IM)
- Metoclopramide (10 mg PO)
- Promethazine (50 mg IM)
- Promethazine (50 mg PO)

At 30 minutes after parenteral or 1 hour after oral administration of above, administer dihydroergotamine (DHE) (0.5 mg by slow IV push).
Vital signs should be monitored and adverse effects assessed before dose and for 30 minutes after the dose.
Subsequent doses should be given every 8 hours for a total of nine doses.
Doses 2 through 9 are for 1 mg DHE.
Steps 2 through 4 are repeated with each dose.
Adverse events may be reduced by dilution of DHE in 50 mL of normal saline and administration as intravenous drip over 30 minutes.

amounts of adjunctive opiates and barbiturates that are required, clinical observation has indicated the equivalent dose of parenteral meperidine is more than 500 mg/day. Methadone given intramuscularly is generally used to avoid prescribing the habituating agent.

Patients consuming excessive quantities of barbiturate-containing analgesics may experience analgesic withdrawal and seizures. Precautions must be undertaken when withdrawing patients who use more than six tablets per day because they may experience seizure phenomena. The use of a benzodiazepine as a substitute for a phenothiazine may reduce the potential for serious withdrawal effects; unlike phenothiazines, benzodiazepines do not reduce the seizure threshold. If the dosage is in excess of 10 tablets per day, management protocol may include a sequence of a long-acting barbiturate, such as phenobarbital, tapered over an interval lasting from days to months. If seizures occur in a patient withdrawing from barbiturate analgesics, a prolonged course tapering the phenobarbital should be started.

Some patients with chronic cluster headaches do not respond to standard methods of treatment and require a course of intravenous histamine desensitization. Histamine desensitization was first proposed by Horton et al[23] and reportedly shortened cluster periods in 95% of the patients in their series. The series reported by Kunkle et al[24] was not favorable, but it should be noted that 11 in this group received a series of histamine injections, which had been given previously and had been reported to have no significant benefit. Antihistaminic drugs were of no dependable value in the three patients who had used them.

At the Diamond Headache Clinic, we reported on the efficacy of intravenous histamine therapy for intractable cluster headaches.[25] The study was performed on both a retrospective and prospective basis. The study involved 150 patients (127 men and 23 women) who had previously received intravenous histamine therapy. Headache-evaluable parameters included headache frequency per day, duration of attacks, severity, and presence of associated symptoms. Evaluation was performed before and after histamine therapy. In 64% of patients, histamine desensitization therapy was effective in preventing or reducing the frequency of attacks by more than 50%. Duration was improved in 39%, and severity was improved in 77%. Associated symptoms improved in 45% ($P<.05$). Because of these results, we concluded that intravenous histamine therapy is an effective treatment for intractable chronic cluster headaches, although the technique is not appropriate for all patients with these headaches. Table 23–8 describes the protocol used at the Diamond Inpatient Headache Unit.

Individualized Therapy

Therapy for the hospitalized patient is individualized on the basis of diagnosis and previous response to therapy. The medication used for relief of acute headaches may not be a simple non-narcotic analgesic, an ergot, or a related drug; however, strict limits on intake and total consumption should be emphasized. The agents and methods used in the treatment of the various headache conditions have been discussed in previous chapters.

Rapid transitions in medical therapies are sometimes initiated to reduce the length of

Table 23–8 Histamine Desensitization Protocol

Twenty-one bags should contain histamine phosphate in 250 mL of normal saline or dextrose in water.
The first bag contains 2.75 mg of histamine phosphate.
Bags 2 through 21 contain 5.5 mg of histamine phosphate.
On the first hospital day, give only 1 bag of histamine phosphate solution.
On the second and succeeding days, give histamine phosphate at titrated rates of infusion based on occurrence of cluster headache and drug tolerance.
Initial infusion rate is 10 drops/min.
Infusion rate may be titrated upward every 15 to 30 minutes in increments of 10 drops/min.
Occurrence of a cluster headache while receiving an infusion should be followed by an immediate decrease in the infusion rate to 10 drops/min until the cluster headache attack ceases.
Adverse effects of flushing, dyspepsia, and nasal stuffiness are an indication of excess rate of infusion.
When the patient has been free of cluster headaches for 24 hours, rates may be increased to accommodate a third bag per day of histamine phosphate infusion.

hospitalization and gain control of the patient's headaches. One example is the patient who needs to undergo a rapid transition from selective serotonin reuptake inhibitor (SSRI) antidepressants to monoamine oxidase inhibitor types, or the reverse. Product labeling specifies that in almost all of these cases, a drug-free interval of 10 to 14 days is required before the new agent is started. This is not a practical solution for patients who have profoundly disabling headaches, and a more rapid transition with a shorter eradication period should be initiated. In general, this type of transition is safe for most patients, although on occasion this type of therapy is potentially dangerous; warning signs include the serotonin syndrome with elevated temperature, agitation, and other serotonergic indications. If left untreated, a potentially morbid situation could occur. Careful observation of these patients is essential during this transition period.

Nearly all patients admitted to the inpatient unit have complicated headache problems; previous single-drug therapy may not have provided adequate prophylactic treatment. For example, patients with coexisting migraine and tension-type headaches may respond to the concomitant use of propranolol and a tricyclic antidepressant. These complicated regimens increase the likelihood of adverse events and drug interactions. The use of more than one medication in the prophylactic treatment of migraine or coexisting migraine and tension-type headaches is best termed *copharmacy.* Initial observation and management within the hospital environment facilitate prompt treatment of complications that may result from copharmacy. Alterations in medical therapy to avert side effects and adverse reactions are also possible.

Close monitoring of physiological processes, laboratory parameters, clinical response, and adverse drug effects is necessary to optimize the outcome without substantial compromise of the patient's functional abilities during the initiation of therapy. For the vast majority of patients, significant adverse events related to the complex regimens may occur during the first 7 to 10 days of treatment. Although the therapeutic effects are far from being maximally achieved, in most patients the results are evident to determine how controlled the headaches are after discharge and what types of therapies may be needed for ongoing care.

Psychological Intervention

Chronic pain, including headaches, may be a manifestation of psychological problems. Accurate diagnosis by qualified psychologists and psychiatrists is essential if development of a long-term treatment program is indicated. The psychological manifestations of chronic headaches are similar to the characteristics of other chronic pain syndromes. Treatment for the chronic headache patient includes attempts to identify specific components of suffering and pain behaviors. The Seattle model of pain[26] may be used to formulate a treatment program; this model is based on the increasing complexity of pain adaptation, from the perception of painful stimuli (nociception) to pain, suffering, and pain behavior. Encouragement of *well behavior* is a vital aspect of this treatment. During hospitalization, patients are expected to wear street clothes, eat their meals together, and participate as a group in a variety of therapeutic and recreational programs.

Specific psychological intervention occurs on two levels. Group therapy sessions, such as assertiveness training, are conducted with a focus on problems common to patients with headache. If indicated, individual psychological counseling is also initiated during the first few days of hospitalization and continued, as necessary, during and after hospitalization. Psychological tests are performed in accordance with the initial diagnosis of the physicians and psychologists. These tests may contribute valuable information and enhance both the initial evaluation and long-term outpatient care.

Levels of proficiency have increased in the management of patients with headache, providing substantial benefits for levels of care. Patients with refractory headaches almost always have psychological issues that have an impact on their ability to respond to treatment. In many patients, the headache process is obscured by personality characteristics, coexisting depression, or other major psychiatric disorders. After an initial assessment and basic psychological intervention, it is imperative to establish a pain management program to help patients deal with the varied aspects of their conditions.

Other Treatment Techniques

Biofeedback techniques have proved to be useful in the treatment of migraine and tension-type headaches; however, biofeedback is only part of the therapy and should not be considered the single criterion for hospitalization. Physical and recreational therapy are vital aspects of the inpatient program. The physical therapy department provides an exercise program for the inpatient, specific physical therapy treatments, and instructions in specific exercises that are incorporated in the patient's individual program. A recreational therapist encourages the patient to participate in arts and crafts sessions, as well as art therapy, stress management, relaxation exercises, and leisure planning. These techniques are useful because they alter the pain behavior of the patient as well as provide alternative methods of coping with discomfort. Art therapy enables patients to gain a new perspective on their pain by transferring vague emotional images into more identifiable mental concepts and viewing pain through inanimate objects. Guidance regarding the use of leisure time enables patients to participate in planning for their eventual discharge.

Education of the headache patient, as provided by physicians, psychologists, pharmacists, and dietitians, is essential in enhancing the patient's understanding of the headache problem and ensuring a successful treatment program. A discussion group, chaired by one of the staff physicians, highlights the general aspects of the headache treatment. A meeting with a staff pharmacist focuses on the actions of the specific medications, their side effects, drug interactions, and expected results. A class is held with a dietitian who discusses the tyramine-free diet, with special instruction for patients on monoamine oxidase inhibitors. Menu planning for the headache patient is also described.

Family members are encouraged to be involved in the program. Often, they may not be able to comprehend what the patient has been experiencing and become frustrated and angry with the patient. In other situations, family members may be a contributing element of stress on the patient, thus aggravating the headache. Family group sessions conducted by a certified social worker or psychologist can help provide other methods of helping the patient. Encouraging well behavior should also be stressed to spouses and other family members because they often are "facilitators" of chronic pain behavior.

A weekly staff meeting is attended by representatives from each department, including nursing, psychology, biofeedback, dietary, pharmacy, physical therapy, recreational therapy, social services, and utilization review. Each patient's diagnosis, therapy, and management are discussed. Other vital issues regarding the unit, such as patient concern about hospital regulations, are also reviewed at these meetings. Interesting cases of hospitalized patients, which may include a rare diagnosis, are presented. On occasion, the case of a patient with an organic headache or with abnormal diagnostic studies is presented, and neuroradiological scans or surgical reports are discussed by the professional staff.

Outcome Measures

In Europe and Australia, inpatient treatment programs for patients with intractable headaches have demonstrated substantial success in providing long-term benefits.[27–30] In the United States, several independent studies have been undertaken to evaluate long-term outcome of inpatient hospital care for headache. The first survey conducted by Diamond et al[31] reported that the mean reduction in headache indices was 42% at 1 month after discharge and 46% at 1 year after discharge; these indices were calculated values evaluating the frequency, severity, and duration of headaches over 30-day periods. Fifty-four percent of the patients reported at least a 50% reduction in the frequency, severity, and duration of the headache attack. Ten percent of the patients had a complete remission. Only 6% of the patients failed to obtain benefit. In another study, 50 patients were surveyed who had chronic daily headaches associated with rebound headaches.[32] The study used outcome parameters such as frequency, severity, and duration of the headaches. At 3 months, 44% of patients had at least a 50% reduction in two of the parameters or a 75% reduction in one of the parameters. Lake et al[33] found that a 55% reduction in headache frequency occurred at the first appointment after discharge and that at long-term follow-up, this increased to 63%.

On the basis of our original study,[27] it was possible to gauge which patients would experience the most favorable outcomes. Patients with migraine and chronic cluster headaches are most likely, based on the parameters used, to have a favorable outcome. In contrast, patients least likely to obtain a successful outcome include those with post-traumatic headaches who may have secondary gain and those with chronic tension-type headaches due to depression. In our evaluation, we were able to see the effects on headache outcomes with the use of caffeine, ergots, barbiturates, and non-narcotic and opiate analgesics. We noted two effects from the chronic use of these agents on the underlying headaches: (1) the agents appeared to increase the frequency and severity of headaches, compared with those without dependency problems; and (2) habituated patients were more likely to experience an exacerbation of their headaches with or without a relapse related to acute therapies during the 6 to 12 months after discharge.

In this age of health care cost containment, a second evaluation involved the study of patients on an ongoing basis and has revolved around the use of expensive health care resources. Specifically, we examined emergency department utilization and hospitalization. Our ongoing studies have found that emergency department utilization drops by 66% after a comprehensive headache treatment program. Hospitalization for headache has been reported by approximately 72% of our patients before their first evaluation at the Diamond Headache Clinic; the mean length of stay was 5.5 days. Of these recidivist patients, only one third required inpatient care, for an average length of stay of 4.6 days. When readmission occurred after inpatient care in the headache treatment unit, in almost all cases it was due to status migraine requiring intravenous DHE therapy. As noted in a previous study,[7] improved performances in the workplace with reduced absences from work as well as increased days of full productivity are also garnered by treatment in the headache specialty environment.

A specialized headache clinic and inpatient unit may provide the last beacon of hope of many patients with intractable headache problems that have been refractory to therapy. Comprehensive evaluations beginning with a carefully elicited history are of utmost importance. Therapeutic measures can then be initiated that use an effective concept of inpatient headache treatment for patients who have not succeeded with conventional outpatient therapy. This type of well-integrated multidisciplinary approach has resulted in a substantial improvement after discharge.

References

1. Saper JR. Perspectives from a headache center with an inpatient unit. *In* Adler C, Adler SM, Packard RC, eds. Psychiatric Aspects of Headache. Baltimore: Williams & Wilkins; 1987:340–384.
2. Clouse JC, Osterhaus JT. Healthcare resource use and costs associated with migraine in a managed healthcare setting. Pharmacoeconomics 1994;28:659–664.
3. Blau JN, MacGregor EA. Migraine consultations: A triangle of viewpoints. Headache 1995;35:104–106.
4. Essink-bot ML, Van Roen L, Krabbe P, et al: The impact of migraine on health status. Headache 1995;35:200–206.
5. Dalessio DJ. Headache games: Dealing with difficult headache patients. Headache Q 1993;4:240–244.
6. Oates LN, Scholz MJ, Hoffert MJ. Polypharmacy in a headache centre population. Headache 1993;33:436–438.
7. Stang PE, Osterhaus JT. Impact of migraine in the United States: Data from the National Health Interview Survey. Headache 1993; 33:29–35.
8. Scopp AL, Peters KS, Li M. Comprehensive headache treatment cost and treatment effectiveness. Headache 1996;36:277.
9. Fitzpatrick RM, Hopkins AP. Effects of referral to a specialist for headache. J Roy Soc Med 1983;76:112–115.
10. Spierings ELH, Miree LF. Non-compliance with follow-up and improvement after treatment at a headache center. Headache 1993;33:205–209.
11. Diehr P, Wood RW, Barr V. Acute headaches: Presenting symptoms and diagnostic rule to identify patients with tension and migraine headache. J Chron Dis 1981;34:147–158.
12. Ziegler D, Hassanein R, Couch J. Characteristics of life headache, histories in a non-clinic population. Neurology 1977;17:147–158.
13. Soges LJ, Cacayorin ED, Petro GR, et al: Migraine: Evaluation by MR. Am J Neuroradiol 1988;9:425–429.
14. Sharff L, Marcus DA. Interdisciplinary outpatient group treatment of intractable headache. Headache 1994;34:73–78.
15. Fordyce WE, Fowler RS Jr, Lehmann JF, et al: Operant conditioning in the treatment of chronic pain. Arch Phys Med Rehabil 1973;54:399.
16. Fordyce WE. Behavior Methods for Chronic Pain and Illness. St. Louis: CV Mosby; 1976.
17. Williams AC de C, Richardson PH, Nicholas MK, et al. Inpatient versus outpatient pain management: Results of a randomized controlled trial. Pain 1996;66:13–22.
18. Leser JD. Perspectives on pain. *In* Turner P, ed. Clinical Pharmacology and Therapeutics. Baltimore: University Park Press; 1980:313.

19. Rapoport A, Stang P, Gutterman DL, et al: Analgesic rebound headache in clinical practice: Data from a physician survey. Headache 1996;36:14–19.
20. Breslau N, Davis GC. Migraine and major depression and panic disorders: A prospective epidemiologic study of young adults. Cephalalgia 1992;12:85–90.
21. Raskin NH. Repetitive intravenous dihydroergotamine as therapy for intractable migraine. Neurology 1986;36:995–997.
22. American Academy of Neurology. Practice Parameter: Appropriate use of ergotamine tartrate and dihydroergotamine in the treatment of migraine and status migrainosus (Summary Statement). Report of the Quality Standard Subcommittee of the American Academy of Neurology. Neurology 1995;45:585–587.
23. Horton BT, MacLean AR, Craig W McK. A new syndrome of vascular headache: Results of treatment with histamine: Preliminary report. Proc Staff Meet Mayo Clin 1939;14:257–260.
24. Kunkle EC, Pfeiffer JB Jr, Wilhoit WM, Hamrick LW Jr. Recurrent brief headache in 'cluster' pattern. Trans Neuro Am Assoc 1952;77:241–242.
25. Freitag FG, Diamond S, Bambhvani S. IV histamine in chronic cluster headaches. Clin Pharmacol Ther 1997;61:141. Abstract.
26. Sternbach R. Pain Patients. New York: Academic Press; 1974.
27. Isler H. Die behandliung der schmerzmitelkopschmnerzen therapeutische. Umschau 1986;43:221–225.
28. Dichgans J, Diener HC, Griber WD, et al: Analgetika-induzierter dauerkopfschmerz. Dtsch Med Wschr 1989;109:369–373.
29. Jauslin P, Goadsby PJ, Lance JW. The hospital management of severe migrainous headache. Headache 1991;31:658–660.
30. Schnider P, Aull S, Baumgartner C, et al. Long term outcome of patients with headache and drug abuse after inpatient withdrawal: Five year follow-up. Cephalalgia 1996;16:481–485.
31. Diamond S, Freitag FG, Maliszewski M. Inpatient treatment of headache: Long-term results. Headache 1986;26:189–197.
32. Silberstein SD, Silberstein JR. Chronic daily headache: Long-term prognosis following inpatient treatment with repetitive IV DHE. Headache 1992;32:439–445.
33. Lake AE, Saper JR, Madden SF, et al: Comprehensive inpatient treatment for intractable migraine: A prospective long-term outcome study. Headache 1993;33:55–62.

Index

Note: Page numbers in *italics* refer to illustrations; page numbers followed by t refer to tables.

B

C

Q

R

S

ISBN 0-7216-6999-9